Skills of Clinical Supervision for Nurses

A Practical Guide for Supervisees, Clinical Supervisors and Managers

Second Edition

Meg Bond and Stevie Holland

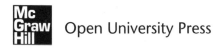 Open University Press

Open University Press
McGraw-Hill Education
McGraw-Hill House
Shoppenhangers Road
Maidenhead
Berkshire
England
SL6 2QL

email: enquiries@openup.co.uk
world wide web: www.openup.co.uk

and Two Penn Plaza, New York, NY 10121-2289, USA

First published 1998, this edition published 2010

A catalogue record of this book is available from the British Library

ISBN-13: 978-0-33-523815-6 (pb)
ISBN-10: 0-33-523815-7 (pb)

Library of Congress Cataloging-in-Publication Data
CIP data applied for

Typeset by Aptara, Inc., India
Printed in the UK by Bell and Bain Ltd, Glasgow.

Fictitious names of companies, products, people, characters and/or data that may be used
herein (in case studies or in examples) are not intended to represent any real individual,
company, product or event.

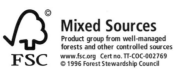

Mixed Sources
Product group from well-managed
forests and other controlled sources
www.fsc.org   Cert no. TT-COC-002769
© 1996 Forest Stewardship Council

The McGraw·Hill Companies

Contents

Series editors' preface

We welcome this exciting second edition of Meg Bond and Stevie Holland's excellent book on *Skills of Clinical Supervision for Nurses*. The first edition was the second book in our series *Supervision in Context*, which looks at the particular supervision needs and issues in the various helping professions. In the first edition the authors provided a timely contribution to the recent but growing literature on clinical supervision in nursing at a time when the rhetoric of clinical supervision was well ahead of the reality of practice in most organizations. The core focus of their book was to close the rift between the rhetoric and the reality by providing more emphasis on the understanding and training of effective nurse clinical supervisors. Since the first edition in 1998, many people in a number of countries have been successfully using the book to train, develop and support clinical supervisors, and have benefited from the practical models that it provides. The book has also played a major role in moving forward the approaches, thinking and policies applied to the practice of nurse supervision.

Since then, the demands and expectations on health systems have continued to grow as have the complexities of the systems needed to meet those demands and expectations. Successive governments, in many of the countries where this book has been read and used, have attempted complex health care reform, but the focus has nearly always been on such areas as structures, economic efficiencies, business processes, workforce planning, etc. After a period of large increases in spending on health budgets the world has suffered a major global recession and the rallying banner in many countries' public sectors has become 'How to do more with less'. Human life expectancy, patient choice and the expectations of health professionals continue to rise, but the economic resources required to meet these needs cannot keep pace. One of the many ways that this is being tackled is the movement of a lot of health practice from within hospitals into the community, and the growth of 'hospitals without walls', 'telemedicine', community matrons, peripatetic nursing and nurses taking on jobs previously reserved for doctors, psychologists and other professions.

In the midst of these challenges, what easily gets lost is the centrality of the patient–nurse relationship which is so crucial to the quality of patient experience, patient choice and health outcomes.

Peter Block (2004) puts this very powerfully in his reflections on nursing leadership in the USA where he writes:

> Nursing, more than almost any other profession, defines the meaning of service. The nurse is the front line, what we might call the touch labor, of the U.S. health care system. The job represents the heart and soul of authentic health care.
>
> Why, then, is there a shortage of nurses and why do so many nurses find the job so stressful? The crisis is not about the work itself, but how to create more fulfillment in the work. The problem is not primarily lack of skill or motivation, but the context in which the work is done.
>
> The agenda for health care reform does not focus on those delivering the service; it's mostly reduced to a problem of cost and restructuring how the system is managed. Reform has become an issue more of politics and economic interests.
>
> Those providing the care—physicians and nurses—occupy only a small part of the conversation. This is tragic for a nation that outspends any other country on health care and ranks barely in the top 10 in effectiveness.

The best way we know for focusing on and improving the nurse–patient relationship is quality supervision, because the capacity of a nurse to provide quality relationships for the great range of patients and patient needs is most affected by how much they themselves are listened to, supported and helped to reflect on their work and to constantly grow their emotional, clinical and professional capacity.

Having made a strongly argued case for regular clinical supervision for all nurses, Meg Bond and Stevie Holland show that establishing the supervision structure is not enough, for without trained and skilful supervisors effective supervision will not happen. The core of this book takes the reader through the key skills of effective clinical supervision and does so in a way that could be of great value not only to nurse supervisors but to supervisors from all the helping professions. They usefully adapt John Heron's model of six categories of possible interventions and show how they can be used, misused and abused in supervision. They also take the reader through steps to increase their own skills in each type of intervention.

The authors are extremely well placed to write this second edition. As well as the experience of being practitioners themselves, they have both spent many years running training workshops for nurses and nurse supervisors. It is from these workshops and the questioning and needs of those attending that the models and approaches in this book have emerged. The book's strength lies in the fact that it stems from contact with real patients, practitioners, managers, professional support workers and educators in real settings and the frameworks have sprung from the authors' heartfelt responses to the needs and concerns of nurses who care about their work and who want to make clinical supervision effective.

This new edition sits proudly alongside the other books in this series, which include:

Supervision in the Helping Professions by Peter Hawkins and Robin Shohet (now in its third edition)
The Social Work Supervisor by Allan Brown and Iain Bourne
Psychotherapy Supervision by Maria Gilbert and Ken Evans

Shortly we will adding to this series with *Supervision in Medical Settings*, edited by David Owen and Robin Shohet, *Supervision in Schools* by Elizabeth Holmes and *Supervision in Coaching and Mentoring*, edited by Tatiana Bachkirova, Peter Fleming and David Clutterbuck. The whole series focuses on how to create, develop and sustain helping relationships, through providing quality supervision to those who work broadly in the people and helping professions. Quality supervision is the key link in helping practitioners connect what they learn in theory with what they learn and do in practice and is therefore at the heart of all continuous personal and professional development. At its best it serves and benefits the professional being supervised, their clients, the organization in which they work and the development of the profession. In today's world no helping professional can afford to be without supervision and this book also provides an excellent frame for nurses to understand what they should be demanding as part of sustaining the quality and development of their practice.

We are confident that this new edition will surpass the first edition in being one of the world's leading textbooks on how to provide, deliver and receive supervision across the nursing professions.

Professor Peter Hawkins and Robin Shohet, May 2010

Introduction to the second edition

In this second edition we have retained a great deal of what we have been told continues to be relevant and works well, while updating, adding and adapting where necessary.

Since the first edition, concerns about the quality of care have increasingly focused on person-centred and joined-up multidisciplinary care. The Care Quality Commission's report (2010) highlighted these two main themes, wanting to give people more choice and control (including protecting their rights) and joining up health and social care.

For staff to be in a position psychologically to really provide compassionate person-centred care in an increasingly complex world, a parallel process must apply: they need themselves to have the ongoing experience of the person-centred support and development that clinical supervision can offer. In order to work with other professionals, they need to understand other professionals as people, get under their professional shield and discover what makes them tick: multidisciplinary clinical supervision can provide an opportunity for this. We offer many ideas in this book for more integrated, multidisciplinary supervision as well as clinical supervision within the nursing specialties.

One thing that hasn't changed is the fundamental style and commitment of this book to offering within its pages a place to think and reflect, shift your own learning positions and try out different ideas. You may not find them all relevant. You may not like them all. You may find some uncomfortable. But then some degree of discomfort is part and parcel of challenging established ways of thinking and doing.

We want to continue to incorporate what we have learned from innumerable nurses from diverse specialisms and settings around the country, as well as from other related professions within multidisciplinary workshops. All of the developments within this edition have in different ways been 'sanctioned' by them. This is what gave this book its initial popularity and accessibility and we see this as a strength that has warranted renewed emphasis in this new edition and is found particularly in the expanded and adapted chapters in Part II. This is where the practical, down to earth way that ideas and strategies for developing thoughtfulness and skills in clinical supervision can be integrated into the realities and complexities of practice. We are impassioned about this essential ethical core of the book – to let the understanding and meaning that nurses have co-created in clinical supervision workshops 'speak again' within these pages.

Bradbury *et al.* (2010) offer a compelling critique of once radical tools for creative learning becoming desiccated dogma rather than living, breathing tools for engagement and curiosity. They focus on rescuing and re-enlivening the more radical aspects of reflective practice. They suggest that 'the original idea of reflection as a tool for critical praxis is reversed and instead becomes a tool for control and orthodoxy' (p. 5). This critique makes sense to the two of us, especially as reflection is a crucial part of clinical supervision and indeed other areas of supervision as well, including line management supervision and in the dilemma-filled balance of meeting individual and organizational needs. Bradbury *et al.* (2010: 3) also suggest that 'there has been little or no acknowledgement of the material reality in which the individual works' and we hope that we continue to redress this by encouraging exploration of the tensions and conflicts in real-world settings.

During the last 10 years or so, we have been increasingly concerned with the hit and miss approach to educating the workforce for effective clinical supervision. There have been many lost opportunities to make it a more integral and organic part of clinical effectiveness and continued professional development (CPD) and there has been an overall lack of courage from the leaders of the profession to model and support this. We have witnessed the difference in areas that invest in their workforce by ensuring more effective training and those who prefer the tick-box culture and a superficial receptivity to it, with minimal investment and related lukewarm payback and rewards. Clinical supervision, as well as reflective practice, is in danger of becoming one of the many taken for granted assumptions or rituals of professional practice, so eloquently outlined by Wright (1997) in one of those classic critiques that sadly seems as relevant today as when it was first written. Bradbury *et al.* (2010: 3) refer to these assumptions or rituals as 'procedural recipes', in contrast to the need to develop more curiosity, questioning and challenging – the hallmarks of professional practice. We want to reassert the crucial importance of effective clinical supervision as a more radical tool for curiosity and connection as well as a tool to fulfil the organization's aim to improve clinical care. A creative juice rather than a stagnant puddle.

Feedback to the first edition also included an appreciation that our approach was not just a 'pursuit of the holy grail' or our own defensive hark back to ' the good old days' when radicalism was perhaps less blunted by the speed and intensity of short-term change in both policy and related practices. It remains our intention not to stir up blame of self or other or to foster regret and grievance, but rather to continue to promote an understanding of what can turn curiosity off, and what emotional and psychic processes affect our ability to learn, to connect, to change and even our desire to learn, connect and change. We explore this in Chapter 2 of Part I and then throughout the book when exploring the pitfalls as well as the strengths of trying to implement ideas and related skills.

In Part III we also seek to place the individual firmly in the bedrock of the organization and pursue rather more an understanding of the dilemmas and conflicts of the line management and organizational context. We continue to place CPD at the heart of our philosophy of clinical supervision, but in the first edition we neglected the impact of the organizational domain, especially in relation to risk and audit, and this edition seeks to rectify this. Perhaps it was also too early then and it needed 10 years of application before this could be explored more effectively, although sadly a lack of research, measurement and evaluation still prevails. We offer ideas for a code of ethics for clinical supervision in this final section of the book.

We believe that the overall approach we take in this book is even more important than it was when we wrote the first edition, but that the dated elements are addressed as well as the need to integrate clinical supervision more fully into organizational audit, without losing its essential creative essence. We hope you find these additions valuable and that you will let us know either way.

You may now choose to move on to an adapted overall Introduction, which contains important signposts for the use of the book and its overall aims.

Introduction

This book is about the interpersonal and personal skills involved in clinical supervision in nursing, taking an approach which highlights focused growth and support as the vehicle for developing and sustaining quality clinical practice. We suggest that clinical supervision provides a route to developing and maintaining emotionally healthier individuals in an emotionally healthier workforce culture. We welcome the impetus towards developing and maintaining clinical supervision in nursing and echo Swain's sentiments that this may be overdue:

> It beggars belief that we have, for so long, failed to incorporate [clinical supervision] as a defined component of practice. Any one of us looking back at the human pain and social distress of others to which we have been exposed – not to mention our own – must surely question what makes us suppose we can practise effectively without such a regular conscientious examination of our work, of what might improve it, what might impede it, and of our own feelings about it.
>
> (Swain 1995: 12)

Effective clinical supervision can bring benefits not only to practitioners but also to the organization and its clients when it fulfils the aim of improving and developing clinical practice. Clinical supervision has to be seen to have an impact on all aspects – teamwork, clinical care and patient well-being, organizational targets and development. It is a place where individual needs can meet organizational needs in a creative way, or a place where tensions and a clash of needs, responsibilities and accountability, abound.

In our work as education and training consultants in the National Health Service (NHS), we still find that some of the most frequently asked questions about clinical supervision are 'What exactly *is* it?' and 'How do we go about doing it?'. From those who have begun to use clinical supervision, we are asked, 'Are we doing it properly?' and those with more experience ask, 'Why has it taken so long to get going in nursing?'. The map of clinical supervision is still very patchy – thoroughly implemented and maintained in some areas, threadbare and minimalist in others. While participants on our skills training courses find some answers to these questions during the courses, many other practitioners have been frustrated with lacklustre implementation and development in some areas, and a lack of will to understand the complexity of what is needed. Our own search for practical guidance to help us with our confusion and uncertainty about clinical supervision in the nursing context has also been frustrating. Much work has had to be done by us and our course participants to sift through and adapt theoretical models to make them practicable. This book attempts to share the results of this work by focusing on the *skills* of clinical supervision, thus giving a picture of what actually happens or could happen. While no single page or chapter will adequately define clinical supervision or provide enough answers for everyone about how to do it well, the book as a whole will offer a sound practical basis for understanding, getting started and reviewing how you are progressing in using clinical supervision. Although our main focus is on practical frameworks which can help, we also want to be realistic and place them within the organizational context of what we know may be helpful or unhelpful to the development of clinical supervision.

Clinical supervision has been referred to consistently within policies and professional codes of practice as being vital to CPD. Experienced nurses who have survived many changes in nursing and management practice in recent years often view this emphasis with a certain amount of healthy cynicism: over-enthusiastic promotion of clinical supervision can make it sound like a holy grail. As with all holy grails, it attracts both devotees and non-believers and it is the search for it that can often attract the most attention and noise. Many pilgrims flock to support it, some out of genuine belief, some because it's the fashionable thing to do. Many may pay lip-service to the creed but, either wittingly or unwittingly, will be highly selective or shallow in putting it into everyday practice. Many will view it simply as the unearthing of old relics and scriptures which they had problems worshipping the first time around. Many more will be indifferent to the entire pilgrimage, preferring to conduct their working lives without recall to any other image.

Although we are obviously enthusiastic about clinical supervision, we would like this book to be a realistic, practical guide, rather than a heroic crusade. We include the reality of the difficulties that you may encounter in developing clinical supervision, signposting some of those challenges that cannot be spirited away. As nurses ourselves, we know well the foibles of our profession, such as the tendency to strive for perfection, with the inevitable discouragement that ensues from not achieving it. Other professions, which implemented clinical supervision decades ago, have not achieved perfection and neither will we. The 'good enough' clinical supervision referred to by Hawkins and Shohet (1989) requires a balanced view, both of the very real potential benefits of clinical supervision and of the limitations and barriers it might face. Some of these barriers come from within ourselves as individual nurses and from within the culture of our profession and the pressures and dilemmas faced within it. It is difficult to keep the lens on reflection and personal and professional development when the pressures on so many nurses at the sharp end of practice seem to be more geared to everyday survival. Our deep concern is to ensure that clinical supervision works well enough in nursing to provide the support and growth opportunities that nurses deserve in doing a difficult job in a difficult political and organizational climate. Our clients deserve to be cared for by people with the backup of 'good enough' clinical supervision.

Who this book is for

This book is aimed at every nurse, midwife and health visitor and their managers, professional support workers and educators who have an interest in the practical implementation of clinical supervision. This is potentially a vast number of people within a huge diversity of contexts and experience. We are conscious of the fact that nursing encompasses a very wide range of settings and that nurses can sometimes be insular within their own discipline. The book focuses on the principles and skills of developmental clinical supervision that can be applied, sometimes with local adaptation, across the board. The examples given will illustrate the type of issues that frequently emerge in our workshops. However, we accept that we cannot describe specific application of the principles of clinical supervision to every setting in nursing, midwifery and health visiting, and we trust that you will be able to use your imagination to relate what we offer in this book to your own specialty. As it is a skills-based book, it also lends itself to adaptation and extension to other related professionals and support workers. This has already been the case with the first edition: social workers (some from overseas) have been interested in our advocating separating clinical and line management supervision, as have family support workers in parenting organizations, and the first edition has also been on the reading list for supervision courses for counsellors.

Just a note about line management supervision: the midwifery profession has developed a specific system of clinical supervision that differs from many of the principles we put forward in this book and is more akin to line management supervision. However, midwives who wish to extend and deepen their use of their clinical supervision system will also find the emphasis on skills in this book useful. Hopefully it will be useful to all readers who identify themselves as offering line management supervision, because those managing risk in more acute areas of care need to have a particularly sensitive understanding of the importance of reflection at the heart of the complexity of professional practice.

Terms used

Usually when one wishes to be inclusive of all branches of the profession, one uses the full title of 'nursing and midwifery' (or alternatively 'nursing, midwifery and health visiting' if working with health visitors who retain that job title rather than 'public health nurses'). In an attempt to be succinct, we will use 'nursing' as shorthand, meaning to include all nurses as well as health visitors/public health nurses, midwives, managers, professional support workers and educators. The term 'practitioners' is used to include all nurses, midwives and health visitors who work directly with patients or clients. We use the term 'clients' in a generic way to include patients, clients, service users, relatives, carers and any client groups.

If we cannot find a non-clumsy, non-gender-specific way of referring to people of both sexes, both practitioner and client will be referred to as 'she' (which reflects the statistical preponderance of women in both these groups).

How to use this book

The breadth and depth of the human skills involved in clinical supervision are potentially vast and it is only humanly possible to explore one or two aspects at a time. Therefore each chapter in this book is designed to enable you to explore a very limited part of the overall picture. The analogy of gymnasium exercises could be useful here. In the gym, you focus on specific groups of muscles and ligaments at a time, to stretch and strengthen them, so that back in the world outside the gym you have more physical strength, flexibility, coordination and self-awareness of your physical abilities and limitations. Likewise with the skills approach in this book, we focus on specific aspects to help you to stretch and strengthen your awareness and understanding of the specific skills of clinical supervision and to recognize your strengths and weaknesses. As a result, we hope that you will be able to apply your learning to the real-life clinical supervision situation with greater skill, flexibility, confidence in your abilities and knowledge of your limitations.

We are alert to the points highlighted in Alison Norman's summing up of a National Health Service Management Executive's workshop on clinical supervision, in which she said that a one-dimensional, inflexible approach to clinical supervision would be a tragedy for nursing: 'we have a history in our professions of having very good ideas and trying to put them in tablets of stone, when they should be fluid and instilled within each individual organisation' (Norman 1995: 24). There may be more specific guidelines in this book than is usual in the clinical supervision literature, where writers are cautious in being over-prescriptive about such a variable interpersonal process. However, in offering our ideas, practical guidelines, structures and ways of identifying skills, we encourage you to use them selectively and to adapt them to your own situation. We do not see them as definitive: there are no tablets of stone.

Frameworks rather than models

We have attempted to apply the discipline of describing each of our ideas as 'a framework for . . . ' rather than 'a model'. The use of the term 'model' implies a replica, giving a fairly detailed impression of the shape and colour of the finished product, perhaps like an architect's model of a proposed building. We prefer the term 'framework', since we offer our ideas as mere frames upon which to hang your work: more like a weaver's loom, with no expectation of the colours and textures that you will create; we merely hope to make it easier for you to weave your own pattern. We have great concern about the proliferation and interpretation of 'models' of clinical supervision in nursing. We find on the one hand that nurses with an academic interest in clinical supervision can tend to collect 'models' of supervision without getting round to erecting the building. Some discussions on courses can degenerate into a 'who can quote the most models?' competition, with avoidance of taking the first step of putting anything into practice. Some nurses, desperate to get started with clinical supervision in this time of great need, adopt one model and try to apply it universally to everyone and every issue ('We are using So-and-So's model of clinical supervision'). We hope that this book will enable you to say, 'We are doing clinical supervision our way and each selecting which frameworks and approaches to use, as and when', rather than paying us the dubious and unwelcome compliment of 'We are using Bond and Holland's model of clinical supervision'. So, we expect you to select and adapt any of the ideas and structures which illuminate, help you to understand and enable you to put into practice some aspect of clinical supervision, or assist you in reviewing your use of it more effectively. We hope that you will ignore those ideas that are not useful to you now, and that perhaps you will revisit them at another time if appropriate.

Contents of the book

Part I, 'The context of clinical supervision in nursing', sets the scene for understanding the special context of clinical supervision in the profession, the organizational impetus for the development of clinical supervision and the factors which have blocked its progress during its first 15 years or so, and may continue to do so if not attended to. There are two chapters in Part I, which, although they interlock, explore similar themes from different perspectives.

Chapter 1 gives the surface picture of clinical supervision, outlines its key principles, its roots in other professions, their influences, the early developments and writings related specifically to nursing and the ideological and organizational factors which are a spur to the development of clinical supervision, as well as its confusion with other support initiatives. In short, the good news. We look at why the need to implement clinical supervision has become so important in nursing. What is its purpose and value? We wish to place clinical supervision in the current organizational, educational and clinical milieu as we see them, by exploring parallel processes and emphasizing the importance of self-disclosure as part of the need for in-depth reflection for effective clinical practice. We particularly wish to examine the debate between non-hierarchical and line management supervision, and place clinical supervision within a strongly ethical framework. We emphasize the importance of clinical supervision for not just surviving ever-increasing organizational and practice complexity, but also for the potential to develop more creatively. We end by exploring what sort of 'frame' this 'picture' might need.

Chapter 2 introduces you to the more 'hidden' picture – the pitfalls, resistances and difficulties the development of clinical supervision may meet on the way, both from individuals and from the prevailing culture of the health service itself: the bad news. We address the questions: why on earth has it taken so long and why is it taking longer still, to implement effectively? The key word here is *effectively*. Some areas of nursing have invested in clinical supervision very thoughtfully and thoroughly, others have paid lip-service to it, and ticked the box with as much meaning as the easily forgotten sound bite. We explore how and why some of its principles may be less well received than others within the complex folds of our huge profession, as well as for reasons of political expediency. We view these blocks as being a matter of individual and organizational psychology.

Our intention is to place the emotional life of clients, practitioners, supervisors, managers and the larger organization firmly in the centre of this book, and this chapter sets the scene. We don't intend that you should become a 'barefoot therapist', but wish to avoid a shallow 'sound-bite approach' to clinical supervision which pretends it can be implemented by knitting on additional practical strategies without reference to what really makes people (and organizations) tick. This superficial approach would result in your emotional feelings about your clients, your colleagues, yourself and about how you practise staying 'out of mind' while retaining their power. It behoves us all to acknowledge the very real dilemmas and contradictions that front-line professionals face, illustrated in the conflicting demands of accountability, particularly in areas of risk.

Chapter 2 explores how practitioners in health care have cultivated their defences against recognizing the emotional underpinning of many of their interactions with others. It also seeks to identify how unconscious emotional responses are mirrored and transmitted between all participants in health care, and outlines the impact and influence this can have on the relationship in clinical supervision. Everyone who has some role in implementing clinical supervision needs to understand how unconscious forces can impact in different ways on the entire process.

We also explore more fully how the 'frame' around this picture may change depending upon issues of risk in clinical practice, and its relationship with the many facets of accountability and the way that this accountability is interpreted. Is there a culture of having a more authoritative or a more facilitative frame and what real practice dilemmas do practitioners face when contained or constrained by such frames?

The pitfalls identified in the skills chapters in Part II are linked to these hidden restraints.

Part II, 'Specific skills of clinical supervision', is the largest part of the book as it is concerned with clarifying and encouraging development of specific skills of clinical supervision and highlighting the possible pitfalls. It builds on Part I by illustrating what can lead to 'good enough' clinical supervision and what can hinder it or make it ineffective or even abusive. It has grown from thousands of hours of workshops with a range of nursing and non-nursing practitioners, debating and applying ideas in the context of their everyday experience.

We begin in Chapter 3 to set the scene for the clinical supervision relationship and offer some frameworks for building and sustaining a working alliance. We suggest some ways of structuring the clinical supervision relationship to enhance its quality and prevent and deal with some of the hidden problems which can emerge to sabotage the process. We are aware that this interpersonal dimension is a vast arena and have therefore selected frameworks that have proved to be in most demand and of most use to our course participants: clarifying the rights and responsibilities of supervisee and clinical supervisor; choosing a clinical supervisor; negotiating a working contract; reviewing the progress of the working alliance; and dealing with criticism.

Chapters 4, 5 and 6 examine the specific skills required to do the work that the clinical supervision relationship is set up to achieve. In Chapter 4, the process of in-depth reflection in clinical supervision is described, and the issue of self-disclosure is examined as well as dealing with the unknown. The skills of the supervisee in preparing for and using the time for in-depth reflection on practice are outlined, and we take a practical approach by offering some frameworks for thinking that have helped nurses get started and review their progress. The chapter does not claim to be an exhaustive account of the vast literature on reflective practice in nursing: this has more usefully been done elsewhere – for instance, Butterworth *et al.* (2008).

Chapter 5 emphasizes the importance of the non-directive skills of support and catalytic facilitation, which are the basis of the help that the clinical supervisor can give the supervisee. While there are commonalities with the use of counselling skills, such as highlighting parallel processes, we put these in the context of clinical supervision rather than counselling sessions, with some possible pitfalls signposted.

Chapter 6 attempts to clarify the importance of the authoritative (not authoritarian) or directive aspects of clinical supervision. Skills of challenging the supervisee are placed alongside the skills of offering support towards change, and the skills of giving information and advice are set alongside catalytic skills of enabling the supervisee to use the information to make their own informed decisions.

Chapters 3, 4, 5 and 6 tend to focus on and illustrate the one-to-one clinical supervision scenario, while Chapter 7 extends the frameworks offered in these chapters to the group clinical supervision context. Additional frameworks for understanding the skills involved in group clinical supervision are offered, along with some structures to enhance the quality of group work and prevent and deal with some of the additional hidden problems which can emerge to sabotage the process of a group. The aim is to ensure that effective clinical supervision can occur in the relationship dynamic of the group setting.

Part III, 'The big picture', is a three-chapter section exploring the implications and challenges for the larger organization. It provides guidelines for managers and coordinators to set up, monitor and develop more effective clinical supervision delivery frameworks. We identify the position of clinical supervision within the range of types of supervision and emphasize the vital role of managers: they are key to supporting clinical supervision systems and encouraging the vital training for clinical supervision. We distinguish between clinical supervision and management supervision, by identifying some of leadership characteristics and the supervsee/supervsior interaction and how they differ between the two types of supervision. We urge all supervisors, whatever their ultimate management remit, to embrace the important balance between authoritative and facilitative approaches.

Chapter 8 explores what has worked most effectively within established initiatives in the UK and abroad, identifying what future initatives may learn from this, as well as critiquing some of the studies of clinical supervision and their limitations. Suggestions are made for methods to monitor and evaluate clinical supervision, within the limitations of the difficulties of finding the relevant evaluation tools for assessing such a relationship-based system, which is notoriously difficult to measure.

Chapter 9 suggests some conditions that are necessary for the development of effective clinical supervision relationships into working alliances and some options from which to choose an appropriate delivery framework for clinical supervision in your organization. It focuses on the important practicalities of enhancing and supporting clinical supervision systemically.

Chapter 10 highlights some issues that need to be addressed for the future success of clinical supervision in nursing. We see clinical supervision as providing an essential complementary process to the establishment and growth of clinical nurse leadership. We propose a code of ethics to be addressed in setting up and maintaining a clinical supervision system and a framework is offered to guide you through the steps involved, which will hopefully in turn mirror and facilitate more ethical supervisory relationships.

Having read the Introduction and got a feel for the philosophy and approach of this book, how you continue to use it will depend on your learning style. On our courses we find that some people need to have a rationale and context-setting introduction before trying out the skills-building exercises, while others learn better by getting on with the practical side and addressing the questions that arise as they go along. Likewise, some may prefer to begin reading this book at Part I and then look at the more practical sections. Others will prefer to go straight to Parts II or III and then flip back to Part I when they begin to wonder why we use a particular approach. Of course, the choice is yours.

Background to the book

The strength of this book lies in the fact that it stems from our own commitment to and experience of our own clinical supervision and our own supervisees, as well as extensive contact with qualified practitioners, managers at various levels, practice development facilitators and educators in real workplace settings. It is based on thousands of hours of in-depth workshops with various combinations of qualified practitioners all over the UK, with unidisciplinary group of nurses, multidisciplinary groups of nurses and multiprofessional groups that include nurses. These nursing staff have been employed in the NHS and also in the local authority, private, voluntary, armed forces and prison sectors, and the nurse educators in universities. The principles and skills frameworks lend themselves well to all these settings. Our interactive, experiential workshops and consultancy work in various NHS Trusts attempt to mirror the interpersonal principles espoused in this book. Thus the frameworks on offer here have sprung from our responses to the needs and concerns of people who attend our courses and who (mostly) want to make clinical supervision work. The relationships we have made with these people have included brave disclosures of their own feelings, thoughts and experiences. We have studied the theoretical background to clinical supervision in nursing and we were involved with some early attempts to develop clinical supervision when we were working in clinical nursing practice. However, we have learned immeasurably more about the realities of clinical supervision in practice, and about its true potential, from the truths that these people have shared about their working lives and the part they play as human beings in their work.

In an attempt not to abuse the trust and openness of these people, confidentiality has been maintained in the use of real-life examples and quotations in this book (all the case examples and quotations come from our workshops, consultancy work and experience of giving and receiving clinical supervision). We have changed names, settings and often amalgamated other details so that individual client, nurse and organizational confidentiality are not compromised. All the examples or quotations were witnessed or heard within the confidentiality contracts of skills training courses or consultancy within Trusts; we are therefore not at liberty to reveal sources.

We could not have written this book without our own unique experiences of receiving clinical supervision to ground the theory and ideas into our own inner as well as external reality. We have both received clinical supervision for many years and are grateful to the supervisors and groups involved. For two decades we have also provided clinical supervision for supervisees from nursing and a variety of professions and have learned much from these working alliances.

We would like to thank our own supervisees, clinical supervisors, clinical supervision group members and the participants in the hundreds of courses we have facilitated for working so generously with us.

Part I

The context of clinical supervision in nursing

1 The surface picture: the development and value of clinical supervision

This chapter gives a brief overview of the context of clinical supervision in nursing. We focus on the sources and development of ideas within the profession and the perceived value of implementing clinical supervision for both individual practitioners and the organization as a whole. Fuller accounts of the principles, aims and models of clinical supervision are given elsewhere (e.g. Butterworth and Faugier 1992; Kohner 1994; Fowler 1996; Cutcliffe *et al.* 2001; Sloan 2006; Stuart 2007). Our aim is to highlight aspects of this development, which we believe will ensure fundamental and effective change and a healthier, more responsive work environment. This includes:

- distilling what is important in in-depth reflection;
- ensuring that reflective processes are applied meaningfully rather than mechanistically;
- a balance between emotional and cognitive thinking;
- allowing for self-disclosure;
- building professional and clinical confidence within the complexities of organizational as well as individualized care-giving;
- understanding the parallel processes between the effectiveness of clinical supervision and the delivery of clinical care.

What exactly is clinical supervision?

Since clinical supervision is a relationship between human beings, it is difficult to pinpoint exactly in one succinct definition what it is about. The variety of helping relationships has much in common, from work-based relationships such as practitioner/client and support between colleagues, to personal relationships such as friendships and family interactions. They all aim towards meeting basic human needs, and when reduced to their basic components, have similar criteria.

There are as many written definitions of clinical supervision as there are published books and papers on the subject: each author highlights the elements that are most important to them. Before we add our own definition, we would like to highlight some of the loaded meanings that the term clinical supervision seems to have for nurses. These loaded meanings come to the fore fairly soon in any discussion between nurses about clinical supervision and we feel it is important to acknowledge them before presenting an ideal alternative.

First, 'clinical' may be an uncomfortable prefix for many practitioners engaged in health care, who may believe it to be too embedded in a medical model approach. Minimalist interpretations of 'clinical' may ensure that only the 'what' and 'how' of immediate technical aspects of care are emphasized; it could be used principally in a reactive way to maintain baseline standards. For some, the term 'clinical' obscures a more critical overview of the broader complexities and context of practice, as well as the wider and more important remit of personal and professional development.

Second, the term 'supervision' may also be met with suspicion. Its general meaning is concerned with 'keeping an eye on someone', checking that work is being done appropriately and effectively and, as such, its more context-specific application in nursing can result in its being tainted with a negative image. For some, it automatically smacks of being looked at critically through a magnifying glass, a one-way process of observation and control. In an early example of the clinical supervision process in health visiting, health visitors and their manager in Stepney were clearly antagonistic to the term 'supervision' for these reasons (Kohner 1994). Such negative views perhaps reflect the very real experiences of many practitioners who have worked in a predominantly non-supportive and hyper-critical climate (Bond 1986; Woodhouse and Pengelly 1991). Although on a rational level many practitioners may realize that clinical supervision is supposed to be a helpful and supportive process, it is important to acknowledge that more jaundiced and confused perceptions exist, and these may distort initial understanding and assimilation of the ideas related to it. Many nurses, particularly at the more senior end of the profession, have found the term 'coaching' more amenable and have sought help from coaches rather than engage in supervision per se. Coaching has gained momentum in recent years and many are seemingly attracted to it as it is deemed to have less of an image problem, particularly in terms of perceived power relationships within it. People tend to see it as less of a threat, but this is ironic when the diversity of definitions and aims is very great, and the training for coaching and the efficacy of its practice are open to as much or even greater caution, critique and concern.

So, many begin their exploration of clinical supervision confused about its meaning and about how it compares to and differs from other support initiatives such as preceptorship, mentoring, coaching, supervised practice or peer support. This is not surprising. Due to the nature and speed of change within the NHS and our profession, there have been many pressures to implement clinical supervision quickly. Despite the absence of clinical data about implementation and effectiveness, initially criticized and mourned by Fowler (1996), many are exploring how clinical supervision can be translated and applied within our vast and diverse profession. The task is a large and daunting one and many have rushed ahead without first really examining the ideas within clinical supervision and their attitudes to it, to see which feel most appropriate and applicable to their specialty or location.

We offer our own, inevitably incomplete, attempt at a definition, though we emphasize that it cannot stand alone without an examination of the principles behind it:

Clinical supervision is regular, protected time for facilitated, in-depth re-flection on complex issues influencing clinical practice. It aims to enable the supervisee to achieve, sustain and creatively develop a high quality of practice through the means of focused support and development. The supervisee reflects on the part she plays as an individual in the complex-ities of the events and the quality of practice. This reflection is facilitated by one or more experienced colleagues who have expertise in facilitation and the frequent, ongoing sessions are led by the supervisee's agenda. The process of clinical supervision should continue throughout the person's ca-reer, whether they remain in clinical practice or move into management, research or education.

We would like to expand on this definition by addressing some simple yet con-tentious questions.

- What are the key principles that underpin clinical supervision?
- Who should offer clinical supervision?
- Who should receive clinical supervision?
- How does it relate to other support mechanisms endorsed within the orga-nization of nursing?

Principles of clinical supervision

We would like to begin by identifying some key characteristics of clinical supervi-sion. We will be highlighting those characteristics which are most congruent with our own values as outlined in the Introduction and which will be fleshed out later in the 'practical' part of the book. We refer to the writers whose work has most engaged our attention and that of the practitioners with whom we have worked. We also highlight some of the ambivalence as to how these principles may be put into practice.

For many, the importance of clinical supervision is that it focuses its lens clearly on clinical practice – how practitioners engage with clients for the benefit of clients, to improve care and standards and to develop personal/professional skills and sat-isfaction. Butterworth (1995: 4) states that his preference is for a definition that encapsulates the 'heart' of clinical supervision – 'that which talks clearly about sustaining and developing nursing' – and that the focus for this should clearly be the clinician actively engaged in clinical practice: '[clinical supervision is]...an exchange between practising professionals to enable the development of profes-sional skills...We must jealously guard our excellence and skills in clinical prac-tice, and sustain and develop them' (1995: 12). By placing a microscope on clinical practice Butterworth goes on to suggest that clinical supervision offers protection to independent and accountable practice, but only if it is built into professional life – 'it requires time and energy and is not just an incidental event' (1995: 4). The National Council for the Professional Development of Nursing and Midwifery (NCNM) (2008) also alludes to the need to 'stimulate debate and discussion about the role of clinical supervision in supporting CPD in the interests of improving quality patient/client care'.

It is clear that if the importance of clinical practice needs to be restored, then it requires personal commitment from individuals as well as commitment from the organization to ensure its effectiveness and enshrine it within the structure of professional life. Swain (1995: 19) asserts that 'the prime aim [of clinical supervision] is to restore the centrality of professional clinical practice to the health service'. She suggests that for too long the shifting political games have blurred and distorted the picture of service provision away from this central purpose. The 'lens' of clinical supervision may be used to magnify specific features of clinical practice or to make a wide-angled sweep of the context of practice.

This lens analogy can be carried to another concept nurses find helpful. Houston's (1990) simple suggestion of highlighting the *super* in clinical supervision serves to emphasize the far-seeing element and unhook it from the more negative emotional loading alluded to earlier. *Super*vision helps to shift the perspective from a more 'myopic' vision, focusing only on what we can spot right in front of our eyes, which tends to become concentrated into what has not been achieved, or on errors in judgement or practice. A broader view then allows for an overview of past, present and future professional work, as well as an in-depth exploration of specific interventions, feelings and reactions in particular situations.

The interpersonal qualities needed within the clinical supervision relationship should be highlighted, to ensure that it is both effective and humane. Faugier (1992: 24) endorses and writes sensitively about the need for a 'growth and support' model: 'The role of the supervisor is to facilitate *growth* both educationally and personally in the supervisee, whilst providing essential *support* to their developing clinical autonomy'. She goes on to suggest the qualities needed in the clinical supervision relationship to enable this, namely: generosity, openness, willingness to learn, encouragement, intellectual stimulation, humanity, sensitivity and uncompromising rigour. Swain (1995: 19) is particularly eloquent about the need for nurses to develop a more nurturing and truly supportive climate for each other, one that might be more compatible with the aims of their role:

> Something more is clearly needed to help practitioners . . . attention to the
> needs of staff themselves: to their workloads, their professional practice
> and concerns and anxieties about it: to their feeling state and health state;
> to their capacity for creative work, and its encouragement, and to estab-
> lishing a place of safety where disappointment or failure in practice can
> be examined honestly; prejudices challenged constructively, and success
> and good work owned and applauded.

As Faugier (1992) suggests, clinical supervision should be about empowerment and not control, hence emphasizing that the route to professional accountability is through building confidence and self-esteem, which in turn requires careful, supportive feedback. Swain's view seeks to challenge the lack of congruence between the caring vocabulary used by practitioners in their treatment of clients and the distinctly unsupportive if not harsh attitudes and actions reserved for each other.

Reluctance to 'admit' stress is endemic at all levels in the NHS. It may be argued that there is often a huge gap between the concept of empowerment and its true espousal and implementation. Clinical supervision may offer a practical mechanism and forum in which to practise and develop these skills and enable the growth of clinical leadership, which has suffered such erosion in recent years (Rafferty 1993). In an address at King's College in 2008, Rafferty continued to emphasize the need for more creativity in the development of nurses that would feed leadership within both nursing and health care. There are many international initiatives and organizations making the links between effective clinical supervision and improving nursing leadership, particularly in the community, such as the Victoria Healthcare Association (2006).

The capacity for, and skills in, reflective practice are established key components of clinical supervision and contribute to its essential educational function. However, the reality is that there has been a marked lack of time or will for this to happen in practice. Our experience and that of many qualified practitioners with whom we work suggests that instances of good reflective practice are much more scarce than the literature might suggest. Clinical supervision potentially provides the medium in which to structure space and time for reflection, although it still needs personal and organizational commitment to protect it from the erosion of *other* competing organizational commitments. Critical reflection enables a balance and an alliance between feelings, intuition, emotional skills, cognitive insights and theoretical links. It has the capacity to inform and assist both personal and professional development.

Many have referred to the all important need for both players in the clinical supervision relationship to develop skills in self-awareness. Woods (1992) emphasizes the emotional underpinning of clinical supervision and the therapeutic use of self within the clinical supervision relationship. He also rightly examines the organizational and cultural context in which this takes place, and the limited extent to which permission is given to both acknowledge and develop emotional skills. Platt-Koch (1986) tries to balance the educational function of clinical supervision with the therapeutic nature of the relationship. However, there is some ambivalence as to how this might be achieved. For example, Faugier (1992: 19) highlights the therapeutic origins of clinical supervision and the therapeutic intention and outcomes implicit in her 'growth and support' model, but she then seems to water the message down: 'The real purpose of supervision . . . is the promoting of learning about nursing, including some personal growth content'. She suggests that it is neither possible nor desirable for all nurses to shift their philosophical orientation from nursing to psychotherapeutic, social or educational models. We would suggest that these are all part of the clinical supervision relationship and all part of nursing. However, it is very important that attention is paid to boundaries for and skills in their application. There seems to be the viewpoint that if too much attention is given to these subterranean emotions, they might undermine the educative function of clinical supervision completely. That confusing mixed messages exist here is not surprising. Despite nurses, midwives and health visitors working in the highly emotional and vulnerable arena of health and ill-health, where the fear or reality of illness and disability can challenge personal autonomy and the very sense of who we are, there can be a deep reluctance to give space for emotional expression. The extent to which clinical supervision can provide this opportunity remains highly contentious. We will explore the reasons for this deep ambivalence and resistance, as well as the real difficulties in achieving an appropriate balance between the personal and professional components of clinical supervision, in Chapter 2.

Some authors suggest a combination of principal purposes, which try to bring together and provide a more composite picture of the personal and professional developmental model of clinical supervision. For Platt-Koch (1986), the aims of supervision are to expand the knowledge base, develop clinical expertise and proficiency, and develop self-esteem and autonomy. The Department of Health (1993d: 15) defines clinical supervision as:

> the term used to describe a formal process of professional support and learning which enables practitioners to develop knowledge and competence, assume responsibility for their own practice and enhance consumer protection and the safety of care in complex clinical situations. It is central to the process of learning and to the expansion of the scope of practice and should be seen as the means for encouraging self assessment and analytic and reflective skills . . .

To this we would add *emotional skills*. One of the most widely quoted integrated descriptions is Proctor's (1986) trio of formative, normative and restorative functions. The formative function of supervision is about developing the skills, understanding and abilities of the supervisee through an in-depth reflection of the supervisee's work with clients. The normative function highlights the importance of professional and organizational standards and the need for competence and accountability, while with the restorative function clearly acknowledges the supportive remit of supervision:

> [it is] a way of supporting workers who are affected by the distress, pain and fragmentation of the client and how they need time to become aware how this has affected them and to deal with reactions. This is essential if workers are not to become over-full of emotions, or alternatively heavily defended against the distress of the client, therefore lacking empathy and good-enough care.
>
> Proctor (1986: 24)

We adapt Proctor's framework in Figure 1.1, which emphasizes that the means by which the normative function is addressed is through the medium of the restorative and formative functions. This diagram incorporates the principles we have outlined so far in this chapter.

It is also vital that ways can be found to measure the impact of any change ensuing from these functions, in terms of patient care and organizational performance indicators. Driver and Martin (2005: 16) intertwines and explains these many strands succinctly when she writes of supervision being at the interface between disciplines:

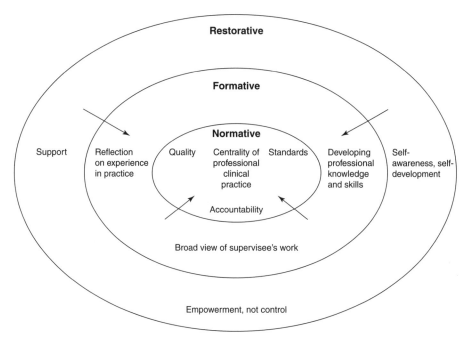

Figure 1.1 The restorative and formative functions of clinical supervision are the means by which the normative function is addressed

Its task is to enable learning but not to teach directly. Its task is to enable internal shifts of perception and awareness in order to understand patients . . . and yet not become therapy. It incorporates, in Piaget's terms, both accommodative and assimilative learning as well as working with, and understanding, the dynamics of unconscious processes. It requires an understanding and awareness of the impact of organisational issues as well as requirements for assessment, ethical practice, clinical responsibility and the development of clinical work.

We will be exploring the main influences on the development of clinical supervision in the last part of this chapter – the 'push factors' that have ensured their frequent, if erratic, appearance in the literature. Chapter 2 will outline the 'blocking' factors that get in the way of effective application of these principles. The rest of the book will focus on the skills necessary to actualize them.

These principles provide practitioners in diverse health care situations with a flexible framework of clinical supervision that can benefit the practitioner, their practice and ultimately the client. They may explore and harness each principle to an appropriate degree, achieving the balance needed to meet very different situations and requirements. There may be a very different balance required by practitioners in accident and emergency who have come through a major critical incident, compared to community paediatric nurses supporting families with chronically sick children at home. Clearly the balance may be affected by the location and nature of service provision – from acute high-tech, public health to acute low-tech community practice, cottage hospitals, general practitioners' surgeries, learning disability teams, hospital and community midwives, secure units and so on – and by the degree of practitioner experience and stage of their career, not to mention the myriad different personal histories and needs of staff in these diverse fields of practice.

All these underpinning principles need to be acknowledged and worked with in the clinical supervision relationship, although some principles may predominate at some times more than others. What we are suggesting is that acute imbalances make for a very different total experience of clinical supervision and the person selected (or volunteering) for the role of clinical supervisor may serve to shift the balance of this entire framework. If the person in the role of clinical supervisor is also a manager then the normative elements could easily attain prominence, while the supervisee's (and indeed the manager/supervisor's) vulnerabilities, stresses and support needs may disappear or go into hiding. This is why we are strongly recommending that managers do not assume a clinical supervisor role with any of their own staff. This theme will reappear throughout the book.

Who should be clinical supervisors?

Qualified senior staff, with more than or equal experience to that of the intended supervisees, should be selected. Although managers may play a role in identifying appropriate clinical supervisors, there should not be any enforced conscription for this role as it involves a great deal of commitment. Supervisors should usually (although not always) be from the same clinical area or have sufficient recent experience of relevant clinical practice. These clinical supervisors need to undergo further skills training to equip them for this role. (These skills will be explored fully in Parts II and III.) It needs to be said that seniority does not always denote appropriate levels of experience. Sadly, expertise is not a quality automatically distilled from years of service. We can all think of people who would consider themselves to be wise elders, and yet whose attitudes are stuck in a bygone age and who seem to have learned little from the intervening years. Maturity, genuine experience based on reflective capacity and a flexible approach to change are needed in what are recognized to be increasingly complex demands of care (Calder 2005).

We are clearly emphasizing the need for clinicians in the role of clinical supervisor and strongly endorse the inappropriateness of having line managers in this role: 'Management supervision and clinical supervision are different functions and should not be undertaken by the same person', Margaret Buttegieg declares (in the introduction to Swain 1995: 5) in a clear message on behalf of the Community Practitioners and Health Visitors Association (CPHVA). Many from other nursing specialties in both acute and community settings have echoed this and it was endorsed initially by the United Kingdom Central Council for Nursing Midwifery and

Health Visiting (UKCC 1996). Senior managers have an extremely important role in facilitating the development of supervision systems by identifying and providing resources for training, in its evaluation and in making a case for its inclusion within service contracts (see Chapter 9). But any embodiment of clinical supervision within line management will be liable to cause confusion and mistrust and lead to mixed messages about its aims and potential.

Management-led clinical supervision could lead to restrictive practice rather than reflective and growthful practice, although of course non-managers can achieve this too. We realize that some practitioners and managers may disagree with this, although almost all practitioners on our workshops supported this view and most managers who have participated have returned to base to rethink their intended implementation locally. Hawkins and Smith (2006: 6) warn that:

> we need to be wary that [the transformational potential for change] is not going to become a tool that can be used to coerce individuals and groups to someone else's will, a will they have no real chance of resisting, because it is dressed up in the clothes of performance efficiency and benefit to the organization, or more directly impacts on whether they stay in their job.

In specific areas of practice, notably throughout midwifery and in some instances in child protection, a form of management-led clinical supervision is already in progress. We know that many in reality will also follow this approach. We hope that even if your views differ, you will find ample ideas in this book to aid your role and allow the developmental rather than the punitive aspects to flourish. Specific guidance for managers is given in Chapters 8, 9 and 10.

Who should receive clinical supervision?

We believe that all qualified practitioners in all clinical areas need clinical supervision to maintain proficiency in practice, to ensure their accountability and to aid their specific personal and professional growth and development. This includes those who have had additional training to become clinical supervisors. We believe that no one has achieved such a hallowed status that they are above needing clinical supervision. We also believe that all related personnel – teachers and managers – should also be in receipt of the equivalent of rigorous non-managerial clinical supervision, although they may tend to call it 'mentoring' or 'coaching'. This acknowledges the challenge made to all professionals – that their initial qualification is only a passport to practice and that it is necessary to endorse mechanisms that ensure continued professional competence (Jarvis 1983).

Clinical supervision can contribute to this lifelong need to update, improve and develop, and does so by being firmly rooted in the work context. As Hawkins and Smith (2006: 13) suggest in one of their 'golden threads', 'Learning is for life, not just for courses. The moment we stop learning is the time our effectiveness at work starts to decrease'.

Few are 'qualified enough' or expert enough never to need help and guidance with their own developmental process at some time. We are aware that in such a large profession as ours, the means for achieving such extensive clinical supervision networks will take the form of carefully planned and layered training programmes and will take a lot of time, effort and resources. However, universality is crucial.

Not until recently has clinical supervision been seen as the right and responsibility of every practitioner. However, many may still find it more comforting to regard it as appropriate only for those who are in difficulty, those who are not maintaining standards or those who are encountering particularly stressful, acute or complex situations. This emphasis on 'problem' versus growth and development in nursing can be difficult to let go of, just as the espousal of illness rather than health has been for many within the NHS.

Comparisons with other structured organizational support mechanisms

The principles of personal and professional support and guidance have been more easily endorsed for new practitioners and for those returning to practice after a break. This is possibly why clinical supervision is frequently confused with preceptorship and mentoring schemes. 'Coaching' is also starting to creep into the terminology, rippling the water still more. There is an added history here of the blurring of terminology and confusion in the teaching/assessing and general supportive aspects of these roles. How is clinical supervision similar to and how is it different from these and other more informal support schemes? (See Table 1.1.)

Preceptor support

Preceptorship is aimed at facilitating the sometimes stressful transition from student to newly qualified practitioner and helping build confidence in that new role. The preceptor has an educative and modelling function, enabling the new practitioner to develop new skills and aiding the application of theory to practice. Ideally this 'allows for a smooth transition from learner to accountable practitioner' (Morton-Cooper and Palmer 1993: 99). The difficulties of applying what was originally a US-grown model of preceptorship, which was akin to an apprenticeship learning system, to different educational and service models in the UK has been well documented (Butterworth 1992; Morton-Cooper and Palmer 1993).

The UKCC's (1993) guidance on preceptor support differs in that it emphasizes that it is a relationship between two qualified practitioners, both of whom are accountable for their practice. The more experienced participant works in partnership to guide the newly qualified practitioner in adapting to their new role. The preceptor needs to have had at least 12 months or equivalent experience within the same clinical field. The guidance stresses the support required from the preceptor to assist in the 'beginner's' adjustment to new responsibilities. The Commission on the Future of Nursing and Midwifery in England (2010) endorses the setting up of a nursing preceptorship framework (Department of Health 2009) to enhance

Table 1.1 Distinguishing between some structured support systems in nursing

	Mentorship	Preceptorship	Coaching	Supervised practice	Structured peer support	Clinical supervision
Supervisee	Student nurse	Newly qualified nurse or qualified nurse entering a new field	Senior nurse specialist or manager	Student health visitor on final fieldwork placement	Any nurse	Any qualified nurse
Period of time	Throughout training especially on practical placements	During the 6 to 12 months of adjustment	Short-term, tends to be problem-focused	The final three months of the HV course	Varies; support groups have a reputation for petering out	Throughout entire career
How widespread	Integral part of the course	Varies; likely to become more widespread	Very patchy	Integral part of the course	Patchy; not widely accepted	Patchy
Assessment function	Mentor often has a part to play in assessment of practical work	Preceptor may report to supervisee's manager	No assessment function, coach does not report to anyone unless there is evidence of unsafe or unethical practice	Supervisor has a defined assessment role: HV cannot qualify without passing this part of the course	No assessment function, colleagues do not report to anyone unless there is evidence of unsafe or unethical practice	No assessment function, clinical supervisor does not report to anyone unless there is evidence of unsafe or unethical practice

this earlier stabilization of professional confidence in the role of nurse. Unfortunately this was not echoed explicitly in relation to clinical supervision although it is essential if many of these recommendations are to be achieved.

The earlier work of Kramer (1974) had outlined the 'danger zone' period of transition as one which could create the stressful burden of 'reality shock'. Ironically, as our own work with returners to practice suggests, part of that reality shock may involve dealing with the intransigence and poor role-modelling of those in a preceptor role (Holland 1994). The difference between the intended remit of the preceptor role and the reality of the joint experience depends upon the quality of preceptor selection and the training available. Morton-Cooper and Palmer (1993) refer to the resource difficulties in obtaining enough willing practitioners for this role and the likely problems of coercion in what should be a creative and sensitive learning relationship. Words of warning indeed for those setting up clinical supervision systems or those being persuaded to become clinical supervisors before they are ready.

It is interesting to note that some of the early references to supervision in health visiting (see Fish *et al.* 1989) seem to refer to the period of supervised practice towards the end of this post-registration course. These are more reminiscent of the need to guide and support the newly-qualified practitioner than clinical supervision per se.

Mentor support

Mentor schemes have gathered momentum in the last decade in the UK and have gained increasing prominence particularly within nurse education programmes, specifically within Project 2000, to assist with educational input and support in the practice setting. Much of the research stems from North America with, as Butterworth (1992) suggests, dubious applicability to nursing in the UK. The role of mentors has been subject to much debate. Some suggest that they possess very similar characteristics to preceptors; the two terms have been used interchangeably. Morton-Cooper and Palmer (2000) allude to the confusion in terminology now being added to by the additional concept of clinical supervision. Mentoring involves experienced practitioners who nurture and guide students in clinical placements but also have an active educational element. There is some contention whether they also have a role in assessment (Stuart 2006). Mentoring is based on a one-to-one method of teaching and facilitation, the content and direction of which should be negotiated by both parties in joint planning (Brockbank and McGill 2006). It has been suggested that assessment is not compatible with the supportive functions of the mentor:

> Mentoring concerns the building of a dynamic relationship in which the personal characteristics, philosophies and priorities of the individual members interact to influence in turn the nature, direction and duration of the resulting, eventual partnership. What lies at the heart of the process is the shared, encouraging and supportive elements that are based on mutual attraction and common values. These ... facilitate the personal development and career/professional socialization for the mentoree – leading to

eventual reciprocal benefits for both parties. A mentoring relationship is one that is enabling and cultivating; a relationship that assists in empowering an individual within the working environment.

(Morton-Cooper and Palmer 1993: 59)

Morton-Cooper and Palmer advocate that the person with the role of mentor needs a repertoire of helper functions – adviser, coach, counsellor, sponsor, teacher, resource facilitator – a menu to be mixed and matched. Their buoyantly enthusiastic and flexible model suggests that those within a mentoring relationship need to be personally matched – individually tailored to suit both parties. Whether those within the relationship should select each other or be chosen by a third party may also prove to be a contentious issue within clinical supervision. There could be a danger of collusion as well as the potential for reciprocity. The advantages and pitfalls of choice in clinical supervision will be developed in Chapter 9.

Mentorship schemes have demonstrated a range of comparative problems: their degree of effectiveness has depended upon individual motivation, sufficient resources, selection and training, to name but a few. Burnard (1988) has also highlighted the role-modelling function implicit in the role and the assimilation by the mentoree of elements of good practice.

New practitioners from pre- or post-registration courses need specific guidance and support in their transition, additional practical help with adjustments to practice, as well as broader educational additions to their developing knowledge and skills in this new arena. Some will require more authoritative monitoring and assessment to ensure that standards are met. This is the main difference between mentoring and clinical supervision, which needs a more delicate balance between the authoritative and facilitative approaches.

Clinical supervision refers more to an exchange between practising professionals, in which there is far less of a power divide between clinical supervisor and supervisee than, say, between student and mentor, although there may be some recognition of seniority and experience. We prefer to see preceptorship, mentoring and clinical supervision more as a continuum rather than acting as appendages or substitutes for each other. They all need to provide a range of opportunities for guidance, learning and support which should reflect the different degree and complexity of the needs of practitioners at different stages in their career and development. Many of the issues covered in this book, especially the skills development section, are equally relevant to those engaged in preceptorship and mentorship, as they centre on the skills and pitfalls of purposeful interaction common to all. There are some core similarities, such as the need for a nurturing and supportive relationship. The differences are more ones of emphasis in the educative and authoritative functions of respective roles.

Coaching

The world of coaching has developed at an astonishing speed and in many directions, and we have been a small part of this process. Its background is partly from the competitive arenas of sport and business, combining with elements of the personal growth movement of the 1970 and 1980s, and it has developed and branched out into the management of many types of organization, including the upper layers of health care. One of the authors of this book (MB) taught coaching courses to senior consultants within a large management consultancy in the 1990s, and those course participants applied coaching in their work at Trust board and senior management levels in the NHS (and many other organizations, including high levels of government departments).

Starr (2008) defines coaches as working alongside individuals to help improve their performance at work, regardless of whether the coach could do that work themselves. Rogers (2008: 7) offers a simple definition that nevertheless she says conceals complexity: 'The coach works with clients to achieve a speedy, increased and sustainable effectiveness in their lives and careers through focused learning. The coach's sole aim is to work with the client to achieve all of the client's potential – as defined by the client'.

Many emphasize 'goal-setting', 'performance measurement' and 'behavioural' or 'tangible outcome' gain. As this is an area still to be developed within evaluations of clinical supervision, perhaps it has more of an appeal to those who want more justification for it organizationally. As Bluckert (2006: 3) suggests, 'for coaching to be seen as relevant and a positive intervention, it must go beyond the facilitation of learning and development and translate into more effective action and improved performance'. He emphasizes from an executive perspective the importance of organizational dynamics and systems issues.

Clinical supervision in nursing is often criticized for being too individually focused, and wider systemic team and structural issues may serve to bolster its case. However, although both Rogers (2008) and Starr (2008) offer a very thorough grounding in the skills needed for coaching, many publications come over as a little thin, mechanistic or overly sound-bite laden and optimistic. However, many link it to more reflective practice (Brockbank and McGill 2006; Hay 2007) or the need for more emotional and psychological underpinning (Bluckert 2006). Hawkins and Smith (2006) suggest that the need for supervision has come to prominence recently within the diverse practice arena of coaching, largely due to its huge and unregulated growth.

Comparisons with peer support

Illustrations of good practice in peer support undoubtedly exist (Holland 1987), and many more have been highlighted in the initiatives of the National Association for Staff Support. However, problems with peer support have been endemic within the NHS (Booth and Faulkner 1986). Despite clear guidelines existing (Bond 1991), many peer support groups have petered out through lack of structure, ideas, facilitation, group skills, leadership or just motivation. Blame has been fairly evenly directed at management or peers. Clinical supervision, on the other hand, offers the potential for more structure, clarity and boundaries than many of the more unstructured support mechanisms that have limped on ineffectively or have petered out. It also serves to endorse the principle of support within the fabric of the organization rather than leaving it open to the enthusiasm and energy of a few. However, as Swain (1995) reminds us, the support provided by clinical supervision is different from that which can be experienced within effective staff support groups, counselling and therapy services, and should never *replace* these services. They are needed now more than ever and should sit side by side with clinical supervision networks.

It is now important to explore some of the overt and covert driving forces towards the development of clinical supervision in nursing to understand why it may be interpreted so diversely. Many different viewpoints and motives propel its implementation. We need to look at some of these key influences, both those from other professional groups outside nursing and in terms of earlier attempts to implement a form of clinical supervision within nursing. We will then seek to identify further influential driving forces from within the profession.

External influences: what we can learn from other professions about clinical supervision

Many clinical supervision models being developed in nursing draw on the theory, development and experience of supervision in other disciplines. Many nurses themselves have had experience within these other professional groups, leading to them being strong advocates for clinical supervision within nursing. This impetus has been vital, but nursing needs to be wary of accommodating models in their entirety, because they are built out of different professional philosophies and cultures. We need to select or adapt some of their component parts to fit our own professional orientation and organizational culture (see Table 1.2.)

Psychotherapy and counselling

The term clinical supervision originally stems from the training and practice of psychotherapy (including psychoanalysis) and counselling. Trainees in these professions are expected to have weekly supervision for their work with clients, and some may be required to have two clinical supervisors during the training period. After qualification and registration, many continue with at least one clinical supervisor on a weekly basis and even the most experienced of practitioners would be expected to seek supervision for specific cases or emergent difficult clinical issues, if not for monthly ongoing monitoring and the development of creativity in their work. All counsellors, psychotherapists, trainers and supervisors are required to have regular and ongoing formal supervision/consultative support for their work (BACP 2010). Clinical supervision is built into the counselling and therapy culture; it is a prerequisite not a choice, and it is universally accepted as the norm and as a necessity.

Supervision in this context is as much about the therapist/counsellor as the client. It not only focuses on the 'inner' and 'outer' world of the client and on clinical techniques within the therapeutic relationship, but also on the conscious

Table 1.2 What we can learn from clinical supervision in other professions

	Psychotherapy and counselling	Social work
FEATURES	• Built into professional culture and structure: compulsory for students, expected for newly qualified psychotherapists and counsellors, compulsory for all practising BAC-registered counsellors, most experienced psychotherapists continue throughout career • Considerable emphasis on surfacing and learning about the unconscious processes which help and hinder the work with the client, including those of the therapist/counsellor • Emphasis on building the 'internal supervisor' skills of the counsellor/ therapist (i.e. in-depth self-monitoring and self-appraisal) • Non-hierarchical: most non-NHS counselling/therapy organizations separate clinical and line management supervision • Qualified practitioners choose their own clinical supervisors • Most practitioners satisfied with their clinical supervision	• Built into professional culture and structure • Immediate intensive backup in acute situations, without stigma • Widespread dissatisfaction may stem from lack of skills-training and the power differential: supervisor is usually the supervisee's line manager • Practitioners usually unable to choose own supervisor
LEARNING POINTS TO APPLY TO NURSING	• Aim to build into structure and culture, possibly making clinical supervision compulsory • Develop the self-awareness element of clinical supervision by using structures and methods, not just vague rhetoric	• Allow flexibility so that a supervisee can receive increased clinical supervision sessions in acute situations, without stigma • Ensure supervisor is not supervisee's line manager • Ensure adequate skills training for supervisees and supervisors

and unconscious processes of the practitioner, their prejudices, blind spots and inner difficulties. The alliance between clinical supervisor and supervisee is analogous to that in the so-called 'therapeutic alliance' between therapist/counsellor and client as many of the dynamics being tussled with clinically in practice may resurface in supervision. This allows for some of the more hidden dynamics in the practice-based relationship to be focused on in the present and so enables a clearer understanding of what is really going on. This parallel process is applicable to clinical supervision in nursing and is developed later in this chapter. The clinical supervisor may support the therapist/counsellor just as they try in turn to provide what is often referred to as a 'holding' environment, for the client to explore emotional difficulties and blocks to understanding and feeling. Supervisory support is also needed to help therapists/counsellors to 'work with the unknown' or to stay with the state of 'not knowing' (Casement 1985); this may also have important lessons for many nurses, who may have become too controlling or directive in their role. Casement's (1985: 19) influential work on the 'internal supervisor' – building the therapist's skills in self-monitoring and appraisal – may also resonate with those keen to see clinical supervision promote professional development and accountability in individual practitioners in nursing.

Many of the functions of clinical supervision in therapy/counselling have parallels in nursing. Nursing is essentially about relationships, with both clients and colleagues, and there are similar needs for practitioners to develop self-awareness and interpersonal and emotional skills to cope with the often stressful nature of their work. As Hawkins and Smith (2006: 13) say, when referring to their 'golden threads' within organizational learning: 'All real time learning and development is relational'. Swain (1995) suggests that clinical supervision in nursing could provide a similarly containing and holding environment – what Winnicott (1991) called the 'facilitating environment' – and so contribute to the lessening of professional anxiety and defensiveness. As Faugier (1992) warns, however, this approach in unskilled hands or, rather, unskilled mouths, could so easily become intrusive or exploitative and lead to relationship 'traps'. She also suggests that this might lead to a confusion between 'therapy' and 'clinical supervision'. It would indeed be inappropriate if this were to happen in nursing, yet there tends not to be a confusion between these two distinct yet related areas in psychotherapy and counselling. Nevertheless, what is required in nursing is at a very different depth and intensity, especially regarding the highly complex world of unconscious motives. But to deny and devalue their application to clinical supervision in nursing is perhaps more dangerous than trying to adapt and use some of these 'relationship dynamics' from supervision in therapy and counselling. Nursing literature includes many references to the need to develop more self-awareness – easy to write and rather more difficult to do – in order to help practitioners delineate clearer boundaries between themselves and others, to see the difference between their own needs, motivations and wants and those of others. The human capacity to distort where oneself ends and another begins is notorious – almost as notorious as the human's capacity to deny that this happens. Hopefully, clinical supervision in nursing can help provide this relatively 'safe space' to nurture practitioners' capacity to disentangle the complexity of their interpersonal relationships, while not losing sight of their wider professional principles and clinical aims.

Social work

Clinical supervision has a long history in social work, although it has often been supervision based on casework rather than a process which embraces some of the broader principles outlined earlier. Although some supervision focuses on the best allocation of resources for client groups, Hill (1989) suggests that it is more to do with providing the 'cornerstone' of professional practice and emphasizes its role in improving the therapeutic proficiency of social workers. She also makes the point that supervisors act as a 'buffer' between social workers on the ground and those in senior management, which Butterworth (1992) suggests might also be a useful function within nursing.

Although Woodhouse and Pengelly (1991: 236) acknowledge that social services have a tradition of regular supervision, certainly when compared to health care, they suggest that 'it is commonplace to find that this has either lapsed altogether or become an arena for anxious case management rather than for reflective understanding'. Brown and Bourne (1996) write about the 'wholly inadequate preparation for this skilled task of supervisor' in social work, which their book is designed to redress, and refer to a range of research studies which highlight widespread dissatisfaction with supervision. They are quick to point out that excellence does exist and that the task is to encourage others to emulate those examples that work well. However, they also add a note of caution:

> Some of the dissatisfaction with supervision is structural and inevitable, stemming from the dynamics of a relationship in which power is not distributed equally and which also provides a focus for the wider frustrations and anxieties that arise in the daily, often stressful and demanding work of practitioners in social work and community care services.
>
> (Brown and Bourne 1996: 6)

Practitioners from nursing who have worked closely with social workers in families where there has been abuse, or where social needs are many and complex, have envied their social work colleagues' access to supervision, whether ideal or not. We should heed these messages about felt and actual power in supervisory relationships, and acknowledge that extensive good practice in supervision is dependent upon the non-managerial nature of clinical supervision in nursing and the coordination of effective training.

Given the type of culture we have in nursing we could look for further learning points from the established systems of clinical supervision within our own field.

Influences within nursing, midwifery and health visiting

Clinical supervision has been in existence in midwifery, mental health nursing and branches of the profession dealing with child protection (mostly health visiting and paediatric nursing) for some time. There are lessons to be learned from these early developments, and we need to take into account the culture of these contexts, in comparison to the culture of psychotherapy, counselling and social work (see Table 1.3).

Table 1.3 What we can learn from early developments in clinical supervision in nursing and midwifery

	Midwifery	Safeguarding children & vulnerable adults	Mental health nursing
FEATURES	• Long-established as management supervision, to ensure safety of clients by guiding and directing to ensure practice is correct • Linked to disciplinary procedures • Early recommendations (1920s) that supervisor is 'counsellor and friend rather than relentless critic' have not been enshrined in the structure and practice of supervision and therefore lost	• Policies require employers to have in place management monitoring of procedures to ensure safety of children and vulnerable adults by guiding and directing to ensure practice is correct • When managers are the safeguarding advisers, they tend to take over the safeguarding work and become overloaded • The safeguarding advisers who do not have a line manager role seen as being more effective	• More contact with psychotherapy/ counselling models of clinical supervision • Long accepted as a concept, not widely established in practice • Usually based on the social work model, i.e. combined with line management • Often with some inappropriate confidence that clinical supervision is 'old hat' • Active use of structured reflection skills in supervisees often under-developed • Support and catalytic skills often not well developed in clinical supervisors
LEARNING POINTS TO APPLY TO NURSING	• Hopeful statements about the growth and support element of clinical supervision are not enough: they need to be backed up with structures to create the conditions for this to happen • Other branches of nursing have similar cultures to midwifery and are therefore also likely to lose the growth and support element of clinical supervision if it is linked to disciplinary procedures • Need for separate management monitoring and clinical supervision	• Need to separate management monitoring of safeguarding procedures and clinical supervision	• Need for re-evaluation of clinical supervision in areas where it has been established • Not to assume that clinical supervision is happening effectively in areas where the concept is well accepted • Be alert for any tendency to inappropriate psychotherapeutic interventions into personal life • Ensure adequate skills training, even for those apparently experienced

Midwifery

Supervision has been an integral part of midwifery practice since 1936 when the role of inspector of midwives was changed to that of supervisor. The supervisor of midwives is designated by a local supervising authority and Bent (1992: 7) suggests that she is a key worker in the implementation of a principle which is at 'the very heart of supervision – the safety of mother and baby'. The route to this safety appears to embrace a specific model of supervision which links it firmly to managerial supervision and emphasizes standards, accountability, professional misconduct and the legislative framework, all of which are clearly very important. Supervision in midwifery is often felt to be more of a management tool for staff appraisal and disciplinary procedure. This very singular version of supervision has been challenged both inside and outside midwifery, and the UKCC's guidelines (1996) implicitly deter others in the broader sphere of nursing from following this approach. Others have been more explicit in their criticism:

> The role [supervisor in midwifery] however has not developed into one of empowerment or professional development; rather one of guidance and direction to ensure practice is correct. It is also used to discipline when practice goes wrong. One would not wish to see clinical supervision within nursing and health visiting developing in this way.
>
> (HVA 1994: 4)

Midwives, like those within other specialties within health care, may feel themselves to be incompatibly different from colleagues in nursing and thereby indifferent to such criticism. Indeed, the history of their own legislative framework has fuelled that difference. Yet concerns over the way clinical supervision has been translated exist within midwifery itself. The tension between those who wished to promote more of a growth and support model and those who insisted on maintaining the managerial directive approach was witnessed during the development of the controversial 'professional development' module, in material aimed at the preparation of supervisors (ENB 1992: Module 4). The organizational emphasis is clear:

> As we have seen, whilst the supervisor is specifically concerned with safe practice and clinical competence, the manager is concerned with broader organisational goals such as the overall quality of services and the effective use of resources . . . The manager's interest in professional development is . . . a means of improving current performance at work and of making the most effective use of immediate human resources.
>
> (ENB 1992: 16)

This document goes on to suggest that 'individual performance review' is a tool that can help identify these staff development needs. This may not necessarily augur well for the principles of creativity, growth and support suggested earlier in this chapter. It illustrates the warnings of Hawkins and Smith (2006), alluded to earlier.

Other branches of nursing have similar cultures to midwifery and are therefore also likely to lose the growth and support element of clinical supervision if it is linked to management monitoring and disciplinary procedures.

It is, however, interesting to note that in the preface to this material in Module 1, Bent (1992: 7) reminds us that a departmental committee in 1929 had recommended that: 'an inspector of midwives should be regarded as the counsellor and friend of the midwives rather than a relentless critic... and make them feel that there is always someone to whom they can look for sympathetic understanding'. However, these sentiments seem to have been mislaid during the intervening years, possibly due to midwifery becoming incorporated in the NHS in 1948 and into a hierarchy modelled on that of the military at that time.

The current predominant language of service requirements and 'resource commodities' overshadows the human needs suggested in this early document in midwifery, and since then endorsed by the UKCC as being essential for the implementation of clinical supervision in the rest of nursing and health visiting. We can learn from this that hopeful statements about the growth and support element of clinical supervision are not enough: they need to be backed up with structures to ensure they are incorporated as central to the process of clinical supervision.

We hope that those supervisors of midwives who would like to balance their supervisory contact by developing more of a professional and support component to their role will find the rest of this book useful, and that it could bolster rather than dilute the unique statutory and professional aspects of midwifery practice.

The safeguarding of children

The uneasy alliance of clinical supervision and management supervision is not unique to midwifery but also exists in a more limited way within child protection work. For many community practitioners, clinical supervision is totally associated with managerial supervision when children are at risk, but this is only a part of the role, for many an extremely small part, albeit a stressful and anxious one. In areas where child protection numbers are higher, some have already questioned the logistics of this system as well as the narrowness of its focus and approach.

Every Child Matters (Department of Health 2003), The Children Act (2004), *Working Together* (Department of Health, Home Office, Department for Education and Employment 2006) and *Support for All* (Department for Children, Schools and Families 2010), as well as biennial analyses of serious child review cases, have led to policies requiring managers to ensure regular review and monitoring of all aspects of work in this context. However, the increasingly attacking scrutiny by press, politicians and public makes it understandable that those who are involved in this complex, difficult arena are subject to more intensive managerial monitoring within supervision. When a child is killed, the urge to find a professional scapegoat is very great. There is a mistaken and hugely omnipotent belief that child deaths can be avoided if only professionals were more vigilant. Of course rigour in the assessment and monitoring of risk, as well as punctilious communication, both written and verbal, between all professionals and family members concerned, are vital. Where reviews of serious cases demonstrate that there have been professional or systemic failures or shortfalls, then action to try and minimize re-occurence needs to happen. Sadly, the related feelings of anxiety, and the huge fear of making mistakes, can lead to a mechanistic approach which does not seem to have been able to contain the mistakes that are reported so repetitively within serious case reviews. Interprofessional policies are clearly vital to the effective management of safeguarding, but if applied defensively and punitively, they can add to defensiveness in turn, and result in a lack of transparency rather than the desired openness.

Once again it very much matters *who* provides the supervision. An early but still relevant example mirrors current concerns. Parkinson's (1992) study of local policy in the London Borough of Tower Hamlets led her to challenge its effectiveness:

> The impossibility of carrying out this policy without excessive management workload...precipitated a management crisis...The policy document also seemed to be one step further towards restricting and controlling community nurses, rather than enabling, empowering and supporting them to take professional responsibility for their own work.
>
> (Parkinson 1992: 41)

Parkinson challenged the Department of Health's guidance to senior nurses on supervision in child protection work. She raises important points about whether line managers can meet the full supervision needs of community staff who are working with abusive families and whether a line manager can provide a safe environment in which to discuss feelings about child abuse.

This experimental study, which compared earlier manager-led supervision with the extended supervisory function of new child protection advisers who had no managerial responsibility, found the personal and professional benefits of the latter to be enormous. Parkinson also suggests that it was felt to enhance the individual's own responsibility and accountability: 'Some staff explicitly contrasted this with the situation before the project, commenting that they felt managers took on, or took over, responsibility for child protection work once they had been brought into contact with it...One manager also thought that a large number of staff felt "safer" in their work' (Parkinson 1992: 49). The subsequent development of named child protection specialists is in line with legislation, public inquiries, government reports and guidance documents. However it is acknowledged that in some areas it is nevertheless 'not within some Trusts' capacity' (Calder 2005).

This example again supports the premise, endorsed originally in principle by the UKCC but not adhered to fully by the Nursing and Midwifery Council (NMC) in 2001, that the line manager should not undertake the role of clinical supervisor for those staff for whom she holds management or disciplinary responsibilities. The NMC suggests that local areas have to be allowed to develop clinical supervision in their own way.

As Swain (1995: 40) states passionately: 'Any moves to establish links between clinical supervision and formal disciplinary process should be challenged. This is not to say the two should never touch. Clinical supervision is integral to good management which in turn is integral to an effective, healthy organisation'. Both the need for clarity of separation of management–supervisor roles, and the need to communicate with and integrate into managerial systems, will be addressed in Part III.

Mental health nursing

Presumably due to greater links with the worlds of therapy/counselling, the concept of clinical supervision has been part of mental health nursing for some time. White (1990) and Ferguson (1992) suggest that clinical supervision is more developed among nurses working in psychiatry, particularly in community settings, and yet as Thomas (1995: 27) has candidly admitted, 'it is indeed a very mixed bag' and it may be happening to some extent in some areas but certainly not in others. This is also emphasized by Carson *et al.* (1995: 54): 'Although the concept of clinical supervision is well accepted in mental health nursing, it is a less well established reality for most practitioners. It is clear that clinical supervision is certainly not yet the norm for the majority'.

Our experience in workshops has tended to support this view, where there is a tendency for some mental health practitioners to show a rather bored 'been there, done that' attitude. Yet it is clear within the skills component of the courses that many aspects of clinical supervision have often been poorly thought through and practised (with some outstanding exceptions). The tendency to over-'therapize', pathologize and use non-responsive listening or interpretations by way of support is also more apparent in this group than in others. As a result, many supervisees we have observed have been (understandably) defensive against the self-disclosure required for in-depth reflection on practice. Faugier's (1992) warnings of inappropriate therapeutic interventions may need to be heeded. Our observations indicate that skills assessment and training are necessary for many experienced supervisees and clinical supervisors. The experience of clinical supervision for mental health nurses highlights the need for re-evaluation of clinical supervision and the need not to assume that clinical supervision is happening effectively in areas where the concept is well established. One area of useful difference is that mental health lends itself to a more multidisciplinary approach to clinical supervision and the advantages of this are explored by Mullarkey *et al.* (2001).

The explicitly espoused aims of established clinical supervision systems could be viewed from the perspective of the professional cultures in which they are situated. Psychotherapy has explicit emphasis on valuing the 'therapeutic use of self', along with in-depth reflection on oneself and the part one's own personal qualities, abilities and feelings play in the professional care of the client. There is little or no managerial monitoring of psychotherapy practice since most of it is done outside institutions and it is impossible for managers to observe practitioners at work. Social work also has a degree of explicit valuing of therapeutic use of self, but within a definite (and necessary) managerial structure for monitoring practitioners which tends to increase standards of procedural safety but inhibits the development of therapeutic use of self. Mental health nursing has some degree

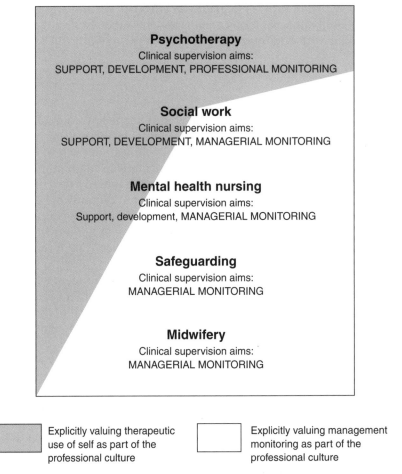

Figure 1.2 Main aims of clinical supervision related to various professional cultures

of explicit valuing of therapeutic use of self, within a management monitoring system. Child protection in nursing has less explicit valuing of therapeutic use of self and even greater explicit managerial monitoring, while midwifery has very little explicit valuing of therapeutic use of self enshrined within the culture, with considerable emphasis on managerial monitoring. Notable exceptions do exist in these nursing examples whereby explicit valuing of therapeutic use of self coexists alongside rigorous managerial monitoring. However, we are taking a broad general view here. Figure 1.2 highlights these comparisons.

So, specific examples of clinical supervision have existed in the profession for some time but all of them either offer a limited vision of its potential or have been inconsistently implemented. More recent developments have made it imperative for all practitioners and their managers to adopt more extensive and better thought-through systems of clinical supervision within their organizations. The last part of this chapter will briefly describe this.

The impetus for clinical supervision from within nursing

Continuous developments along major themes have provided the impetus for clinical supervision to become an urgent agenda item in any discussions and initiatives aiming to sustain and develop nursing practice. These developments include:

- broad organizational changes that mirror increasingly complex social changes;
- related policy directives;
- concerns about accountability and the related need for nurses to be more authoritative and develop a stronger voice;
- quality initiatives for improving standards and measurement of care;
- concepts of person-centredness, patients' rights, empowerment and partnership becoming integrated into nursing philosophy;
- educational drives towards reflective practice and lifelong CPD;
- concern about practitioner health and preventing burnout linked to concerns about workforce profiles and attrition;
- increased value placed on the dynamics of professional relationships, therapeutic interventions and concomitant requirements for self-awareness and an understanding of parallel processes.

We emphasize these positive factors which are contributing to the 'push' towards developing clinical supervision. However, in this section we also point to some of the ambivalence which can block this development and upon which we expand in the next chapter.

Some of the main 'pushing' factors for clinical supervision are outlined in Figure 1.3, forming the first part of a 'force-field analysis' diagram. We will complete this force-field analysis in Chapter 2 by examining the blocking factors which have so far impeded and may continue to impede the effective development of clinical supervision in nursing.

Broad organizational changes

Health care is becoming increasingly complex and more demanding of everyone. Technological change is only one part of this. Much of it is due to extensive change within the organizational structure of the NHS and in the philosophy of health care provision, with the impact falling heavily on clinical nursing staff. Intensive and extensive organizational change over 30 years has had unprecedented influence on how all practitioners deliver care to clients, and how they themselves are managed. Our workshop participants are steeped in organizational change, and sometimes are weary and cynical of it. As Swain (1995: 14) puts it: 'Repeated organisational changes tax even the most flexible of practitioners. Continuing

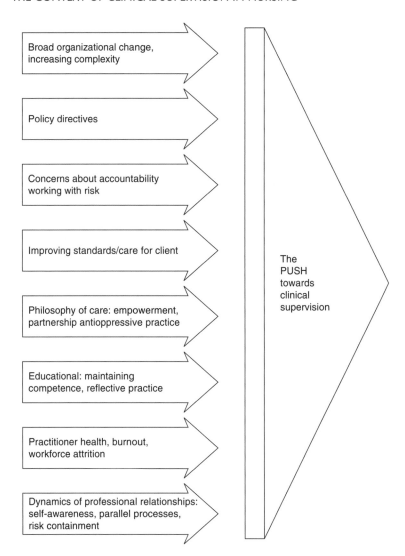

Figure 1.3 Factors which have contributed to the present impetus towards developing clinical supervision in nursing

clinical work while at the same time practising creatively through the development of imaginative ideas for future practice requires professional stability, boundaries and containment'. There is increasing recognition that clinical supervision can be a system for providing this stability, boundaries and containment to enable practitioners to cope with and positively adjust to organizational changes.

However, clinical supervision cannot be viewed in isolation from other key government agendas on health care. For the purposes of this chapter we have decided to speak generally, unlike in the first edition when illustrations and examples were out of date as soon as the ink had dried. The dilemma is that as soon as a book is printed the political fabric of health care delivery changes its language, dating so quickly the terminology and initiatives that were once so new – well, new-ish. Although the language can change, ideas are not so much 'new', as 'evolving', albeit in a cyclical fashion, and actual mutation is slow. You know that the main developmental changes in the last 20 years or so have involved themes of measurement, quality, standards and efficiency alongside more philosophical accounts of how to engage and include patients in their own health and care, an emphasis on public health and prevention, and a related interest in the more visible role of the nurse in clinical leadership.

The demands of market forces, the need for standards to measure efficacy and efficiency and the relocation of power and management in the NHS have all put pressure on every single practitioner to rethink how they perform their work, and how they must skew or adapt their priorities. Purchasing contracts with commissioning authorities have to be adhered to. Future contracts depend on it. In the current economic climate there is a need to ensure that best practices, including supervision, address the needs of all stakeholders, while staying ethical. And yet practitioners who are closer to client groups have often had little say in the early negotiation of contracts and have seen the quality of their health care interventions sacrificed for quantity. Because of this, many initiatives exist to encourage practitioners to develop the necessary skills of marketing, skill mix and campaigning to influence purchasing decisions (Department of Health 1994; HVA 1994). *High Quality Care for All* (Department of Health 2008) highlighted the need to encourage a culture of innovation and speed up the 'mainstreaming' of good ideas. The Commission on the Future of Nursing and Midwifery in England (2010) decries the lack of nurses involved in such initiatives, suggesting that they are the lynchpin for innovation.

Primary care and public health has had its fair share of organizational shifts – for example, backwards and forwards in the employment, role and responsibilities of GPs, guided by specific measurement and evaluation tools which are contentious. The NHS and Community Care Act 1990 addressed divisions in health and social care, and there have been subsequent developments in further integration in training and practice and multidisciplinary working. If you have been around for a very long time you may be struck by the fact that this is not such a novel idea, particularly the health visitors among you.

The community care part of the Act has also been subject to extensive criticism from all client groups. Its honourable rhetoric about caring for people in their own homes has not been matched by the resources to do so (King's Fund 1997), leaving community practitioners at the very sharp end of care. Greater numbers are being discharged earlier, so that one set of colleagues meeting targets puts increasing pressure on others.

As Watkins (1993: 436) has said, 'Community care should be a philosophy not a place'. Sadly it is often viewed more simplistically and pragmatically as a place – a cheaper place. The main carers here of course are not even community practitioners, but those who have always provided the bulk of care in the community – families and carers, and usually women. Wynne (1994) and others have recorded how community care policies have placed an additional burden on women carers. As the majority of our nursing workforce are women, this may impose a dual burden, professional and personal, on them.

The restructuring of management has led to a reduction in nurses in more senior positions within Trusts and there are very few in purchasing positions. The Commission on the Future of Nursing and Midwifery in England (2010) highlights its concern at this and seeks ways to redress it. This has led many nurses to feel under-represented and marginalized in negotiating crucial decisions for service provision. The flattened management structure in nursing has put pressure on the role of clinical team leaders to provide this leadership and to implement the changes, while still fulfilling their clinical responsibilities without additional resources. Broader restructuring of skill mix, where it has been done with the full involvement and negotiation of staff, has resulted in a better utilization of appropriate skills all round. But it has often been implemented solely with cost-cutting in mind, more 'What grades do we choose to afford?' than 'What skills do we need to meet the health needs in our specialty?'

The Patient's Charter (Department of Health 1991c, 1993c), which led to developments in person-centred care, advocated patients' rights and their own expertise in and understanding of their own health issues, made more promises than the resources given to match them. Although most practitioners would heartily agree with complaints procedures introduced to challenge shortfalls in service provision, many feel that they have been left to face understandably angry and upset clients with both hands tied behind their backs, unable to offer the services that grand mission statements have promised to provide.

Inequalities in health care continue to grow. Some of these affect not just client groups 'out there' but many practitioners in nursing who in turn may become recipients of health care; we are all potential clients.

Racial and sexual inequalities are mirrored particularly well within the layers of the employment hierarchy, despite attempts to address equal opportunities in the workplace. Such attempts in the 1990s included *A Programme for Action* (Department of Health 1993b) to increase the numbers of ethnic minority staff and *Opportunity 2000* (Department of Health 1991d) to increase the very low numbers of women in leadership positions (Rafferty 1993). Many believe there to be a mismatch between rhetoric and reality in the development of equal opportunities. Robinson (1992) argues that some developments in nursing, notably in primary nursing, actually serve to reinforce sexual and racial divisions and this is backed up by a much later study which highlighted that senior management in the NHS is seen and experienced as a 'brutal' environment within which to work, not softened by four reorganizations of leadership development within 10 years: see NHS Confederation (2009). Hence senior management is not a very attractive working environment for anyone from a disadvantaged group who may have had to struggle more than most to be acknowledged. Again, one of the main recommendations of the Commission on the Future of Nursing and Midwifery (2010) is the need to nurture and fast-track leaders within nursing, and generally build damaged self-esteem and the image of nurses.

These perceptions or realities of differences in class, race, culture, age and sexuality can be mirrored within the supervisory relationship and will be addressed later.

In reworking a theory of critical reflection, Fook (2010: 40) states, 'I would now articulate critical reflection (for clinical supervision) as involving the ability to understand the social dimensions, and political functions of experience and meaning making, and the ability to apply this understanding in working in social contexts'. Clinical supervision is not – and must not be – isolated from this context of broad societal and organizational change.

Ironically, although buffeted by all these organizational changes which increasingly affect the way practitioners think, make decisions and prioritize their work, many say that direct contact remains the same, in that people are still scared and vulnerable when ill, carers still want the best they can get for their loved ones and babies still assert their right to be born and cared for. This makes for growing tensions between the demands of the client and the sometimes conflicting demands of employers. Clinical supervision is needed not only to help practitioners cope with the pressures of all these many changes, but also to enable them to face the ethically demanding nature of some of these tensions and the ensuing dilemmas. The clinical supervisor may herself feel that she is in the centre of a triangle of often competing demands – those of the practitioner, the organization and the client. She needs to have the skills and resilience to work with the clinical dilemmas that emerge. In today's NHS the clinical supervisor is required to have an understanding of the needs of both the provider and the purchaser: nurse and client.

Policy directives

Although there has been a growing professional impetus towards clinical supervision, it required political endorsement to give it additional potency and weight. Policy directives continue to ensure that clinical supervision will become a national concern rather than being left to areas of good practice. Although in the short term this may mean that the implementation of clinical supervision in some areas is based on compliance rather than commitment, and may be interpreted and introduced in a minimalist way, the directives nevertheless provide an essential long-term lever to improve clinical supervision systems.

A Vision for the Future (Department of Health 1993d) was the first document officially to recommend that the concept of supervision should be explored and developed, so that it is integral through the lifetime of practice, thus enabling practitioners to accept personal responsibility for – and be accountable for – care, and to keep that care under constant review. It mirrored the UKCC's emphasis on the parameters of safe practice and the educational requirements for greater professional autonomy and accountability within *The Scope of Professional Practice* (UKCC 1992), as well as the potential extension of this practice, when it announced that it 'is central to the process of learning and to the expansion of the scope of practice' (Department of Health 1993d: 15).

In its statement on clinical supervision for nursing and health visiting, the UKCC (1996) suggested that clinical supervision should assist all practitioners to develop a deeper understanding of what it is to be an accountable practitioner in the context of the realities of clinical risk management. The document emphasized the potential organizational benefits to be accrued from this, linking to the NHS Executive six medium-term priorities: 'to develop NHS organisation as good employers with particular reference to workforce planning, education and training, employment policy and practice, the development of teamwork, reward systems, staff utilisation and staff welfare' (UKCC 1996: 3).

The UKCC placed clinical supervision firmly in the context of the profession's need to develop lifelong learners and made an important assertion that 'Clinical supervision is not a managerial control system' and should be 'non-hierarchical' in nature (1996: 3).

Although the NMC has continued to echo earlier statements (see Table 1.4), it has dropped any reference to clinical supervision being non-hierarchical and therefore we consider it does not go far enough in supporting non-managerial supervision as distinct from line management supervision. The open-endedness of these guidelines leaves the possibility for anything to be called 'clinical supervision' and for claiming this falls within the NMC guidelines and ticking the box. We have seen this happen in a number of organizations: examples include a complaints procedure, management by objectives, a disciplinary procedure, a chat with a colleague in the corridor, a debriefing after an incident. Most of these examples were disingenuous. While we welcome leadership in strengthening the authority of line management supervision, we advocate integrity in maintaining clinical supervision as regular, facilitated, in-depth reflection on practice, delivered within an ethical framework which is sensitive to the self-disclosure issues involved. We expand on this in Chapters 8, 9 and 10.

Table 1.4   NMC's (2008b) statement on the principles of clinical supervision

- Clinical supervision supports practice, enabling registered nurses to maintain and improve standards of care
- Clinical supervision is a practice-focused professional relationship, involving a practitioner reflecting on practice guided by a skilled supervisor
- Registered nurses and managers should develop the process of clinical supervision according to local circumstances. Ground rules should be agreed so that the supervisor and the registered nurse approach clinical supervision openly, confidently and are aware of what is involved
- Every registered nurse should have access to clinical supervision and each supervisor should supervise a realistic number of practitioners
- Preparation for supervisors should be flexible and sensitive to local circumstances. The principles and relevance of clinical supervision should be included in pre-registration and post-registration education programmes
- Evaluation of clinical supervision is needed to assess how it influences care and practice standards. Evaluation systems should be determined locally

Concerns about accountability and risk

The UKCC's code of practice, and related guidance on the concept and practice of accountability from the initial *Exercising Accountability* (UKCC 1989) and *The Scope of Professional Practice* (UKCC 1992) to expansions within the NMC code (NMC 2008a), have all challenged practitioners to focus on maintaining clinical standards and to link this with the growth and development of their own competence and educational progress. The latest NMC code has also emphasized the importance of being able to assess and contain risk and situations of potential risk. Future codes will no doubt expand upon this, based on further developments in organizational and practice complexity that impinge on professional responsibilities and accountability.

Professional accountability is, however, only one aspect of legal accountability. Dimond (1990) highlights the different types of accountability when she compares and contrasts it with accountability to the client, to society as a whole and to the employer. Although to maintain accountability in one arena may automatically ensure accountability in another (for instance, accountability to clients based on confidentiality is part and parcel of our professional accountability), many dilemmas in practice can result from a clash between professional accountability and accountability towards an employer (Holland 1991). Pressures on employers to curtail and limit resources can have both a direct and an indirect impact on the ability of individual practitioners to maintain even their current scope of practice. Practitioners need help and support to clarify the implications of the many-faceted nature of accountability in everyday practice and there is increasing recognition that clinical supervision can provide a forum for this. They also need to develop a more authoritative voice within these debates to draw attention to these dilemmas as they affect client care. The training for the extension of the role of Approved Mental Health Practitioner to include mental health nurses is a more specific example of the need for this, as are the additional areas of risk when working with all vulnerable adults and children.

In an increasingly complex organizational picture of different multidisciplinary settings, there is also a related growing need for clarity about roles and the boundaries between individual practitioners, especially when philosophies and approaches to client care, needs assessment and service delivery may clash. Shifts in power within work systems and partnerships all demand a shrewd grasp of accountability principles in practice. As Johnson (1995) has suggested, clinical supervision can allow for the development of role clarity without which teams cannot collaborate effectively. Mullarkey *et al.* (2001) have referred to the potential for this in multidisciplinary approaches to clinical supervision.

The actual process of clinical supervision may on occasion also provide a challenge to the clinical supervisor's practice of accountability. We have endorsed a non-managerial approach to supervision, but there is much concern about what happens when it is clear to the clinical supervisor that the supervisee's practice is not 'good enough' and may even be unsafe. This link between clinical supervision and accountability in practice is found in the section on clinical supervision contracts in Chapter 3 and in the section on authority in Chapter 6.

Concern to improve standards of care for clients

Although many initiatives in nursing have been motivated by a desire to improve client care and service delivery, it is also sadly true that clients may become lost behind grand professional posturing and a plethora of theories and concepts. We live in a sound-bite age. We would do well to be reminded that 'the first principle of clinical supervision must be that clients should benefit, individually and corporately, directly and indirectly' (Swain 1995: 22). Standards of care need to be at the root of clinical supervision (Department of Health 2004). It is about what we do for our clients, how we listen to, talk to and relate to clients, what the outcomes of our contact with them are and what the overall clinical effectiveness is. It is about efficient and effective use of our time. Maintaining and enhancing standards needs to be placed and viewed in its political, social and educational context, and the centrality of client care in the organizational and educational context has been at the heart of all continuing education initiatives (UKCC 1993). In reality it is hard to do this effectively without maintaining and demonstrating thoughtful curiosity about, and emotional empathy with, the people in our care and others we work with. Forming relationships feeds this curiosity and empathy, and this needs the nurturance and challenge of the clinical supervision relationship. This links to the emphasis on 'compassionate' care in the document *Front Line Care* (Commission on the Future of Nursing and Midwifery in England 2010), while emphasizing the importance of demonstrating effectiveness and good practice in the maintenance of standards.

Changing philosophies of care: partnership, empowerment and working with diversity

The last 20 years have witnessed a gradual demedicalization of nursing and a slow maturing of nursing as a profession, moving away from a practice based on the biological/medico-sciences towards ideas from sociology, psychology and educational theory, and a general push towards higher education. The growth of notions of nursing independence, epitomized by process-based nursing, has resulted in a related emphasis on individual autonomy and accountability which, some suggest, has left many practitioners adrift between theory and the shifting sands of clinical practice, without some of the defensive mechanisms of the past. Butterworth (1992: 5) suggests that clinical supervision can offer some protection, 'giving nursing the necessary support it needs to mature into greater independence'.

Movement towards a more person-centred approach (Care Quality Commission 2010) has led to demands for client advocacy rather than direct intervention and for working with clients in partnership, aiming to empower rather than 'do to or for' or 'talk at or about'. The move towards health promotion and prevention, even in the acute branches of nursing, and albeit slow and incomplete (Department of Health 1995), has challenged us to retreat from crisis ad hoc responses and to reflect on the possible range of long-term choices, encouraging the essential involvement and participation of clients en route. For Faugier (1995), clinical supervision and patient empowerment are very closely linked. Yet despite the numerous advantages of working to involve and empower rather than control, outlined by many commentators and practitioners such as Pearson (1988) and Chavasse (1992), this shift in approach presents a threat and a challenge to practitioners who are reluctant to let go of time-honoured ways of relating professionally (Bond and Holland 1992). Kendall (1991) is one of many researchers who have found that working collaboratively with clients is more of a myth than a reality, even when practitioners earnestly believe that this is what they are doing. There is a need to disentangle the realities of working in partnership from the more superficial rhetoric associated with the term; its true implications for both client and practitioner could be teased out within clinical supervision. There is increasing recognition that the true development of partnership and empowerment requires the kind of backup support and challenge provided in the clinical supervision relationship.

This is also where we can integrate awareness and responsiveness to inequalities in health through explorations of difference, working towards anti-discriminatory and anti-oppressive practice (Burke and Harrison 2010). Although we are also aware that using difference can be a defensive ploy, the long-standing grievances from those who have felt invisible or avoided within the health care system are justified. There are many accounts of individual and institutionalized racism, as well as prejudice towards those from specific cultures or different sexual orientations. You can't work in partnership if you cannot even be seen. This adds yet more layers of complexity and takes courage and skill for all parties to both name and explore (Kareem and Littlewood 1992; Dalal 2002; Morgan 2007).

Developments in education

There have been both direct and more subtle changes in educational philosophy and approach in nursing, shifting away from control of the content of clinical material and towards encouraging ownership by learners of their own educational process. The emphasis is more on *how* people learn, on encouraging a diversity of learning styles and needs, and on achieving a better educational balance between authoritative and facilitative teaching styles. It has been important to encourage safe, experiential learning (Kolb and Fry 1975) to allow for an emotional and personal engagement with the theory. This approach to adult education is more likely to encourage practitioners to take responsibility for their own 'lifelong learning' and to use clinical supervision as part of this within education standards. However, for many teachers and learners, these have been painful shifts. Once again there is a reluctance to let go of much safer scripts, to focus on regurgitating the 'what' rather than asking why, and to be more directed and directing than enabling in its broadest sense. This is the antithesis of the 'thinking and curious' culture that clinical supervision seeks to enable. It also needs to be said that not all higher educational experiences offer this either: education is not a place but is part of a relationship, and the encouragement to learn is subject to many subjective relational experiences.

Reflection has become firmly established in educational theory and practice since Schön's influential work in the 1980s (1983, 1987), when he developed ideas and differentials between 'reflection on practice' and 'reflection in practice'. Reflection has been used as a tool to bridge the divide between theory and practice. Many different models have been devised and some are discussed and adapted in Chapter 3 as frameworks to guide and supplement reflective thinking. However, there is a growing awareness that the value placed on reflection in the nursing literature is not always mirrored in practice. Swain (1995: 9) suggests that 'We speak and write of reflective practice, yet experience out in the field suggests a very different reality. Time for reflection is in fact a very rare commodity indeed'. Boud (2010) also suggests that the teaching of reflection within universities and professions has become mechanized, with an over-emphasis on model formats creating a 'tick box' superficiality, rather than applied meaning. So reflection needs to be done, but it needs to be done well.

Later in this book we adapt ideas on reflection to link more with the picture of growing complexity in health care, when dilemmas and tensions imposed by many different sociocultural and organizational demands, as well as anxieties about risk and accountability, can lead to minds in retreat rather than minds that can engage and reflect.

Reflection is not a simple process – not as simple as looking in a mirror. Even that is not really simple. We imagine that, depending on mood, and how you feel that day, you do not always want to look in the mirror; do you choose the ordinary mirror or the magnified view? Do you choose to see flaws or not? Are flaws the only thing you see? The result also depends on the angle of the light and where you stand.

Clinical supervision may offer just such a place for space and reflection, helping practitioners to integrate theory to practice, increase awareness of research findings, understand what can be done and cannot be done, contain anxieties, and develop curiosity and a more confident nursing voice.

Evidence of the importance of paying attention to practitioner health

Evidence of the advantages of promoting supportive cultures in the workplace abound. Cooper's (1981) and Hingley et al.'s (1986) work refers to the economic and efficiency benefits to the organization of reduction in sick leave and reductions in the mobility and attrition of the workforce. Butterworth et al. (1997) suggested that nurses were experiencing a time of increasing stress levels in the 1990s, as compared to other projects carried out in the 1980s using the same measure (the Nurse Stress Index). Using standardized instruments, they also found that clinical supervision could stabilize, and in some cases reduce, these measurable stress levels. In their work on preceptorship (but equally relevant when applied to clinical supervision), Morton-Cooper and Palmer (1993: 31) suggest that 'if we can become more understanding and supportive of our colleagues, then similar values could be carried in our day to day work and help us to communicate more fully (and perhaps more honestly) with those people who place such faith and trust in us at times of crisis and transition in their lives'.

Swain (1995: 29), humane as ever, reminds us that practitioners need help for themselves first and foremost, before they can be of help to others: 'We need to take our own grief and stress somewhere, express it and deal with it'. Johnson (1995: 22) also refers to the managerial and organizational benefits of clinical supervision. She states that it could help practitioners develop 'their emotional responsiveness so that they don't become burnt out and so that they remain able to offer a high quality service in a climate of rapid change'. Research by Edwards *et al.* (2000) suggests a positive correlation between clinical supervision and reduction of burnout, as does that of Brunero and Stein-Parbury (2008). However, it takes Australian initiatives to explore how clinical supervision might address workforce development for the purpose of retaining staff (National Centre for Education and Training on Addiction 2005; Victoria Healthcare Association 2008).

Swain (1995) suggests that some of the low priority given to strategies that might aid emotional support or give time to reflect is due to the realities of a very pressured external world which result in practitioners marginalizing their own physical and emotional health. She and many others suggest that the impact of tremendous organizational changes has created a more non-compassionate culture, superceded by demands for targets and measurement. There was a vibrant anti-professional political culture in the 1980s and 1990s in many diverse service professions such as education, social work, probation, police and prison services, and many have shared similar feelings of resentment and loss, resulting in low morale and attrition of the workforce. The nursing literature is full of references to 'support' and the need for nurses to develop more emotional skills, yet self-care has not in general featured highly in the nursing agenda, nor is it truly just a product of more recent political change, although this has undoubtedly exacerbated it. Lip-service is frequently paid to the need to support each other but the lack of extensive support networks indicates the poverty of both organizational and individual commitment to it.

Increasing value placed on self-awareness as a therapeutic skill

When the work itself is intrinsically highly charged and makes emotional demands, and when this is added to by the pressures of rapidly changing organizational demands and limited resources, there is a need not only to offer more extensive structures for support but also to encourage individuals to build their own skills in survival and growth. The current push towards helping nurses to increase their self-awareness is essential if they are to look after themselves more and contribute to a healthier, more caring workforce culture. Self-awareness will also allow for more sensitive and effective interventions in nurses' work with clients and will improve clinical standards and care.

Yet Guggenbuhl Craig (1971) reminds us that our unconscious drive towards helping others can in itself lead to unhelpful ways of being and relating. Heron (2001) refers to these as 'degenerative interventions' and you will be exploring many of these pitfalls throughout the skills chapters of this book. Much of Hawkins and Shohet's (1989, 2006) work on supervision focuses on the concept of the 'wounded helper', which we shall explore in the next chapter, and although they rightly suggest that our 'wounds' or vulnerability can be a strong asset if recognized and supported, they can also lead to unconscious interventions that are not helpful to others or ourselves. Therefore our capacity to understand, respond effectively and help is more likely to be genuine, appropriate and centred in the client if tempered by understanding of ourselves and our motivations. As Hawkins and Shohet (1989: 5) state: 'our experience is that supervision can be an important part of taking care of oneself, staying open to new learning, and an indispensable part of the helper's on-going self development, self awareness and commitment to learning'.

This links to the need to build your own 'internal supervisor' (Casement 1985) which can be used in reflective learning in practice and brought back to your actual clinical supervision session for further honing, clarification and help. In this way we can learn to watch, listen to and understand ourselves as well as our clients and so 'stand back' from the relationship to assess and monitor it as well as take part in it. Taylor (2007) suggests that this can be thought of as a triangular space in the mind in which the subjective self is observed having a relationship with an idea in relation to the clinical 'other' – a client from the clinical context, or what/whoever the focus of concern is, and the internalized capacity to think about it from a different position (the external supervisor position). This is linked to the importance of shifting position in reflection, explored earlier. This is essential for the sophisticated ability to reflect 'in' practice (on the job) as well as 'on' practice. It is not the same as being emotionally distant or aloof from another or from ourselves, but it is a way of building inner resources and awareness to improve and develop our work and is a vital part of mature CPD and lifelong learning.

The parallel process within clinical supervision

This capacity to think on the job, develop, internalize help, and experience and build your own inner supervisor needs of course a relationship with a real supervisor first, and it is important to understand the parallels between the nurse and their clinical relationships with clients and colleagues, and the nurse-as-supervisee and her supervisor. This dynamic can be transferred and can impact for good or ill. For good – because if understood correctly it can offer a very immediate way to understand what might be going on and allow it to be felt and thought about differently. The supervisor is the third 'other' – standing at a distance and outside the relational and practice focus of the supervisee, and so may be able to encourage a different view. The capacity of both parts of the supervisory relationship to do this, and so bring more oxygen and thoughtfulness to a situation, demands that they are able to:

- observe and be observed;
- think and be thought about;
- help and be helped.

For many this may prove difficult: too revealing, too open to perceived criticism. The converse possibilities for disruption and misunderstandings will be addressed in the next chapter. However, a more analytic approach to this parallel emotional dynamic can make the supervisory task multi-layered and complex, but rich in its potential. As Woods (2007: 25) suggests, clinical supervision 'takes place in a tension between the potential for pleasurable learning and the potential for anxiety, confusion and concern'. Part II of this book attempts to address this by exploring the skills necessary for this complex relationship – those that encourage rather than diminish learning, and where anxiety can be more contained.

'Framing' the picture of clinical supervision

We see the 'frame' of clinical supervision being made up of intertwining elements from both the supervisory dyad, the team, and the managerial and organizational structure. The frame needs to provide firm, durable supportive boundaries to preserve the protected space of supervision. But like all frames, it can vary. Think of a visit to an art gallery. Do you ever remember loving a particular painting but wincing at the surrounding heavy, ornate gilt frame that seemed to suffocate it, and wishing for something less intrusive? Or how some others may have a rather minimal, bland surround that does little to bring out and highlight the image and colour within, or may be so tatty that it appears to be falling apart. Sometimes, however, the frame can be just right – and that is when you are probably not even aware of it at all. It does not detract from its inner picture, and so the creative work is all you see. Someone has been quite clever choosing and making the frame to go with the picture, to achieve this effect.

A good enough frame for clinical supervision might be something like this.

A commitment to boundaries in supervision 'offers a secure frame . . . this may enhance a sense of safety and containment, and allows the exploration of sensitive, personal anxiety-provoking material . . . Regularity, privacy and reliability contribute to the necessary sense of safety' (Wood 2007: 25). All layers of the organization have a responsibility to be committed to this. Establishing a frame is what is needed first and foremost (Thomas 2005) and it is also what can go so desperately wrong. We write more about establishing the frame in Chapters 2, 3, 8, 9 and 10.

Summary

Well thought-through and resourced systems of clinical supervision could indeed help meet many of our own unmet professional needs, which are both a part of these forces pushing for change as well as a byproduct of some of the more positive forces. Practitioners need an uncontaminated, supported and supportive space to share, reflect and analyse what they do and how they feel. This will provide a focus for developing skills for effective practice, so contributing to improvements in practice. However, there is also a great danger in viewing clinical supervision as a universal panacea for existing shortfalls or ills. As we explored in the Introduction, it is as effective as the commitment, training and resources allocated to it. Managers in the organization have to be convinced that it will add to efficiency and effectiveness in order to justify developing and maintaining it. Practitioners and managers have to be open to the language and meaning of clinical supervision to the other. Chapter 2 presents the other side of the coin, already identified within the ambivalence of some of the 'push' factors in this section. It explores some of the more resistant elements to this change and focuses on the vital emotional underpinning of clinical supervision.

2 The hidden picture: resistance to clinical supervision and implications for the clinical supervision relationship

Although the momentum towards implementing clinical supervision has been growing in recent years, there is also concern about why it has taken so long to become accepted in nursing and how it can really take root and grow in a culture that can be so resistant to major change, particularly change which is dependent upon encouraging more meaningful and transparent professional relationships. Undoubtedly there is sufficient political will to support it in principle but it remains to be seen how extensively and effectively it will become an organic part of nursing life and be truly instrumental in helping support and develop clinical practice.

Maybe during your reading of the first chapter you also felt your cynicism rising as the old mantras reappeared. Don't we know enough already, you might think, about the need for accountability, for working in partnership, for improving standards of care? We are all trying to survive great organizational change and have been for some time. There has always been an imperative to balance individual and organizational needs. Prevention of burnout through developing self-awareness has been acknowledged for more than 20 years, so why are we still going on about it? The repeat button seems to be stuck. And yet we are all destined to keep on repeating ourselves, both individually and collectively as a profession, until what is being aimed for is felt to be understood, accessible and attainable.

This cannot happen until the powerful processes which inhibit us from understanding and reaching our perceived wants and goals are also acknowledged, accepted and understood. In so doing we can divest them of their power to sabotage the process and identify more realistic ways of being effective. We have to bring the unacknowledged and therefore unknown unconscious processes between ourselves and others, be they clients or other colleagues, into our awareness; we need to bring them to the surface where they can be seen and coped with more easily. Similarly we have to understand that within the organizational culture we may also be affected by the systemic unconscious processes belonging to the organization as a whole, which although they are not directly part of us, can still impinge on our capacity to work in the way we would like to, and can confuse and distort how we ourselves act and think (Obholzer and Roberts 1994; Huffington *et al.* 2004).

All of this is part of the crucial emotional underpinning of clinical supervision and indeed all human relationships. But it is particularly important in a professional supervisory relationship which espouses the principles of growth and support and centres on reflective practice as a way of improving the care of ourselves as well as our clients. Towards the end of the last chapter we explored the factors influential in 'pushing' towards clinical supervision. As a means of counterbalancing this we will start with an overview of the forces within ourselves and the organizations in which we work which will unconsciously try and resist this major force for progress and change. We will then link this more directly to the implications for the clinical supervision relationship and the types of unconscious communication that can take place within it. From this we will distil some of the practical implications for developing clinical supervision to allow for its valuable potential to mature rather than wither.

Resistances to clinical supervision

Although the potential value of clinical supervision is extolled, the literature is also full of anxiety and misunderstandings about it. Some of these anxieties have real components to them: pressure on time, staffing levels and resources are factors of life in the NHS and will have an impact on the frequency of, and commitment to, clinical supervision. And yet many nurses have always used these factors defensively to avoid thinking about and applying aspects of professional change. Given the history of defensiveness in nursing, it is not surprising that clinical supervision may be viewed with suspicion.

Clulow (1994) refers to the ambivalence generated by the term and the fear of either being overly controlled or nannied – 'We were struck by the negativity about supervision' (1994: 181), resulting in lip-service being paid to the need for it, without any real conviction or active commitment to it. Platt-Koch (1986: 7) has said: 'confusion about and resistance to clinical supervision could be depriving nurses of one of the most valuable tools in existence for learning and refining skills of assessment and treatment of patients'. Hill (1989) suggests that practitioners tend to think of their supervisors as authoritarian and that the whole concept of clinical supervision is linked conceptually to an authoritarian figure. Hill goes on to decry this 'because clinical supervision is much wider and generous in its intention' (1989: 9). Fear of being disempowered in the clinical supervision process led community nurses from one neighbourhood nursing team, in Kohner's (1994) overview of clinical supervision in practice for the King's Fund, to reject the concept. They preferred to describe what they received as advice, support and professional guidance rather than clinical supervision. Although their reluctance to embrace the term may be understandable, their reason for doing so is more worrying. They seemed to want to protect their own autonomy and control over particular areas of practice and expertise: 'it feels uncomfortable and threatening to have someone supervise you. Most community nurses have picked this sphere of nursing to get away from control and lack of autonomy over their own practice' (Kohner 1994: 31). Clinical supervision is clearly seen here as a critical intrusion rather than a positive relationship.

Both individual and organizational defences may serve to block the establishment of clinical supervision and/or be destructive to its effectiveness once
established. These resistances, rather like many of the push factors in Chapter 1, in-
terlink with each other and it is difficult to see where one begins and another ends.
They impact on and leak into each other, and yet each has distinctive characteristics and roles to play. We need to ask what they are protecting us from, and why.

The simple question to ask to start with is why do we need to defend against
clinical supervision? We develop defences as protective devices to prevent us from
feeling anxious, but this anxiety tends to mask other deeper feelings. Defences
serve to protect us in particularly difficult situations when we feel we have to be
seen to cope. Yet both these individual and collective defence strategies in nursing
have also led to ways of working and relating that are counter-productive to effective practice and personal emotional survival. The protection they give is flawed
and may actually cause a range of other problems. Coping defensively (and often
ineffectually) is very different from developing and using skills to manage and
contain our anxiety when we both need and choose to. Then we are more in control within the situation, rather than having unconscious defence mechanisms in
control of us.

In clinical supervision this continuum of resistance, moving from deeply defended to accepting, is shown in Table 2.1. The more hidden underlying feelings
that the defences are trying to protect from are also outlined. We need to explore
these components in more depth.

Table 2.1   Levels of resistance to developing clinical supervision

LEVEL 4 RESISTANCE	LEVEL 3 RESISTANCE	LEVEL 2 RESISTANCE	LEVEL 1 RESISTANCE	NO RESISTANCE
Individual nurse				
Rejection – 'get enough criticism and interference from management as it is'	Irrelevant to me – 'good idea but too busy'	Resignation – going through the motions	Give it a try – tentative testing the water	Commitment
Organization				
Rejection of the real principles – just rename IPR or line management as 'clinical supervision'	Irrelevant to us – 'too costly'	Resignation – paying lip-service	Pilot projects	Commitment
Hidden issues				
Struggle for power, control, autonomy	Fear of relationship	Fear of emotional floodgates opening	Interest, relief	Valuing, seeing effect on practice

First, we will enlarge on the types of defences in nursing, and relate some of these more specifically to clinical supervision. Then we need to identify the main anxieties they are protecting us from, which, for simplicity, we will take from Figure 2.1 and divide into:

- fear of personal and professional power, of inequalities in power, and the impact of this on our own skills and autonomy;
- fear of developing more secure, supportive working relationships and professional attachments when the expectation is more about criticism and attack;

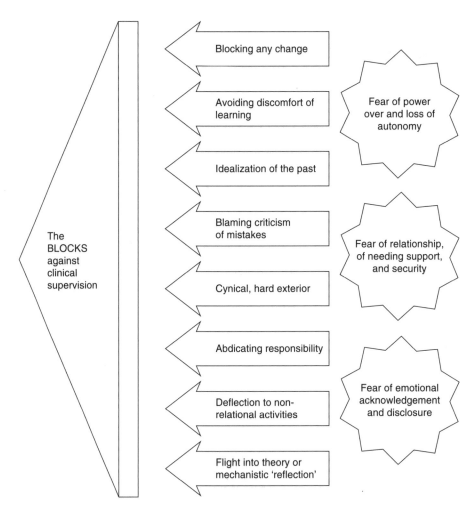

Figure 2.1 Defences which block the effectiveness of clinical supervision and the unacknowledged fears behind them

- fear of emotions, disclosure and expressing feeling – leading to a pervasive anti-emotional climate.

If you were to place these anxieties opposite the push factors in Chapter 1 you might be forgiven for thinking that in logical and practical terms the push factors would have a 'walk-over'. However, Lewin (1972), in his model of force-field analysis which seeks to compare the influence of factors affecting change, warns against such an assumption. He suggests that the resistant factors which spring from our feelings, even though we may be unaware of them, can undermine a greater number of factors which stem from apparent common sense and rationale. The factors which allegedly make 'no sense' can be much more powerful than ones which do. The impact of both emotional life and unconscious processes on our conscious cognitive self is now the subject of intensive research in neuroscience (Damasio 1999; Corrigall and Wilkinson 2003). Watt (2003) explains this well when he argues that emotion has for too long been relegated to the 'back of the bus' in cognitive science and alludes to the strong case emerging from the research for emotion binding together 'virtually every type of information that the brain can encode'. He suggests that emotion is 'the glue that holds the whole system together' (2003: 84). He is speaking of the internal system of mind and body but many would see this as complemented by a more transparent recognition that emotions also affect the rational cognitive dimension in the parallel system within an organization. How do we make sense of these hidden forces?

Anxiety and defences

Individual and collective anxiety

Anxiety is part of the human condition. How individuals respond to anxiety is at the root of much relational research. It is central to managing internal and external conflict. It determines the way we feel about ourselves and how we interpret our experiences. It provides an important alarm system to alert us to situations that we will find stressful. Appropriate and realistic anxiety can be a spur to creativity and growth. However if, in our early histories, anxiety is not able to be contained by another (as it is in 'good enough' mothering), or we are not helped to contain it at other times throughout life, and if we in turn do not learn to use it as a resource, then the internal conflict it produces becomes unmanageable and it works against us. We are then compelled to bury or block it, but it still acts as an 'undercover agent' to distort our perceptions and actions, leading to inappropriate or limited responses. The role of anxiety in organizations and the social defences that arise from it have long been acknowledged to have a major impact on behaviour and attitudes in the workplace. Anxiety increases when the level of risk is perceived to be high, and sturdy social defences may grow to protect or anaesthetize us from these risks. The factors that determine how you identify sources of risk and assess the degree of this risk will vary. They may evolve from your own history of handling anxiety, the role and degree of responsibility, authority and power you may feel you have in your professional life, and both the overt and covert strategies that are employed in the organization to include or exclude, control or motivate others. There is an interplay between organizational and individual anxiety and defences: 'we see organisations as key sites where early anxieties are replayed; and we see the very structures of the organisations as reflections of the apprehensions and frustrations of their members. Organisations are emotional arenas' (Fineman 1993a: 30–1).

The health care organization is a particularly emotional arena where Menzies (1959), in her influential work on social defence mechanisms in nursing, spelled out some of the strategies through which this interplay was enacted. For Menzies these defences develop over time as the result of collusive interaction and agreement, often unconscious, between members of the organization as to what form they shall take. The socially constructed defence mechanisms then tend to become an aspect of external reality to which old and new members have to adapt. For instance, many enthusiastic students or returners to practice, with their imaginations fired by the potential of nursing, often have to face the reality shock (Kramer 1974) of colleagues who have defended themselves by becoming cynical and disinterested. How they too may subsequently inherit the habitual ways of reacting and defending is well expressed by Obholzer and Roberts (1994: 9): 'Newcomers may be able to see more clearly but feel that they have no licence to comment. By the time they do, they have either forgotten how to see, or have learned not to. They too require defending against their anxieties, not least the anxiety of upsetting their colleagues'. Although Menzies' (1959) original study is now fairly old and only focuses on hospital nursing, much of it is as depressingly relevant today as it was then, and her more recent work alludes to this (Menzies-Lyth 1988). Some of the specific examples within the defences have changed but others have replaced them. The Commission on the Future of Nursing and Midwifery in England (2010: 79) recognizes that despite many illustrations of innovative work: 'Many nurses and midwives spoke passionately about the obstacles in their way. Despite lip service to change, their lived experience was inertia and resistance. Some barriers were systemic; others lay in colleagues' attitudes; and yet others lay within nurses and midwives themselves, especially low self-esteem'.

We need to acknowledge that many specialties in nursing have worked hard in both their education and practice to shift some of the more task-oriented, ritualistic and emotionally distant behaviours and explore the value of engaging more openly and directly with the raw emotions implicit in their contact with clients. The most obvious examples of this are within the hospice movement, in work with vulnerable adults and children in the community, and in work with people with HIV and AIDS, but it is implicit in the everyday potential of nursing engagement.

Social defences

Menzies-Lyth (1988: 79) referred to the following defence mechanisms, which determined the culture and shape of the organization of nursing work, and protected the nurses from the anxieties that threatened to overwhelm them. We have enlarged and added to some of them. See how relevant you think that they are to you in your area of practice. You may have to make a distinction between the current jargon of intended practice versus the reality of practice:

- *Keep the nurse and client apart as far as possible as it is the closeness of the relationship that increases anxiety.* Menzies-Lyth cited task orientation, rotas and compulsive paperwork as methods for achieving this. Ironically, improvements in surgery 'throughput' and patients going straight to surgical admission wards has meant that nurses in post-surgical wards do not get to know the client prior to seeing them affected by the anaesthetic and surgery. There are reports of this affecting the nurse's capacity to build a relationship, as do other improvements in the speed of delivery of care.
- *Depersonalization.* Clients are labelled and categorized, often linked to an illness, pathology or problem. The contribution of emotional life, family context and social environment is ignored.
- *The rhetoric of coping and detachment.* A defensive 'don't care' attitude: 'a good nurse must not get too involved'; 'nurses should always cope'. Menzies emphasized how attachment needs are minimized not only between nurse and client but between nurse and *nurse*, referring to the lack of stable, consistent working placement and the practice of moving nurses around wards to fill in gaps.
- *Checks and counterchecks.* This reduces the weight of responsibility about ultimate decision-making about a client.
- *Rituals.* Repeated tasks, lists, non-individualized questions and procedures. We have already illustrated that even the process of reflection can be besmirched by this same mechanistic distortion (Boud 2010).
- *Repression, discipline and reprimand.* A whole chorus of critical feedback responses, which result in a reluctance to seek feedback. This links to a fear of making mistakes, leading to an emphasis on 'playing safe' rather than using initiative.
- *Collusive social redistribution of responsibility.* This leads to projections of blame and irresponsibility onto others.
- *Responsibility and accountability avoided and pushed upwards to avoid fear of retribution.* This minimizes the exercise of discretion.
- *Avoidance of change.*
- *Obsession with tasks, making it difficult to prioritize.* Difficulty letting go of time-honoured approaches in order to try something new.
- *The ultimate detachment of leaving the service.* 'It is the tragedy of the system that its inadequacies drive away the very people who might remedy them.'

We would like to enlarge briefly on how some of these defences may be replayed in our current climate and mention others which we have witnessed frequently within accounts of anxieties about clinical supervision (see Figure 2.1). They may refer both to direct client care and to work with other colleagues (the potential content of clinical supervision sessions) as well as to the nature of the clinical supervision relationship itself and include the following.

- *Being immobilized and stuck, blocking all suggestions for moving on.* There is a strong resistance to problem-solving or even to thinking. We may block and parry all suggestions – with 'we've done that, it doesn't work'. We may emphasize how awful it all is and repeat it endlessly. Many of our actual complaints may be more than justified but we then defend ourselves from the hurt and the loss of feeling unsupported, misunderstood and generally unacknowledged by others and then feel disempowered to do anything about it.

- *Avoiding the inevitable discomfort of learning about new things which may include recognizing our current limitations in some areas.* Anxiety may often be a block to learning, and part of the task in clinical supervision is to enable those involved to test their perceptions in the light of new possibilities. For example, a senior ward manager may be asked to develop some new skills so that she can supervise others. She may feel defensive at first, but given the opportunity to express and discuss her fears, she may begin to value the opportunities for new learning that preparing for role change provides. Others may defensively cling to their years in practice as proof of their experience and the non-necessity of doing additional training. We forget that unless we learn from experience, mere length of time in practice may be meaningless.

- *Idealization of the past or different ways of working.* For instance, some older nurses may be stuck in the myth of the rosy idealization of their own youth and of 'nursing-as-it-was', as a defence against the reality of adjusting to changes and perhaps against the sorrow of loss of their own youth. Woodhouse and Pengelly's (1991) study of anxiety within a group of health visitors referred to their idealization of more 'expert' agencies in dealing with specific problems, and the corresponding diminution of their own sense of personal competence and authority.

- *Projection of everything that is felt to be wrong onto something or someone else.* All the 'bad bits' of our working lives, and the conflict that they arouse, are the fault of someone else – management, other nurses, other multidisciplinary colleagues. To deny that these feelings of conflict reside within us, and to protect ourselves from all that is bad, we have to defend our own righteous position and ensure that the boundaries between 'us and them' are made more and more rigid and impermeable. Woodhouse and Pengelly's (1991) work, which explored the adverse effects of anxiety in working collaboratively in partnership between a range of agencies in the community, refers to the poor collaboration that results from such 'toxic conditions' and to the condemnation and intolerance that can accompany it. This can lead to feelings of being victimized – 'the world is against me' – and of being an innocent partner in the whole mess.

- *Hiding feelings of loss, shame and guilt under a cynical and harsh exterior.* This can lead to an apparent rejection of moral considerations, where another's feelings become irrelevant to personal or organizational survival. This again is visible in the 'dog-eat-dog world' of competition and marketplace survival.

- *In order to defend against fear of getting it wrong, making mistakes and not knowing, some people may divest themselves of responsibility for both the process and outcome of their work, preferring to follow in the slipstream of another.* A supervisee, for example, may expect their clinical supervisor to do all the work involved in setting agendas and later follow-through of action. It is easier for some to sink into apathy rather than run the risk of imagined failure or inadequacy.

- *Deflection or displacement of attention onto a component of work which is less risky and which thereby allows us to distance ourselves from the real source of anxiety (often linked to attachment relationships).* The flight into paperwork and bureaucracy is an example of one such distraction technique. Some deflective strategies, while giving an impression of being very busy, actually result in sabotaging any real involvement with the main task or tasks.

- *Flight into theory.* This protects ourselves from engaging in real emotional understanding, in which we can tap into our own experience and empathy to appreciate what might be being experienced by someone else. It can feel comforting to focus on intellectual understanding. We were once asked to review a book on stress in nursing which managed to cover more than 200 pages without once mentioning how it feels to be anxious and stressed. There can be a similar tendency for some practitioners to focus on endless models of clinical supervision to avoid thinking about how to implement supervision realistically. Casement (1985: 4) suggests that theory also helps to moderate the helplessness of not knowing and thereby is an attempt to reduce anxiety, but goes on to remind us that 'it remains important that this should be the servant to the work . . . and not its master . . . By listening too readily to accepted theories, and to what they lead the practitioner to expect, it is easy to become deaf to the unexpected'. This principle is echoed within an excellent guide on measurement and evaluation tools (Campbell *et al.* 1995) which challenges us to not devalue the totality of our work with clients by being restricted by the current climate's narrow demand for quantitative outcomes, but asserts instead the importance of being open and responsive to unintended contacts and outcomes in the evaluation of our work. Campbell *et al.* admittedly focus on work in the community where unintended outcomes are particularly relevant amidst the complexity of community contacts, and where initial objectives have to be modified to meet more immediate and pressing health needs.

Many readers will either have direct experience of the social defences first described by Menzies or recognize that some elements of them still flourish today, but along with the intervening years has been a growth in those who have challenged and tried to rework some of this unwanted inheritance. Many practitioners in our workshops state that they feel devalued by the social system and deprived of personal satisfaction. They want to exercise their full range of skills with more creativity and responsibility. Many recognize that their capacity for care and concern, compassion and empathy, and for action based on these feelings – the fuel for their initial motivation to work in nursing – has been hampered by these defensive restraints and that the protection they offer is often neutralized by the dissatisfaction and erosion of confidence that they bring. They also recognize that blaming the 'system' is one way of prolonging the feeling of helplessness and that collaborative action to change some of the restrictive practices does work. Let us hope that clinical supervision can provide a forum for this.

Fears about power and autonomy

Initial fears about, and therefore resistance to, clinical supervision are often related to a sense of having to lose control over what you do, of feeling oppressed by having to fit clinical supervision into an already busy schedule, or worrying that, by its very nature, it will involve another person (the supervisor) invading your work. The clinical supervisor tends to be viewed as a figure of authority and often can be an authority figure in reality, if only by virtue of seniority rather than having a management role. We need to tease out both the real and imagined aspects of power issues in clinical supervision and how they manifest both interpersonally and within the structures of the organization. Broader inequalities in the manifestations of power in society, in the form of gender, race and sexuality, may impact on both of these. It is also interesting that power is often viewed as 'bad' or abusive; there is little room for positive images of authority and influence implicit in having power in nursing, and we wonder how this affects a nurse's capacity to enable, encourage and empower in turn.

Reality of power structures in clinical supervision

Undoubtedly not all the suspicious or protective feelings leading us to resist clinical supervision are solely to do with being defensive or being unable to focus on the positive attributes of supervision. There can be very real, justifiable issues around the use of power in clinical supervision, related to how it is managed within the service or how it is conducted within the working alliance. Brown and Bourne (1996: 32-3) suggest that:

> It is this structural dimension of power that is frequently understated and underestimated in its impact on the clinical supervision relationship . . . These personally, culturally, structurally and institutionally based inequalities of power . . . will have an effect in addition to, and interlinked with the more obvious power issues associated with the relationship between a clinical supervisor and a supervisee.

Sources of individual power in clinical supervision

Having 'power over' rather than 'power to' within a professional relationship has a very different feel to it. Drawing on Kadushin's (1992) different components of

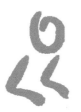

Designated authority

**Agency – the power
to influence**

Access to learning
resources

Personal attributes

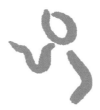

Figure 2.2 Sources of the clinical supervisor's power – the emphasis

power, let's see how it might relate to clinical supervision in nursing and identify when it might be deemed to be controlling rather than enabling (see Figure 2.2).

Kadushin distinguishes between four main sources of power:

- *Designated authority* – implicit in the position/role of the supervisor. As we are explicitly advocating that clinical supervisors are not also the supervisee's line managers this may help to reduce the confusion over status and authority that the merger of these dual roles can bring. Although for many this merger of roles might enhance and legitimate the supervisor's authority, it can also lead to some confusing messages about how the power of the clinical supervisor may be used. It could easily emphasize the normative aspects of the role and allow for a rapid shift into areas of coercion and retribution, and possible disciplinary procedure should certain organizational criteria not be met. The midwifery supervisor has a clearly legitimated normative function within her role. This makes the 'power over' function much clearer and many Trusts would like to see this principle established in other areas of nursing. Some supervisors, of course, who do not have legitimated permission to pursue this aspect of the role, will delight in a more controlling and authoritarian stance even when this approach is not intended in the workplace. In contrast to this, the UKCC (1996) has essentially supported the more formative and restorative functions, preferring to emphasize the need to develop the 'power to' be more effective and accountable, rather than 'power over' to ensure this. The clinical supervisor can still have 'designated authority' but this is reflected more in respect for her seniority, experience and skills. Even though the clinical supervisor may try and promote the latter enabling and collaborative image, some supervisees may not be able to get past their stereotype of the more authoritarian and controlling image of the term 'supervisor'. Whatever power stance is adopted there needs to be clarity about what is to be done if clinical standards are not being met (see Chapter 3).
- *Agency* – the clinical supervisor has the power to influence a supervisee to do something or behave in a certain way. This may involve a more controlling approach such as coercion or the offer or withholding of rewards. A clinical supervisor choosing a more encouraging and self-directed

approach may suggest or make recommendations for further training or a move to another post. Each approach may also include the covert 'reward' of negative or positive feedback respectively, thereby seeking to restrict or motivate supervisees.

- *Resources power* – Handy (1990), writing about managers within organizations, regards this as the most important and potentially influential source of power at one's disposal, in order that change can really be effected. It is more difficult to see the sorts of resources that supervisors have the authority to use, which is perhaps the main disadvantage of divorcing supervision from the management role. Sometimes 'power over' resources can be very enabling! However, resources do not necessarily have to be economic – they may also relate to sources of knowledge and ideas which can be encouraged and shared.

- *Personal attributes* – this may include the force of personality, energy and enthusiasm of the supervisor, and the skills and experience they tap into in their role as supervisor, such as some aspects of modelling which may be positive, or not. For instance, a charismatic and dazzling personal style can unfortunately lead to disempowering the supervisee. These personal sources of power also belong to the supervisee, of course, and the sharing of aspects of experience, skills and personal attributes can lead to mutual exchange and respect for what each has to offer. Hawkins and Smith (2006: 13) have as one of their 'golden threads' the belief that: 'All real-time learning and development is relational. This means that the coach, the mentor, the consultant and the supervisor need always to be learning themselves'.

In Kadushin's (1992) study in the USA, focusing on perceptions of power in the clinical supervision relationship, both supervisors and supervisees found that positional and personal power were the most relevant. Perhaps you might like to reflect on which components best sum up your feelings about where power, in its broadest sense, may lie within your own clinical supervision relationship, and whether its use enhances or depletes your own professional abilities.

Structural power

Attributes of individual influence and power need to be placed in a cultural and organizational context to appreciate additional layers of covert power implicit in the relationship. For instance, how might gender difference affect the relationship; how might it feel to have a clinical supervisor who is white in a practice workforce that is predominantly black? A thorough overview of the complex and important issues related to discrimination/anti-discriminatory practice and oppression and anti-oppressive practice is made by Brown and Bourne (1996). Although their work refers to social work practice, which has a longer history of training and action in inequality issues, it is just as relevant to health care, perhaps even more so as there is a dearth of anti-discriminatory training throughout the layers of the service. The Department of Health's (1991d) response to the Opportunity

2000 initiative attempted to address the lack of women in senior positions at all levels of the NHS first highlighted by Salvage (1985) in the 1980s, although the NHS organizational reforms appear to have increased rather than tackled the problem of gender disparity in positions of influence and power. As Davies (1995) reminds us, it is the masculinization of the whole culture that is even more relevant than statistics related to gender/professional status in the inequality debate (more of this later in the chapter).

Ahmad's (1992) work on the politics of race and health, and Dalrymple and Burke's (2006) insights on the need for anti-oppressive practice, highlight the social and health status inequalities in the delivery of health care in the UK, and the ethnocentric bias and discrimination in mental health are also well addressed by Fernando (1995). These inequalities are mirrored in the workforce profiles in health care and in the comparative paucity of black and ethnic minority staff at senior levels. Increased emphasis on the need for anti-discriminatory practice for both client groups and colleagues has increased over recent years (Department of Health 1993b, 2008a) but there is still much to do in providing training for anti-oppressive/discriminatory practice. It would be much more effective if it were integrated seamlessly into all aspects of education and training.

During recent years, the Royal College of Nursing (2003) has supported an increased awareness of inequality factors affecting gay and lesbian staff in relation to visibility, openness, acceptance, trust, and the comparative need for a reduction in prejudicial, homophobic responses to lesbian and gay clients and their partners. These deficits and inequalities must be tackled structurally by employers, translating anti-discrimination laws into more proactive commitment to action.

How might these wide and complex structural dimensions of unequal power relationships impact on clinical supervision? The clinical supervisor needs to be aware of their own prejudices and assumptions which might distort the time and attention given to the supervisee, and the way the organizational structure may contribute to disparity. They may need to acknowledge the realities of difference, but seek to ensure that the person is treated equally and fairly (avoiding collusion in an attempt to over-compensate), while at the same time recognizing some of the additional blocks and hurdles they may have to overcome to be accepted and effective in their role. The supervisee may in turn be adversely affected by racist, sexist or homophobic reactions from clients and need support in dealing with this. The supervisee, of course, may harbour discriminatory thoughts and attitudes about the clinical supervisor, which may also affect their commitment to the process. But we have focused more on the potential effects on the supervisee, as the clinical supervisor may be perceived to be, or is in, the more authoritative position, and this may enhance felt difference.

Interpersonal aspects of power

Our personal feelings about and behaviour towards people in positions of perceived power often stem from our own childhood experiences, however far away, distant and faded they may seem. Throughout childhood, adult carers exercise enormous power over children and the types of attachments engendered can create lifetime patterns for the way the future adult will relate to others in an authority role. These patterns of course are not immutable; they can change through experiencing and internalizing different ways of relating and so shift our perceptions of how we are 'allowed' to be with another 'parental' figure. But some patterns can be enduring, especially at times of stress and this can lead to transferring our images from the past onto an authority figure in the present.

If the clinical supervisor represents authority in some way for you – and this will be compounded if there is a managerial component to this role and if your experience of authority figures from the past was that they would try and undermine or even demolish you – then you might only focus on certain comments or feedback which seem to you to be critical, dismissive and authoritarian. The term supervision, as Clulow (1994) has suggested, may itself be instantly translated by some into an image of an authoritarian relationship even before the real people in the relationship actually meet each other. Assumptions may be formed and critical projections directed towards the other. These critical projections may take many forms. The other person may be seen in a variety of negative ways – as useless, unhelpful, not trustworthy; they may even arouse envy or competition. They may be seen as too 'mumsy', stifling and suffocating, encouraging you to withdraw in order to find your own independence. Conversely, if there is a pattern of idealizing authority in the past, they may be imbued with equally inappropriate ultra-positive projections – they may assume an all-knowing guru status, always knowledgeable, always right, which leaves the supervisee always infantilized, always looking up to the supervisor. Whether feelings about the authority figure are negative or positive the result is similar – the supervisee can be stripped of their own authority and confidence.

Reality of personal power in the role of supervisor

Brown and Bourne (1996) suggest that supervisors in social work are not comfortable with their authority and power and seek to sidestep it. We would endorse that this is very much reflected in nursing in a great many aspects of the role. Nurses often deny the authoritative dimension of their work and role and are over-diffident when faced with the professional authority of another. There often appears to be a deep confusion between being authoritative and authoritarian. Heron (2001) makes a strong distinction between these two different concepts, which may have the same root but differ substantially in how they might be received and accepted in the long term:

- *Authoritative:* refers to the authority you have by virtue of the experience, knowledge and skills acquired in your role and in your development. You may assert this 'authority' when you feel it is appropriate to do so with varying degrees of emphasis depending on the wants or needs of the recipient. You still respect the other person, encourage collaboration, include their views and perceptions and support their right to make up their own mind and not agree with you. You can admit when you do not know and that some things are not 'knowable'.

- *Authoritarian:* means that you are absolutely sure that what you say is right, based on an expert-knows-best approach. You do not acknowledge the right of the other person to make up their own mind or allow for disagreement. You are really seeking compliance. Sometimes an authoritarian approach may be packaged in the guise of an authoritative approach, but the evidence of the need for control and compliance and the lack of collaboration seeps through.

The authoritative approach tries to encourage a more collaborative, symmetrical relationship based on emphasizing 'power to' rather than 'power over'. If the clinical supervisor believes in the support and growth model of clinical supervision rather than just endorses organizational norms, then the clinical supervision process has to be interactive rather than one-way and should be compatible with the principle of empowerment – it can in fact put the 'power' back into empowerment and so endorse and encourage the confidence and autonomy of the supervisee.

The misuse of the term 'empowerment' has been critiqued by Salvage (1992), who suggests that the move towards professionalization and creating nursing experts may just replicate the older power relationships that doctors had with their patients, this time nurses assuming the mantle and the emotional distance that goes with it. They need instead to let down their restrictive all-knowing barriers and work more collaboratively with clients. Skelton (1994: 417) adds a touch of cynicism about the misuse of 'empowerment' – 'it is essentially about getting you to come round to a way of behaving that I the expert knew in advance was good for you, whilst encouraging you to think that changing your behaviour was your idea in the first place'. This is a salutary reminder for the clinical supervisor with her supervisees and for the practitioner with her clients. Salvage (1992) goes on to remind us that if we are to empower clients then we need to empower nurses, but not give them power to use *over* clients. The clinical supervision relationship could help model this difference.

Power, autonomy and the supervisee

If the clinical supervisor is more comfortable with establishing an interactive, collaborative relationship without the abuse of power, then the supervisee's own professional confidence and accountability can develop. Again this is easier to imagine happening within a clinical supervision relationship that does not have a managerial component.

As Brown and Bourne (1996: 34) remind us, a symmetrical rather than asymmetrical power relationship in clinical supervision can enable:

- recognition of the clearly defined limits of the legitimate power of the clinical supervisor;
- understanding that this power is to be exercised constructively in a two-way relationship between people of equal status and worth as human beings;
- recognition of just how much the supervisee has to contribute to the working alliance in clinical supervision.

We would add:

- the importance of both clinical supervisor and supervisee identifying their rights and responsibilities within the relationship and engaging in two-way feedback as a way of monitoring the process of clinical supervision (see Chapter 3).

It is sad that there is so much misunderstanding of this potential, so much resistance to it, and ways of relating that lead to the abuse of power rather than its constructive use.

The fear of developing professional relationships

Try as we may, it is difficult and, we would suggest, undesirable to divorce our 'external' professional self from the personal 'internal' sense of who we are and how we feel. Our early life experiences are a key to understanding the emotional resources that we have at our disposal in current working relationships. They can provide clues for some of the difficulties we experience in our contact with both clients and colleagues. Attachment theory, when applied to both individual development and the organizations in which we work, can offer a framework for understanding many of the insecurities that occur in working relationships.

In the last 40 years there have been two major developments in nursing practice which have been concerned with allowing closer human relationships to be part of the care of clients: open visiting on children's wards and the individualized patient care/primary nursing/named nurse approach for patients of all ages. In both cases, there was massive resistance in the profession against the introduction of these developments. Being more emotionally involved with patients would get in the way of all the essential tasks that had to be done. Yet now we would be shocked to find a paediatric ward with restricted visiting and which did not address the emotional, attachment and play needs of children; or an adult ward run on a task allocation system: we would consider these approaches as inhumane and detrimental to recovery. The development of attachment theory had a direct influence on changing attitudes and practice in paediatric nursing and, we believe, an indirect influence on increasing the relational component of the organization of adult client care. There is more acceptance that, whatever age they are, human beings need consistency and reliability in relating to other people and that this need is even greater when experiencing the trauma of ill health, when they are separated from those to whom they are attached. Therefore it might be fruitful to borrow some of its concepts to construct a framework for understanding the needs and resistance of nurses as regards clinical supervision.

Early attachment theory

The 'founder' of attachment theory was John Bowlby who, in his famous trilogy on attachment (1971), separation (1973) and loss (1980), suggested that attachment to others was an intrinsic biological human need, which was clearly visible in infancy and childhood but was equally relevant throughout the life span. He emphasized the importance of the child's emotional as well as physical needs and the sort of emotional environment necessary for 'good enough' emotional development. He stressed the need for security and consistency, the need for sensitivity and responsiveness from parents and carers, in order to develop secure attachments that could weather the conflicts and losses that are part of all relationships. His early work outlined the problems that could occur for both individuals and for society at large if these basic human needs were not met and when the lack of a sense of a 'secure base' could result in a poor sense of self; more insecure, conflictual relationships with others; and potentially wider social problems of fragmentation, alienation and antisocial behaviour.

Bowlby's work contributed to James and Joyce Robertson's moving films about children in hospital and residential care in the 1950s, 1960s and 1970s and the long-term traumatic effects of poorly managed separation, especially when combined with lack of consistency from alternative carers (Robertson and Robertson 1989). Although vociferously attacked by many doctors and nurses at the time, their work later led to important shifts in social and hospital policy. Perhaps it now seems so obvious to focus on the emotional needs of sick children and to ensure that parents can accompany them in their care that it is easy to forget how recently these changes occurred, and how strong the professional resistance to them was. Many still have problems in translating some of these principles to the needs of adults at times of illness and stress. The professional resistance to providing regular, consistent support for nurses through clinical supervision is an example of this. The potential impact of current attachment research on social institutions and social policy (Kraemer and Roberts 1996; Cassidy and Shaver 2008) is as relevant today as it was in the 1960s and certainly very relevant for life in large organizations.

Secure and insecure attachment

Attachment theory outlines the conditions in which the learning of social and emotional skills can most effectively take place. It is essentially based on the simple premise that those who are treated respectfully are more likely to be respectful to others, and those who are cared for without being robbed of the sense of who they are can develop, grow and provide, in turn, non-intrusive, sensitive and appropriate care for others. Attachment theory can perhaps most clearly be seen in the early development of attachments between parents and children, and in the ensuing behaviour of children related to their internal sense of self. Under 'good enough' conditions the quality of these relationships becomes internalized (Bowlby's term for this was the 'internal working model') and so coalesces into a coherent personality – someone who feels realistically good and confident about themselves.

Mary Ainsworth's pioneering work with families in the home and, later, in controlled research studies (Ainsworth *et al.* 1978) fleshed out Bowlby's work on early development and provided an important initial framework for highlighting the differences between secure and insecure attachments and types of insecure attachment. This early work has been extensively replicated in numerous samples, many testing its applicability to different cultures (Grossman *et al.* 1985; Miyake *et al.* 1985; Sagi *et al.* 1985). More recent in-depth studies involving intensive observation of infants with parents (Stern 1985, 1995) support much of the early attachment research and add to our understanding of how the development of a baby's internal sense of self is so sensitive to vicissitudes in the relationship with the main carer. Attachment research has also been widened and extended to include many longitudinal studies of children at different ages, and these have highlighted the long-term impact of early attachments on later relationships in childhood and on the child's skills in emotional expression and ability to get on with others (see the Minnesota Studies from the 1970s to the 1990s, Sroufe *et al.* 1990, and more recent work by Fonagy *et al.* 2002).

Adult attachment

Numerous extensive research studies on attachment in adults relate to the durability of many early attachment patterns, and their replication in adult relationships and communication with others. Mary Main's work in particular, in the Adult Attachment Interview (Main and Goldwyn 1985; Main 1994), provides clues for assessing the quality of adults' relational attachments. She focuses on how comfortable adults are talking about adverse experiences, the inner conflict that can arise, and their emotional responses. One of the important outcomes of this work is that it demonstrates that those who develop some awareness and understanding about adverse experiences, those who can 'name them' and talk about them rather than block them off or become engulfed and enmeshed by them, can learn to deal with the conflictual feelings they produce. Attachment patterns are durable, but not rigid templates that are totally resistant to change. They can shift through developing more secure relationships with others.

In nursing, the bereavement studies of Parkes and others (Parkes *et al.* 1991) have been the most influential extension of attachment research in adults, adding to our understanding of separation and loss; but studies into more everyday expressions of adult attachment needs and loss are being developed all the time (Bartholomew and Perlman 1994; Sperling and Herman 1994). Attachment research has become a huge growth area and much of it is relevant to our work in health care and in understanding our own responses, as it spans the 'external' world of what is observable and 'said', and the internal world of major emotions and how we are really coping.

Attachment relationships and clinical supervision

It is important to remember that attachment research is not about categorizing or labelling people, but that it provides a framework for understanding the effects of key relationships in a person's past and present. Attachment patterns can only be seen in the context of relating with others. Although durable, particularly at times of stress and anxiety, and especially when linked to the fear of separation and loss, they are open to change. New ways of relating can be learned.

As clinical supervision is essentially about a relationship between two people, many of our own past ways of relating may be re-triggered within it, either through reactions of the supervisee's relationships with clients or within the dynamic of their own working alliance. It will impinge on all the feelings and reactions to power and authority explored earlier in this chapter. Those with more personal experience of insecure attachments may find establishing closer working relationships more difficult. Those with a history of predominantly insecure avoidant attachment may avoid close contact with others and even choose a specialty which allows for maximum independence. Those with insecure ambivalent attachment histories may become more enmeshed with their clients or with their clinical supervisor but also resentful of the feelings of dependency this may lead to. Both clinical supervisor and supervisee may find it helpful to acknowledge the part their own personal history of relationships may play within their professional relationships, particularly at times of stress. It is also important to remember that those of us with the most secure of histories can be knocked sideways at times of acute stress or trauma, even though our capacity for recovery may be greater. In group clinical supervision, of course, these attachment relationships will be even more layered and complex, rather like they are in families. It is ironic that peer group clinical supervision is perceived as the 'easier option' in this context: in fact, it is only the resourcing of it which may be simpler.

Attachment in organizations

In order to make sense of the influence of attachment histories, we have concentrated on personal attachment relationships between people, but the overall professional and organizational culture can also enable or diminish people's capacity to attach and relate to each other in a meaningful way. Goodwin (2003) explored the relevance of attachment theory to the organization, as well as the practice and philosophy of mental health care. The question you might like to ask yourself is: how well does your organization provide a secure base for you to practise in? The notion of a secure base, first coined by Ainsworth (Ainsworth *et al*. 1978) and then developed by Bowlby (1988), does not mean an ideal environment, but one which provides a 'good enough' supportive context for individuals to explore, try things out and develop their skills and confidence. It develops an independence of spirit rather than dependency, feared by so many. You may find it useful to ask yourself the following questions to assess whether you feel emotionally included and secure where you work:

- Are consistent working relationships encouraged or positively discouraged?
- Is time invested in building teamwork or is your team a collection of disparate individuals who squabble and compete with each other most of the time?
- Are you consulted over major change policies or are they imposed on you?

- Is there a climate of trust or of suspicion?
- Are the main policies that frame your work consistent with the philosophy of your role or are they restrictive to that role?
- Is a major change followed by a period of reflective review and consolidation or are too many changes happening at once?
- Is there regular planned protected time for reflection on your practice that you can rely on?

Holmes (2001) has written extensively about the application of attachment theory and research within mental health, and recognizes professionals' need for a secure base before they can offer a secure helping relationship to their clients.

Many of the major organizational changes in the NHS have tended to heighten insecurity. Business culture is one based on competition rather than cooperation. Some aspects of competition may well be healthy but they can also serve to alienate groups and individuals from each other, and can lead to coercion and threats in order to achieve targets. Many workshop participants have alluded to what seems to them to be the 'divide and rule tactics' within their workplace, leading to the splitting up of good working relationships and a reduction in motivation. Where there is insecurity there can be incapacitating anxiety and the pace of change of recent years has certainly tended to heighten both.

Confusion and distrust are also enhanced when people are asked to work in a culture of mixed and conflicting messages. The emphasis on personalized care is a good example. Many practitioners do desire to work in this way with their clients, but they find that the way they are treated in turn is the reverse of this philosophy. They often feel infantilized and controlled, rather than empowered to empower. Many are left deeply cynical about 'sound bite' management and the falseness and lack of congruence between mission statements and reality. More recent work on the political and organizational aspects of attachment allude to some of these discrepancies: 'The markets depend upon non-market institutions, on trust, on relationships between people and within communities, on norms of good behaviour, on social capital. Destroy that and you not only damage efficiency, you also destroy the conditions for a good life' (Kraemer and Roberts 1996: 1); and: 'A culture with a relentlessly competitive ethos undermines trust and maximises insecurity, and it is hard to believe that this can be healthy for society, even in its economic relationships, in the long run' (Marris 1996: 194). Ironically it is the fostering of secure attachments, rather than the current compulsive drive towards competing forces in the NHS, which will facilitate the creativity, motivation, autonomy, accountability, efficiency and effectiveness needed in the workplace.

The need for a secure base

To hope for a major organizational shift from insecurity to security would be idealistic indeed, in the current climate. But perhaps the main message that we wish to extract from this overview of attachment is that clinical supervision could eventually attempt to provide, even in the most fragmented working environment, a space for stability, consistency and responsiveness where thinking can take place. A relationship built on trust and support could provide the 'secure base' so desperately needed by everyone – an oasis amid the emotional aridity that is so often a byproduct of continual change and confusion.

Attachment theory and its application do not provide all the answers to the complexities of both personal and organizational development, but the ideas within them, bolstered and strengthened as they have been by extensive and varied empirical research, have much to inform us about the way we relate to each other. They also provide an understanding of how and why more defensive patterns may emerge in relationships and why the emotional contact needed for security and support is feared and neglected.

Anti-emotional climate in the nursing profession

Faugier (1995: 8), in selecting a 'growth and support' model of clinical supervision, seeks to counter the lack of emphasis on the emotional effects of nursing work: 'I worked on the wards as a student nurse in psychiatry where people committed suicide and nobody ever discussed it. Nobody ever talked about what had gone wrong, what we should have done, and what we should have all been thinking. I know that still goes on in some settings. That was wrong and it has to stop'.

Nurses from all specialties have had to learn to keep their emotions under wraps. We have a history of creating stiff upper lips. We had to learn consciously how to apply aseptic technique to physical wounds, and unconsciously had to learn how to develop a parallel emotional asepsis to protect our wounds of vulnerability. Messy and wayward feelings must be prevented from contaminating our work. This analogy of linking emotions to the dangers of infection control has been developed by Dartington (1994: 105), who explored the impact of contradictory beliefs in nursing leading to despondency, passivity and an avoidance of emotional attachment to others:

> If for a moment, we consider the institution as the patient, it is as if emotional dependency is experienced as the most contagious of diseases. Everyone is under suspicion as a potential carrier, and an epidemic of possibly fatal proportions is likely to break out at any moment. The only known method of prevention is stoicism, which is administered by example and washed down by false reassurance.

Many of course do acknowledge ambivalent or difficult feelings, but tend to develop personal strategies to deal with the stress they cause. Within the organization as a whole, emotions tend to be marginalized; there is seldom time to deal with them in ways which might help. In the King's Fund exploration of the need for clinical supervision, Kohner (1994: 5) found that nurses did not have mechanisms to talk about successes and positive feelings, let alone the feelings of uncertainty, inadequacy and despair that were commonly expressed. As one of them said: 'In nursing we are not going to get away from the bad things in life...it's what it's all about, to make those bad things a little more bearable for the people involved'. This nurse was referring to her clients, but emotional stress needs to be made more bearable for nurses too. We need to identify how the organizational culture contributes to the denial of emotions.

Organizational suppression of emotions

A great deal of work that has been done on understanding how organizations are structured and how people within them behave has ignored their essential unique human ingredient – feelings. If feelings have been referred to it has tended to be in the context of 'attitudes about' work rather than understanding how the organizational culture itself allows or disallows certain types of emotional expression. The organization often takes the form of a censor and, by pathologizing certain forms of emotions, seeks to stifle them. Hearn (1993) and Parkin (1993) link this to the fact that, in political terms, organizations are masculine arenas where emotions are seen as feminine, uncontrolled and irrelevant, or even dangerous to achieving the main task. However, women, usually of lower organizational status, are often used to deliver 'bad news' and deal with the aftermath of negative emotions. Putnam and Mumby (1993) harness the concept of 'emotional labour' to suggest that our emotions in organizations have been controlled to a far greater extent than is normally recognized. They explore how some emotions may be selected for use and incorporated as commodities for instrumental ends. For instance, a climate which encouraged wariness and fear holds potential dissidents and challengers in check; professional accountability may encourage whistle-blowing to reveal poor standards but employees are often silenced and disempowered for fear of losing their jobs. They suggest that this is not only pernicious for individuals but that also, ironically, it is the key to an organization's ineffectiveness.

Emotions can contribute to healthy growth if they can be harnessed appropriately, or can be unhealthy if they reappear unconsciously in ways which are destructive and harmful. Out of sight may be out of mind for some, but even well suppressed feelings tend to erupt into the open, causing problems in relationships and in our ability to manage stressful situations and change. Fineman (1993a: 15) suggests that feelings are like 'social glue', part of the 'inner wiring' of an organization and that they 'will make or break organisational structures'.

Emotional repression in the organization of health

Many commentators and researchers have alluded to a similar process of emotional suppression in health care, where they are viewed as dangerous and disruptive and as marginal rather than central to life at work. The medical model approach, which has been so influential in our own nursing history, tends to split off aspects of external physiological pathology from a person's own unique history, the quality of their relationships and the impact of their environment. It helps to disengage these external elements from inner emotional life. This mind–body split alienates and fragments individuals. The disturbing power of the emotions is anaesthetized and we can settle down to focus on the much more manageable, compartmentalized bits that have gone wrong.

An enormous amount of both personal and organizational effort can be employed in suppressing emotions so that socially acceptable norms of relating, based on composure and rationale, can happen. Emotions and intuition, in a culture dominated by largely masculine values which elevate rational forms of knowing, can be seen as feminine and deviant. 'Emotional labour' in the helping and caring profession of nursing encourages benign detachment, which disguises and defends against any private feelings of pain, anxiety and distress. James (1993: 114) explored the divisions in emotional labour with reference to disclosure about cancer and managing emotion. She refers to the 'unwritten rules' about status, gender and organizational role in shaping who says what to whom, and how their feelings are expressed:

> The mechanisms through which emotion is controlled during the disclosure of cancer are applicable to a wide range of organisations. The mechanisms may be commonly observed: the use of particular kinds of space and time: more or less public encounters; denial of the emotion; limiting the information released; formal and informal disciplinary rules; gender divided labour; and most importantly, through senior staff setting the context, routines and rituals within which other staff and clients can express their emotions.

Davies' excellent overview of *Gender and the Professional Predicament in Nursing* (1995) again refers to the predominant organizational logic as a masculine one that denies the world of emotions and the need for interdependence rather than fragmentation and conflict (enhanced still more in the development of the competitive marketplace of health care). She summarizes her thesis thus: 'Masculinity fears and feminizes dependency. It handles vulnerability and indeed any emotional expression by handing it over to women, and repressing and denying the need for any discussion in the rational forum of a public space (p. 187). It is why, she suggests, nurses feel so disempowered from asserting the emotional underpinning of their professional caring and the need to see this translated into organizational policy and support.

Trying to voice emotions in nursing

Many fear that if you just let a trickle of emotion out you could soon find the situation veering towards the chaotic. Workshop participants from all specialities voice these fears well:

> Her eyes filled with tears; I could tell she was desperate but the clinic was full, I had loads still to see, so I jollied her along. I feel bad about it now. But I was tired. It had been a long day. And anyway, you never know what you're letting yourself in for. The floodgates could open. Her life is in such a mess. A bit like mine really.

All this stuff about feelings is all very well, but ITU is very pressurized. There's always relatives around and you have just got to stay in perfect control. It's really not good to get too involved. A lot of them aren't going to make it so there wouldn't be any point. If one lot of relatives start to break down then they all start. It's not so bad if they go to the visitors' room but it all gets a bit much if it happens in the unit.

I hate going to visit him. He is always so smarmy and full of sexual innuendo. We have to do quite personal things for him. I dread going in. He makes me squirm. I just have to bottle up all my distaste and anger. There's no point. Anyway he's a friend of the chief exec, so I couldn't say anything anyway.

Quite frankly we are treated like shit by the GPs, they have no idea what our role is, but we have to keep our heads down. Our manager says that if we want to keep our jobs we just have to get on with it and dance to their tune. The service contract is due for renewal soon.

Fears of catharsis, personal retribution and things generally getting out of control can mean that practitioners keep their own emotional lids on tight, and in so doing ensure that the client's needs for appropriate emotional expression are not encouraged either. Yet many have been trying to loosen the lid in recent years, but without everyday supportive strategies and space for this the pace for change tends to be slow. We forget that placing emotions on the map is relatively new in health care. It is only some 30 years ago that the first nursing research linked anxiety reduction to pain relief (Hayward 1975; Boore 1978). It was then a common belief in paediatric circles that babies did not experience pain, and local analgesia was not given for many physical interventions. The therapeutic value of a more holistic approach to care based on partnership did not really gain momentum until the late 1970s and 1980s. However, as the emotional life of clients grew to be recognized it often became a category to be ticked on a form rather than truly integrated into assessment and care. For instance, the Postnatal Depression Scale now used extensively in community nursing can be used minimalistically or creatively depending on the skill of those using it. Confusing mixed messages abound. It can be disconcerting when policy documents emphasize working in partnership at the same time as tighter, more cautious procedures discourage individual practitioners' assessment and initiative. Some Trusts may become so paranoid about not missing signs of child abuse that they create policies which encourage restrictive formats for contact with whole client groups. The compartmentalization of tasks and the increase in the use of checklists – shifts in policy which covertly affect the nurse–client relationship – can reduce individualized care and deplete confidence in the practitioner's own abilities. More recent changes in the organization and delivery of health care and the focus on short-term measurable outcomes have led to even less emphasis on messy affective variables. The feminist research of the 1970s and 1980s, with its focus on 'softer', more subjective, qualitative data, tends not to thrive in such a crude, mechanistic climate.

Although a push towards more affective methods of learning has grown in recent years, Morton-Cooper and Palmer (1993: 119) suggest that we still have a way to go:

> Given that health care is, above all, a human service, it seems reasonable if somewhat overdue, to be looking more closely at the affective domain of learning. In this way we can begin to examine our responses to emotional stressors and perhaps determine new and more acceptable ways of dealing with those that pose us with the greatest problems.
>
> Affective aspects of education could then be perceived as a legitimate subject for study, instead of being relegated to the lower ranking 'qualitative side' of educational theory. Because an approach is qualitative rather than quantitative it is sometimes accused of being too 'soft' or 'unscientific'.

Smith (1992) argues that the values of human connectedness and involvement which are so implicit in caring in nursing need to be both taught in an explicit way and underpinned organizationally. Even Benner's enormously influential overview on the philosophical roots of caring in nursing (1984) alludes to the conundrum of the 'embarrassment of caring' in an essentially masculine culture and the need to assert the centrality of its role.

This resistance to expressing and harnessing the values of emotions requires addressing in both education and practice. This is not to say that our distress should spill out all over the place all the time, but the pressure to redirect anxiety, grief, anger and stress into the deeper, non-reachable recesses of our psyche leaves us adrift from important tools for understanding ourselves and others, and from communicating with them.

Denial of feelings in nursing is particularly ironic when we all work directly or indirectly with illness, disability, threats to self-image, fear of death and pain and all the major emotions of fear, panic, anxiety, anger, sadness and loss that accompany these states. Menzies-Lyth (1988: 46) refers to the emotional ambivalence experienced by many nurses, torn by the pull of opposite feelings: 'The work situation arouses very strong mixed feelings in the nurse; pity, compassion and love; guilt and anxiety; hatred and resentment of patients who arouse these strong feelings; envy of the care given to the patient'.

Emotional well-being contributes to our overall health and satisfaction, and developing emotional skills enables our clients to utilize their own healing resources. Emotions are central and not marginal to our work and this needs to be reflected in clinical supervision. Clinical supervision has the potential for creating a space to discuss the emotional residue of our work, to identify the skills we have and those we need to develop. (See the section on emotional skills in Chapter 4.) Put simply, 'if we do not care for ourselves, we cannot care for others; if we cannot look after ourselves, we cannot look after others; if we do not respect ourselves, we cannot respect others' (Swain 1995: 29).

Implications for the relationship in clinical supervision

These undercurrents of anxiety fuelled by defensive resistance lead to a number of implications which serve to hinder the implementation or effectiveness of clinical supervision, but they could provide a spur to its progress if understood and recognized. The main implications for clinical supervision we wish to highlight are the need to:

- make space for hidden feelings;
- contain anxiety and conflict;
- understand the subtle process of mirroring and reflecting;
- recognize unconscious communication in the clinical supervision relationship and its link to clinical practice and organizational culture.

Making space for feelings in clinical supervision

This chapter seeks to redress a major imbalance in nursing education and practice which denies the power of emotions and the effect of hidden feelings in the way we relate to and communicate with others. We in no way wish to suggest that the clinical supervisor and supervisee will always be engaged in quarrying some deep dark and mysterious pit of the unknown. We are far too practical and fun-loving for that! Many aspects of clinical supervision will not involve you in unconscious processes at all.

All we are suggesting is that there needs to be more space given to explore the unconscious dynamic in education and practice, and that the clinical supervision relationship offers a time and space to incorporate this. We support and endorse Hawkins and Shohet's (1989) image of the 'wounded helper' in order that we can use rather than deny hidden but active feelings to help both each other and our clients. To do this we need to be more aware of our own motives and needs within the helping relationship, both in direct clinical care and in clinical supervision, and acknowledge that we all have the capacity to be healed and helped by the process:

> the wish to heal is basic to helpers and non-helpers alike. We have found that when we have been able to accept our own vulnerability and not defend against it, it has been a valuable experience both for us and our clients. The realization that they could be healing us, as much as the other way around, has been very important both in their relationship with us and their growth.
>
> (Hawkins and Shohet 1989: 14)

As Maroda (1991) also suggests, this belief in the mutuality of the relationship rather than in the expert, non-disclosing authority of the role, allows for some humility, true empathy and the potential for a more meaningful attachment relationship – a secure base from which to explore and try out new things.

If space is given for this then it is more likely that we can understand and so contain some of the key anxieties at work related to role and goals and identify and moderate the use of unconscious defensive ploys. Instead we can really find ways of looking after and protecting ourselves. Many of our defensive strategies grew out of a real need to protect ourselves but became as harmful as the original fears and anxieties they originally protected us from. It is more important to recognize and name what is really causing external and internal conflict and distress rather than attack or collude with it: 'Yet now more than ever, it is imperative to retain the capacity to think and act effectively under threat. If anxiety can be contained, then what needs to be talked about can be named, and some effectiveness recovered' (Mosse and Roberts 1994: 155).

Containing anxiety and conflict

In the sort of supportive, facilitating environment that clinical supervision could provide, where conflict and difference are addressed rather than avoided, the defences can be modified and the likelihood of collusion reduced. With reference to their work with community practitioners, Woodhouse and Pengelly (1991: 222) state that, 'Given time, practitioners could learn from their experience of these phenomena [anxiety and defences] in an environment where conflict and anxiety were accepted and contained rather than condemned or avoided. Practitioners need such detoxifying conditions if they are to modify or appropriately relinquish defences which hinder their work'. Roberts (1994) also emphasizes the need for containing space and time to encourage support and sharing and so repair the contusion created by the ideology of a caring nursing culture and the reality of the uncaring, non-nurturing climate nurses worked in at that time.

The less we are preoccupied with defending ourselves from each other, the more energy we release and the more we expand the field of reliable and secure relationships. This can allow for more collaboration and understanding rather than merely coping or surviving in uncertainty and isolation. It involves us monitoring what the real issues are, their boundaries, possibilities and limitations. This is possible by standing back in the reflective process and helping others to do likewise in order to notice your reactions, assessing when they seem more intense than the situation may warrant, and identifying repeated patterns in the way that you relate which lead to conflict and problems. In later skills chapters we will refer to you using yourself as a 'barometer' to test out your self-reflective and awareness process within clinical supervision, and your assessment of the emotional needs of others.

Communication of hidden feelings

'It is a very remarkable thing that the unconscious of one being can react to that of another without passing through the conscious' (Freud 1915: 194). We are briefly going to explore how this can happen between individuals within the subtle but powerful silent communication of transference and counter-transference and then see how individuals may become mouthpieces for the organization's own defences against anxiety. To acknowledge the power of unconscious communication we have to admit that we do much that is contrary to our conscious intentions, and that we are not altogether in total control of our thoughts and feelings. That is a difficult enough beginning!

We know from our experience of working with nurses that some react to such concepts as transference and counter-transference by feeling overwhelmed at their apparent complexity, and with concern that to apply this to themselves would be intrusive and 'playing counsellor or therapist'. This may reflect the shallowness of much of their previous experience of learning communication skills – teachers can also display and encourage many defensive strategies when teaching these skills. However, many nurses express relief that their experiences at last can be linked to some understandable ideas that fit and explain how they feel and what they know. Some of you may wish to return to this section when you have had further experience of clinical supervision or at a later stage in your development. We have found that with some skills training, nurses can learn to use 'emotional barometer' skills non-intrusively and at an appropriate level for clinical supervision. Perhaps an easier route into this is to refer to the more easily imagined mirroring and reflective process in clinical supervision.

Mirroring and reflecting in clinical supervision

Throughout this chapter and indeed the entire book, although we relate the ideas primarily to the clinical supervision relationship, this obviously does not exist in isolation. Much of what goes on between the clinical supervisor and supervisee is affected by two other main sources:

- *the client:* unconscious enactment in the clinical supervision relationship may reflect the dilemmas between supervisee and client;
- *the broader organization:* the relationship in clinical supervision is likely to mirror fundamental tensions within the organization (Clulow 1994).

These interconnections and the mirroring effect between them are outlined in Figure 2.3. These mirrors can enhance and make things clearer or, like fairground mirrors, distort our image and understanding.

As we suggested in the previous chapter when we explored reflection, it depends what position you take to what is being reflected and what sort of lens you use. The link between the working alliance in clinical supervision and practice relationships has been described as the 'reflection process' (Mattinson 1975) and describes the leakage between the personal boundaries of those involved. When supervisory problems in social work were studied in a nine-year project by Mattinson it was often found that unconscious defensive interactions between the practitioner and client were being mirrored in the interaction between the clinical supervisor and supervisee. Searles' (1955) term 'reflection process' (or 'parallel process' from Chapter 1) was adopted to describe what was happening (not to be confused with the wider use of the term 'reflection' which is applied throughout the rest of this book). Woodhouse and Pengelly (1991) give a clear account of this process in the

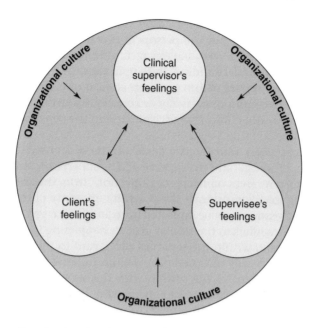

Figure 2.3 Emotional mirroring between client, supervisee and clinical supervisor within the organizational context

wider arena of group case discussion built on principles of clinical supervision in health care practice, where there were clear parallels between both the client's and practitioner's feelings of lack of support and isolation. The peer group then in turn had difficulty in attending both to the practitioner's clinical contact with the client and to the practitioner herself, as their own similar anxieties came into play. These involved the inner conflicts and fears inherent in anxious attachment which were reiterated by everyone, and fears about over-protection and dependency: 'She [the health visitor being supervised] conveyed a crippling sense of helplessness; of being too close and invaded by clients' (Woodhouse and Pengelly 1991: 133); this spread to her peer clinical supervision group.

Similarly, the organizational defences referred to earlier can also become confused, entangled and reflected in the clinical supervision relationship. If used consciously to enable rather than disable, our understanding of the mirroring process can provide us with an effective working distance, neither so close that we are in turn immobilized, nor so out of touch that we are void of insight and unable to help.

Transference and counter-transference

Transference and counter-transference are terms used to describe how human beings use each other for unconscious purposes. Although they originated within the discipline of psychotherapy to describe aspects of the psychotherapeutic relation-ship (from the dynamic within the person in therapy and the therapist respec-tively), they are relevant for everyone engaged in human relationships. Clearly a sophisticated in-depth understanding and application of this dynamic would be untenable and inappropriate within our own clinical discipline, but a simple de-scription of this very common, everyday unconscious process does aid our under-standing of its use within clinical supervision and in the supervisee's own clinical practice.

In clinical supervision, transference relates to the supervisee's displacement of their own internal feelings onto the supervisor. The supervisee, in their direct work with clients, in turn receives transference projections from their clients when they are in the helping role. For instance, the practitioner's sense of the client's frustra-tion, anger or helplessness may be imported onto and felt in turn by the supervisor. Counter-transference refers to the similar process happening in reverse within the clinical supervisor (and within the supervisee in regard to their client). The clini-cal supervisor may not only re-experience feelings imported from their own past which the current content of the session with the supervisee or the supervisee themselves reactivate, but may also be experiencing the feelings from the clinical situation in a displaced form within the relationship with the supervisee. The task for the clinical supervisor is to try and disentangle what belongs to them and what truly belongs elsewhere, but also to use these powerful feelings as a guide to what might be happening even though it has remained unacknowledged and unsaid.

> For example, Chantal has been relating a very full and complicated account of her contact with a client with a multiplicity of health and social problems. Frank, her supervisor, suddenly realizes that he has not been listening, but has instead been thinking about what shopping he needs to pick up on the way home. He has disengaged from the awfulness of her account. He realizes that he has had to escape from listening to any more, and tries to put into words how disempowering this whole situation with the client must feel for Chantal, who with a frank sigh of relief admits that she just wants to run away from the whole awful mess.

Recognizing the numbing effect of these feelings can not only help the practi-tioner know how awful in reality some situations are, which can help them not to berate themselves for not being good enough and instead recognize the bound-aries of what is possible, but it can also help shift blocks and aid more creative thinking.

> Another example: Sally is feeling dismissive of her supervisee Jessica. She thinks that Jessica is hopeless in dealing with a very anxious client and feels suffocated by the 'excessive' demands being made on her clinical supervision role. Again Sally may well be picking up the desperate dependency of the client on Jessica, but Sally also recognizes a very similar pattern within her own responses to demanding relationships within her personal life and personal history.

In this latter example it is easier to see how counter-transference can be a tool for good or ill. Sally may not question these old feelings which are resurfacing but choose to push them down, and distance herself from her supervisee and the problem, perhaps preferring to offer a rational solution to a 'feelings' problem. Or she could use these uncomfortable feelings to appreciate the strong ambivalent feelings for all three of them, herself, Jessica and the client, and so explore the appropriateness of the current type of supportive contact, identifying another approach which might be more anxiety-reducing and containing.

The unconscious use of roles in organizations

Bion (1967) identified the way individuals or groups could become like a 'container' for a problem that was more to do with a larger difficult dynamic within their organization. This enables the 'problem' or 'bad bit' to be singled out but without reference to the larger underlying pathology which is denied. They remain a symptom rather than a cause. Obholzer and Roberts (1994) allude to the stress and social and political pressure within organizations which encourage this dynamic of blame. Sometimes it may lead to personal scapegoating: 'Within organisations it is often easier to ascribe a staff member's behaviour to personal problems rather than discover its link to institutional dynamics' (Halton 1994: 16), so that an individual carries something for the group that everyone finds it difficult to acknowledge and own for themselves. In clinical supervision it may be that the supervisee identifies one particular patient on the ward as a troublemaker, always complaining and asserting their rights. In reality it may be that the standards being provided are inadequate, not because of intrinsic poor care but because the staffing levels are appalling. Fear that the patient will instigate a complaint procedure leads to staff blaming the patient. Conversely a clinical supervisor may view her newly qualified supervisee as a bit of a rebel, far too 'mouthy' and political for her own good, when she really might be saying that she and her older colleagues are too passive and frightened to rock the boat.

Non-helpful use of counter-transference

Knowledge about transference and counter-transference can also of course itself be used defensively and we need to guard against this. It can be used to great therapeutic advantage or else it can be abused. Some practitioners may choose to deny their own responsibility for monitoring their own responses, preferring to place the blame on the other person: 'Well, it's your problem not mine' or 'It's all in your mind'. They protect themselves by refusing to examine the potential reality of their contribution. As Stein (1985: 24) says:

> It is the very ordinariness and unpredictability of the transference dynamic that makes it threatening to many professionals who wish to believe that through our education, experience and will, we are in charge of our affairs – not to mention our ability to influence others. It is one matter to

> acknowledge that patients will transfer their own situationally inappropriate emotions and demands upon the clinician but another to accept that the clinician will do likewise to the patient.

Stein's work relates to health workers and their clients but is just as relevant to the relationship in clinical supervision.

Your awareness of transference and counter-transference can be a very important tool, not only in clinical supervision but also in direct clinical care. An exploration of these everyday unconscious processes has been lacking in nursing education and we lack permission to use our vulnerabilities and the insights we can gain from them in everyday practice. Gregory (1996: 141, 198) alludes to this in her research on the psychosocial education of nurses: 'The professional message seems to be that to be practically competent you need to hide your vulnerability' and 'There seem to be many "shoulds" and "oughts" about splitting the personal from professional work under the guise of professionalism. Bringing in personal content was seen as an inferior way of working. "It could impinge" on your work'.

Woodhouse and Pengelly (1991: 225) found that community practitioners were similarly reluctant to acknowledge and work with the transference of anxieties from clients, especially at times of stress: 'The capacity to use themselves and their knowledge wisely, think imaginatively, be curious, questioning and self observant, could desert practitioners in such situations'. Hawkins and Shohet (1989: 42) refer to the short- and long-term dangers of this. They suggest that workers who are engaged in intimate and therapeutic work with clients are:

> necessarily allowing themselves to be affected by the distress, pain and fragmentation of the client and need time to become aware of how this has affected them and to deal with any reactions . . . Not attending to these emotions soon leads to less than effective workers, who become either over identified with their clients or defended against being further affected by them. This in time leads to stress and what is commonly called burnout.

The 'frame' reassessed: picturing the frame or framing the picture?

So we have the surface picture of positive reasons for encouraging and developing clinical supervision and the ghost-like, hidden picture underneath. These more hidden conflictual or destructive elements may snooze quietly undisturbed to pop up at times when related feelings are prodded, when they can then crash through the millpond surface causing either ripples or tidal waves. If they can be worked with openly, disclosed, their discomfort released, they may not only be witnessed and understood but also contained or transformed into something less harmful – even creative. It all depends on that 'frame' we introduced at the end of Chapter 1.

Will it be over-ornate, ugly, over the top, controlling and suffocating? Or will it be insipid, bland and mediocre in its attempts to provide structure and containment. Both are the antithesis of providing a secure enough base for reflecting, thinking and acting.

Providing a good enough frame allows for real engagement between supervisor and supervisee and time to focus on the picture rather than the frame. What is 'good enough' will change depending on the need to have a more authoritative or facilitative frame to fit in a flexible way the changing purpose of each encounter.

As a final thought, we are reminded of the well-known artist Howard Hodgkin, whose own interesting style is often to paint over the frame as well. The frame structure is still apparent, lending cohesion to the painting, but the creativity goes to the very edge of the frame. We don't want to push this metaphor too far, but it seems to us that if the creativity between what is brought to supervision is matched by what it is greeted by, then a very creative engagement can happen.

Summary

Clinical supervision is a method of offering consistent and reliable backup to people who experience traumatic situations as part of their daily work with patients and clients, and suffer the strain of being employees of a politically traumatized organization. Once nurses understand that clinical supervision is not about management interference or criticism, other hidden resistances can still come into play based on longstanding anxieties related to the emotional elements that are involved in building more responsive, supportive relationships. Yet we hope that in decades to come this book will be redundant, that nurses will see clinical supervision as an essential part of conditions of service and be shocked to hear of areas where it is not in place.

Throughout the rest of the book we will refer to some of these hidden themes in order to see how the pitfalls and resistances can be addressed, and more skilled, effective and collaborative working alliances encouraged in clinical supervision.

Part II

Specific skills of clinical supervision

3 The clinical supervision relationship: a working alliance

The quality of the clinical supervision relationship has more influence on the effectiveness of clinical supervision than any other factor. We acknowledge that many of the elements that make such a helping relationship work are indefinable and are affected by personal and professional histories, perceptions and reactions to each other. However, this chapter attempts to offer you some guidance in clarifying and exploring the skills you can use to create some of the conditions in which the quality of the relationship can develop, and in which hidden unconscious issues which might sabotage its success can be safely acknowledged and contained. We look at some of the elements which most concern the nurses we teach: the rights and responsibilities of the supervisee (especially choosing your own clinical supervisor) and of the clinical supervisor, negotiating the clinical supervision contract and giving each other feedback. Most of the principles and frameworks in this chapter apply to one-to-one clinical supervision, but we ask you to consider that the working alliance can also be between the supervisee and the members of her clinical supervision group: the group becomes the clinical supervisor and the supervisee's relationship is with the group as a whole.

At the end of the chapter we attempt to draw these strands together to ask how the clinical supervision relationship can develop into an effective working alliance. We will link back to themes explored in Chapter 2 and forward to further chapters in the book.

We have found that participants attending courses have reported a wide range of experiences of clinical supervision as supervisees. The worst examples refer to relationships in which power is abused and the mid-range examples indicate some lack of understanding or skill in using clinical supervision. The most positive examples indicate a high level of skills in both the supervisee and clinical supervisor: commitment, ability to accept the support and opportunity for development, and a sense of clinical supervision being integral to good clinical practice. The comments from course participants in Table 3.1 about the quality of previous clinical supervision range from some of the worst to some of the best examples.

Rights of the supervisee

Nurses attending our workshops are often very encouraged by exploring the proposition that the supervisee has specific rights: this establishes a sense of one's own power in the relationship. These rights also need to be set beside the responsibilities

Table 3.1   Some clinical supervision experiences: from worst to best examples

Supervisee's comment	Author's comment
It was confidence-destroying, destructive criticism from my team leader. I realize now it wasn't clinical supervision; it was just a rollicking and a badly handled rollicking at that.	This was not clinical supervision, it was line management supervision (in which the criticism may have been justified but apparently given incompetently).
This psychologist just came in and sat in the circle and said nothing. The silence was unbearable. We ended up getting cross and he said that's what he expected. The session went on like that. Long silences until someone cracked. He gave us nothing: he was only interested when people got nasty with each other. It wasn't my idea of clinical supervision so I didn't go again.	This is a group analytic model, which can be very appropriate for an analytical therapy group but not for clinical supervision, except possibly if all the group members are themselves group analysts.
A mental health nurse coming out of a group session similar to the one above said to his colleague: 'Aha, you cracked! I managed to get through the whole thing without saying a word this time!'	This group had degenerated into competitive silences to protect themselves from an inappropriate format for group supervision.
The practice development facilitator was my clinical supervisor and what I got was all the information management wanted to give us via her, and her collecting all the information management wanted to know about what was going on. There was no interest in what I wanted to talk about. It would have been a better use of her time and mine if we'd done all that as a whole group at the staff meetings.	The facilitator was acting as an information conduit for the line manager, and did not carry out any of the clinical supervisor's role. Practice development facilitators can sometimes be under pressure to take this approach but this needs to be firmly resisted in relation to any clinical supervisor role.
I used to have clinical supervision, the supervisor was nice enough, she did all of us in our team. I found it really difficult to think of something to talk about and sometimes she suggested a few things but they didn't always interest me.	This supervisee had no choice of clinical supervisor and so was probably defended against self-disclosure. She also needed some training in the skills of using clinical supervision, including choosing an appropriate topic.
I belonged to a clinical supervision group and it was quite good, we met once a month for an hour, but the trouble was, each person only got to present a situation every five months, so it wasn't much good for burning issues, you still had to get help elsewhere. It's interesting hearing other people's problems though, you don't feel so alone. And you learn from hearing about how other people do things. But it petered out after about four sessions, attendance dropped, I think because you didn't get a turn often enough.	The time allocated for this group was too short. Each person needs one hour in order to reflect in depth. That's five hours for a group of five. If that amount of time cannot be allocated each month, then group supervision is the wrong choice: one-to-one would be more appropriate.

(continued)

Table 3.1   Some clinical supervision experiences: from worst to best examples (*Continued*)

Supervisee's comment	Author's comment
It's OK, I've only had a few sessions. Usually I go there dreading it a bit and saying I've got nothing to talk about. But I've always ended up talking about something important and being sorry when it's time to finish. It's getting better each time.	This supervisee is learning how to choose an appropriate topic. This might have happened more quickly if she had received some training in supervisee skills first, and if she had discussed her concerns with the clinical supervisor.
Now I know why some of the clinical supervision I have received and given over the last 26 years has been rubbish and some has been brilliant. This is the best supervision course I've been on.	This supervisee has had a lot of experience and training in clinical supervision but skills-based training enabled her to analyse the process clearly and reduce hit-and-miss.
I'm coming up to retirement in a few years and I thought I had nothing more to learn, I was just counting the days until I could retire. In the last 18 months I've been having clinical supervision and quite honestly it's changed my life. I've never enjoyed my work so much as I do now. My clinical supervisor is much younger than me and is a breath of fresh air. The sad thing is that it's taken so long to find out: it wasn't heard of when I started nursing and when it was introduced I kept putting off starting it.	An illustration of how experienced people can assume they 'don't need it', but if they can get through that assumption, and have the humility to perhaps have a clinical supervisor who is younger, clinical supervision is important and beneficial at any point in a career.
We've been combining one-to-one and group supervision, and ours is small group of four from different community disciplines – we met on the course. In the 18 months since the course we've had 100 per cent attendance. It's brilliant and I wouldn't miss it for the world. On top of our own individual learning, we've learnt so much about the other professions and it's improved liaison and teamwork.	This group experienced the benefits of group clinical supervision on their course but realized it was not tenable for them to meet monthly, so they each have one-to-one monthly sessions with a member of their group in between group sessions every six months. They organized it well, making attendance a high priority.
What's all the fuss about? What do people mean when they can't see how they'll fit in the time? I've had clinical supervision ever since I started nursing and to me it's as important as my annual leave: if I didn't have it, I'd be less effective at work, in fact I'd be ill. The same with clinical supervision: if I hadn't had it I'd have left nursing by now, you know what it's been like in my unit. I book in my annual leave and my supervision and the rest of the work has to be fitted around that, but it's not as if we've got plenty of time, we haven't. [Others in the group agreed that the unit had been through a crisis and had been very short of staff.] If I didn't know I was going to have that chance to stop and think, I'd get panicky and my time management would go to pot.	An example of normalizing clinical supervision. This supervisee learned in her training that it is a condition of service that she is entitled to, and in spite of being a very busy ward manager, she prioritized the time for it. She recognized the value of it from the start of her career. Her last comment illustrates the importance of the 'holding' effect of knowing you will have reliable, regular clinical supervision sessions.

Table 3.2 Rights and responsibilities of the supervisee in clinical supervision

Rights	Responsibilities
As supervisee, you have the right to: • Some choice of clinical supervisor • Your choice of topic: to talk about what you want to talk about during the clinical supervision sessions, as long as the issue ultimately has some effect on the way you do your work • Be treated with respect as an equal partner in the clinical supervision relationship – any decisions that affect the clinical supervision are made with your involvement (e.g. mode of clinical supervision) • Confidentiality, with the exceptions of revealing unsafe or illegal practice (or not attending or using clinical supervision, if this is part of your job contract). This includes records: you have the right to have no record made of anything personal you have talked about • Protected time and space for the clinical supervision sessions: support to be able to be released from your clinical responsibilities in order to attend; having the clinical supervisor give your sessions priority and sticking punctually to appointments; appropriate length of 'air time'; no interruptions • Talk about uncertainties and feelings, if you so wish, without being criticized for having these feelings; to set own boundaries to personal self-disclosure	**As supervisee, you have the responsibility for:** • Outcomes in terms of your own learning and development • Asserting yourself in negotiating decisions about clinical supervision; taking the initiative in choosing your clinical supervisor; negotiating the mode of clinical supervision • Preparing for clinical supervision sessions by identifying issues upon which you wish to reflect • Protecting the time for your clinical supervision by giving the appointments a high priority; turning up punctually; arranging cover so that you will not be 'on-call' during the clinical supervision session • Being open to challenge, not interpreting all challenges as personal attacks or discrimination • Giving feedback to the clinical supervisor about their facilitation – e.g. what is most and least helpful • Using the time to reflect in depth on issues affecting clinical practice and avoiding non-productive conversation • Self-disclosure: willing to share thoughts, feelings, mistakes, successes, values related to work • Keeping records of attendance at clinical supervision • Remaining personally accountable for actions and any omissions in your practice whatever the content and outcome of the dialogue you have with your clinical supervisor

of the supervisee in order to get a balanced picture of your role as a supervisee (see Table 3.2).

Anxiety about clinical supervision being a hierarchical relationship in which supervisees have no rights is common. Advocating certain rights for the individual supervisee seems to set the scene for a more empowering relationship in which the supervisee can empower herself. We suggest some rights here, but encourage you to select, write in your own words and add any rights that will help you to feel strong enough to negotiate with your clinical supervisor and to use clinical supervision effectively.

1. *Choice of clinical supervisor.* As supervisee, you have the right to have some choice about who your clinical supervisor is. If you have been allocated a particular person and you do not feel sufficiently at ease with them to be able to reflect in-depth on your clinical practice, then you have the right to set about arranging to have someone else. In particular, you have the right to receive clinical supervision from someone who is not your own manager or team leader, and the literature on clinical supervision supports this. Even if you work in an area where someone is employed expressly to provide clinical supervision for a number of staff, there should be an element of choice built into the arrangement whereby if the clinical supervision pairing is not appropriate or the relationship does not work out, the supervisee can see someone else. However, we are not advocating that you have the right to have total free choice to select your clinical supervisor: this would be impractical, especially in an organization in which there are few skilled clinical supervisors available. Further guidance on choosing a clinical supervisor is given later in this chapter. We also support the right of the coordinator of a clinical supervision system to challenge any choices of clinical supervisor that might lead to collusive misuse of clinical supervision, such as close personal friends or relatives.

2. *Choice of topic.* You have the right to talk about what *you* want to talk about during the clinical supervision sessions, as long as the issue ultimately has some effect on the way you do your work. You should set the major part of the agenda: the clinical supervisor may raise issues that arise from what you have said in the session or in previous ones, but the clinical supervision session is *your* protected time. Should you choose to talk about a personal problem outside work, you will be expected at some time to reflect on how it affects your effectiveness at work and how to maintain quality practice in spite of it: your clinical supervisor will guide you back towards linking it with work if you do not do this spontaneously. Repeatedly focusing on problems outside work might indicate that counselling would be appropriate. Chapter 5 suggests some differences between clinical supervision and counselling and may help clarify how you would use the two scenarios differently.

3. *Respect as an equal.* To be treated with respect as an equal partner in the working alliance is your right. This includes any decisions that affect the relationship being made with your involvement, such as (along with choice of clinical supervisor) mode of clinical supervision, whether one-to-one or group, arrangements such as times, venue and frequency of sessions. It especially means that sessions should be held in a facilitative, non-hierarchical manner which respects you as a person, with no prejudice because of your age, gender, race, class or sexual orientation.

4. *Confidentiality.* You are entitled to have anything you talk about in the clinical supervision session kept absolutely confidential, with two (possibly three) exceptions. These are: first, if you reveal any unsafe or unethical practice and you are unwilling to go through the appropriate organizational procedures to deal with it; second, you reveal any illegal activity. A third exception might be the case where the employment contract specifies attending and making good use of clinical supervision: the clinical supervisor may have the right to contact your manager if this was not the case, though not to disclose anything you have said in the clinical supervision sessions. You would have the right to know that the clinical supervisor was about to break confidentiality and have the chance to deal with it through the normal channels yourself first. Your right to confidentiality extends to any records made of the session: you have the right to have no record made of anything personal you have talked about. We suggest in Chapter 8 that if your employer asks for a record of the session, you provide a record showing the date and time that you attended. If you agree to include a record of topics discussed, we suggest that you write only general topic headings such as 'case review', 'stress management', 'time management', 'team work', etc. If your clinical supervisor breaks confidentiality unreasonably, you would have to right to make a formal complaint.

5. *Protected time.* You have the right to have protected time and space for the clinical supervision sessions. This means that you should have support to be released from your clinical responsibilities so you can attend. It also means that you are entitled to have the clinical supervisor give your sessions priority and stick punctually to appointments. In addition, it means that you should have an appropriate length of 'air time' in which to reflect in depth. This latter point can be a problem when clinical supervision is held in groups: we examine this difficulty in Chapter 8. Your sessions should be in private with no interruptions (except for life-or-death emergencies). You are entitled to have support to arrange cover so that you have no 'on-call' responsibilities that might lead to your being telephoned, bleeped or paged during the session.

6. *Self-disclosure.* You have the right to talk about any difficulties and vulnerable feelings, if you so wish, without being criticized for having those feelings or told that expressing them indicates that you are not coping. You are entitled to have clinical supervision with someone who can accept that your talking about these vulnerabilities is a good coping strategy which enables you to remain professional in the workplace. You also have the right to set boundaries on how personal your disclosure becomes, to not answer questions or probes into your private life or personal history. The decision about how much to reveal about how your personal life affects your work is up to you: you have the right to personal privacy. This links back to your right to have some choice of clinical supervisor in order that you can feel comfortable enough to self-disclose during in-depth reflection.

Responsibilities of the supervisee

The success of clinical supervision depends mainly on the supervisee and it can be useful to look at your responsibilities in this role. Many of the clinical supervisors attending our workshops have found that new supervisees often come expecting to hand over their problems for the clinical supervisor to solve, especially when the clinical supervisor is not seen as a peer, but is of a higher grade. This might be indicative of the dependency culture in nursing, a 'learned helplessness' resulting in expectations of the clinical supervisor as the expert problem-solver.

1. *Learning outcomes.* As supervisee your primary responsibility is for the outcomes of clinical supervision, for your own development and for any actions you take in practice as a result of the sessions. It is your responsibility as a supervisee, indeed as a professional nurse, to be willing to learn and change, however experienced you are. Unfortunately, it is not uncommon for clinical supervisors attending our workshops to report having difficulties with some supervisees who give the impression of having nothing else to learn. Your clinical supervisor would have the right to challenge you if you did not take on this responsibility. It is your task to consider yourself as an equal and to empower yourself to use the clinical supervision session in the most effective way. While you have the right to have the opportunities outlined earlier under 'rights', you also have the responsibility to make the most of these opportunities so that you can use the clinical supervision time effectively.
2. *Choosing/reviewing an appropriate clinical supervisor.* You have the responsibility to take the initiative in choosing an appropriate clinical supervisor. If you are happy to be allocated one, you need to take the initiative in reviewing the relationship and establish whether your clinical supervision is with the appropriate person. If not, you need to speak up and set about arranging for someone else more appropriate to take this role.
3. *Preparation.* It is your responsibility as supervisee to prepare for each clinical supervision session by giving some thought to identifying issues upon which you would like to reflect. At times, this preparation will be easy since there will be burning issues on your mind. At other times, your work may be swinging along and no major events come to mind. In this case there is a danger of wasting the session time and losing an opportunity to take a wider, deeper view of your work. We offer some guidelines about preparation in Chapter 4.
4. *Protecting the time.* Protecting the time for clinical supervision is important and it is your responsibility to give the appointments a high priority in your time management. If you have difficulty with this because of workload, it is your responsibility to seek help from colleagues and your manager. Linked to this is your responsibility to arrange cover so that you will not be on call during the clinical supervision session.

5. *Open to challenge.* Your learning responsibilities include being open to challenge and letting your clinical supervisor know of any special sensitivity you may have about being challenged and about how you prefer to be challenged. While clinical supervision is supposed to be fundamentally supportive, you will also be challenged on your actions, attitudes, values and knowledge and there is the possibility of important learning to be gained from this sometimes uncomfortable process. It is your responsibility to be aware of your tendencies to defend against listening to, taking some account of and learning something from being challenged. You may have a self-image of perfection or be afraid to admit to imperfection, but your responsibility is to see your way through these towards professional learning. Some defences may include interpreting all challenges as personal attacks or discriminatory practice, without examining if there is some validity about what is said. Guidelines for dealing with criticism are given later in the chapter.

6. *Feedback to clinical supervisor.* Giving feedback to the clinical supervisor about their facilitation is your responsibility too. The relationship can build and become increasingly effective as you get to know each other in this special situation, and both learn more about using the time to greatest effect. Letting the clinical supervisor know what is most and least helpful is an essential part of this development. Take the initiative to build in regular review sessions. The evaluation tools shown in Chapter 8 may be useful.

7. *Productive in-depth reflection.* Having set up, prepared for and protected the time and space for clinical supervision, and had a few minutes to settle into your session, it is your responsibility to use the time to reflect in depth on issues affecting clinical practice and to avoid non-productive conversation. This can be especially difficult if you know the clinical supervisor in another role and have other mutual interests to use as red herrings.

8. *Self-disclosure.* In-depth reflection can only happen if you are willing to explore some of your thoughts, values, uncertainties, intuitions, emotions, successes and mistakes in as much as they relate to you as a person in your professional role. However, we remind you of your right to boundaries on personal disclosures and to choose a clinical supervisor with whom you feel comfortable enough to self-disclose.

9. *Action planning and follow-through.* It is your responsibility as supervisee to make action plans or thinking plans after your reflection during clinical supervision, and to follow them through in practice. This links back to the first point: to be willing to learn and do things differently. These plans may be about specific points of clinical procedure or management of clients, or about self-management, communication with colleagues or your own manager, managing other staff and so on. Sometimes you will have not completed your reflection during the session and need to mull it over afterwards: your plan could be to take some more time to think or to discuss it with colleagues. All these action or thinking plans ultimately have a bearing on the quality of patient care.

10. *Accountability.* As supervisee, you remain personally accountable for actions and omissions in your practice whatever the content and outcome of the dialogue you have with your clinical supervisor.
11. *Records.* Keep a record of your attendance at clinical supervision showing dates, times and who was present, and be willing to share this for monitoring and audit purposes. If requested for monitoring and audit purposes, you have the responsibility to keep a record of the value or otherwise of the clinical supervision, without breaking your confidentiality or that of your clients. However, the specific details of what you discuss remain confidential.

Difficulties in asserting rights and taking on the responsibilities of being a supervisee

We find that lack of confidence in confidentiality as a ground rule is a common problem. This might arise from a fear of gossip. Anyone working in nursing will have experienced the extent of gossip among nurses – we have an interest in people, and their life crises and celebrations make fascinating discussion. This is not always a negative phenomenon: gossip can oil the wheels of communication in a community or organization, keeping people in touch with each other. On the other hand, positive gossip can be spoiled by the nurse who relishes behind-the-back criticism of colleagues, and receives any personal information about them as fodder for viciousness, perhaps passing on the information to others in a distorted and damaging way.

There is no foolproof method of preventing breaches of confidentiality, but some measures can help. If you emphasize how important it is to you when negotiating your clinical supervision contract, you may be able to counteract any tendency towards breaking confidentiality by impressing it on your clinical supervisor's mind. Frequent reminders and reviews of the ground rules can help, as well as having your contract visible to each of you during each supervision session.

Difficulties with believing in confidentiality may be tied to mistrust of the clinical supervisor's organizational links, especially when the supervisor is of a higher grade and is within the same unit or locality. Many nurses fear that revealing any personal information or difficulties in doing the job will be counted against them in developing their careers. We spoke with one group of nurses meeting to discuss the dismal career prospects of black nurses in nursing – statistics show a smaller proportion of black nurses in senior positions, compared to the much higher percentage in the lower grades. Many said they felt acutely vulnerable in this respect and were adamant that they could only fully use clinical supervision if it was one-to-one and their clinical supervisor was outside their immediate management structure – i.e. from a different unit, hospital or locality within the same organization, or even a different organization altogether. We believe that this option should be available when setting up clinical supervision.

Fear of being judged negatively can get in the way of really using the clinical supervision time effectively. This fear can be needless or realistic, based on previous experiences of clinical supervision. Needless fears can come from projecting your own worst critic – yourself – onto the clinical supervisor. Many nurses struggle with their inner critic which can destroy their confidence if given its head. One way of dealing with this is to tell your clinical supervisor that you tend to be over-critical of yourself and that you would like help in keeping this realistic and within bounds. Needless fears may also be based on previous experiences of receiving hurtful and incompetent criticism within nursing in settings which were totally different from clinical supervision and do not necessarily have to be replicated within clinical supervision. The structure of clinical supervision that we are advocating in this book may help to build a type of helping relationship which is new to you, and such fears can be gradually diminished through the experience of taking part in it. On the other hand, realistic fears arising from previous experiences of poor clinical supervision may be more difficult to diminish. However, you can bring your learning from these experiences and ensure that they do not happen again, in setting up and following through the clinical supervision contract with another clinical supervisor.

Choosing your clinical supervisor

You are entitled to have some choice about who is your clinical supervisor and we encourage you to take your power and be proactive. There is not usually a wide choice offered to you and it is likely that you will need to seek out a clinical supervisor yourself. If you wait passively to be allocated to someone, this may never happen, or you may be allocated to someone with whom you feel unsafe. In-depth reflection involves disclosure of your strengths and weaknesses, your values and uncertainties, and you need to feel safe enough to speak openly.

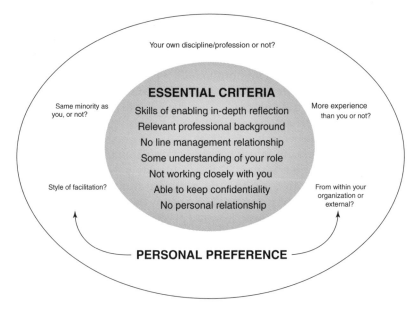

Figure 3.1 Criteria for choosing your clinical supervisor

Essential criteria for choosing your clinical supervisor

We recommend that your bear in mind these essential criteria when searching for and choosing your clinical supervisor (see also Figure 3.1).

1. *Skills of enabling in-depth reflection.* Most importantly, your clinical supervisor needs to have some facilitation skills to enable you to reflect in depth. It does not matter how they got the skills. They might have developed them by any of the following ways: attended a clinical supervisors' course which included plenty of skills-practice experiential exercises; having been a supervisee in non-managerial clinical supervision for a couple of years or so (i.e. had 20 hours or more of their own individual time for facilitated in-depth reflection); being a qualified counsellor who receives supervision for their counselling (but understands the difference between counselling and clinical supervision).

2. *Relevant professional expertise and understanding.* Your clinical supervisor needs to have some professional expertise which would be useful to you. This does not necessarily need to be in your own discipline or profession but she does need to have some understanding of the type of work you do or at least willing to learn about it.

3. *No line management relationship.* We strongly recommend that your clinical supervisor should not be senior or junior to you within your own line management structure (but they could be at a more senior or junior grade to you if from another team). We have made the argument elsewhere in the book about not having your manager as your clinical supervisor, the main reason being that the level of disclosure required to do in-depth reflection is not appropriate to a manager–subordinate relationship. Having someone junior to you as your clinical supervisor, from within your own team, would interfere with your authority and make it difficult for you to be authoritative in day-to-day monitoring and when you have to line manage that person. However, be open to the possibility of having someone who is junior to you but from a different work area, and over whom you are unlikely ever to have a line management role.

4. *Not already working closely with you.* One of the benefits of clinical supervision is to have an outside perspective on your work and this is not possible from someone with whom you already work closely. Objectivity from the clinical supervisor is crucial to maintaining and developing good practice, as collusion can easily happen within teams with, in our experience, potentially fatal consequences. Having your work and that of your team open to benevolent scrutiny of an outside clinical supervisor provides a crucial contribution to quality assurance. There is also a practical issue: it is more difficult for two people to get away from the same workplace at the same time than if they each work in different settings. We have seen this happen in a new unit which had probably the highest staff–patient ratio in its field in the NHS. They felt they were a special new team and wanted to have clinical supervision with each other, partly for team-building. Yet clinical supervision did not get off the ground until they

changed their arrangements and had clinical supervisors from other teams, which also had the effect of reducing their elitist image with other teams and improved cooperation.

5. *Able to keep confidentiality.* Some people find it very difficult to keep interesting details of other people's lives confidential, whether because they have an inability to maintain boundaries, find it too stressful, or engage in such breaches in order to make themselves appear 'in the know'. When you ask other people for recommendations for a clinical supervisor they may be able to tell you if a person has a reputation for being particularly good or bad at keeping confidences. If you have no idea whether the clinical supervisor can do this, you could ask them: this at least highlights the importance of this issue.

6. *No personal relationship.* Lastly, your clinical supervisor should not be a personal friend or relative as the boundaries to the clinical supervision relationship will be too blurred and the pitfalls too numerous, for both your clinical supervisor-supervisee relationship and your personal relationship.

Secondary criteria for choosing your clinical supervisor: personal preferences

Many people assume that their clinical supervisor should be someone more experienced within the same discipline and profession. But we encourage you to think about some wider possibilities.

1. *Same discipline/profession or not?* A person from the same discipline can be an appropriate choice for someone who is recently qualified who needs a preceptor-like relationship, or who works in professional isolation, such as a nurse working in a team comprising mostly social workers and counsellors: a clinical supervisor from your own discipline or profession will quickly understand your situation. However, someone from a different discipline or profession can give a more objective viewpoint and can ask naïve questions such as 'Why exactly is it done that way?' which can be usefully challenging to experienced staff.

2. *More experienced or not?* Early in your career it may be appropriate to seek a more experienced person to be your clinical supervisor. As you become more experienced, you may wish to be supervised by a peer colleague or even by someone less experienced. Someone who trained more recently than you can give a more up-to-date perspective on the theoretical underpinning of your work. If you have caught a dose of 'long-in-the-tooth cynicism', someone less experienced but more enthusiastic than you can give you a 'shot in the arm' and you can be reminded of why you came into the profession. Apart from that, as you get more experienced, it becomes more and more difficult to find someone more expert than you in your own field.

Table 3.3 Examples of appropriate choices of clinical supervisor

---

- Harriet is a staff nurse on a mental health rehabilitation unit. She asks Kim, who is a staff nurse on a different ward in the same unit, to be her clinical supervisor. Kim has recently done the clinical supervisor's course and has started having her own clinical supervision.
- Gerrie is a ward manager of an elderly care ward and chooses Karen as her supervisor. Karen manages an acute surgical admissions ward, and has had monthly non-managerial clinical supervision for three years (though she has not attended a clinical supervisor training course).
- Frank met Carol on the clinical supervisor training course and asked her to be his clinical supervisor, even though Carol only recently qualified and is of a grade lower than him. He knows from working with her on the course that she is good at enabling reflection and he hopes to pick her brains about up-to-date theory.
- Michael is a nurse specialist who has tended to confide in Ranjit, who is also a nurse specialist but in a different type of work. Michael's clinical supervisor leaves and Michael asks Ranjit if he would agree to become his supervisor. Ranjit has not attended a clinical supervisor course but this gives him the spur to enrol for one.
- John is a charge nurse on a renal surgical ward. He asks Janet, the manager of a district nursing team based in a nearby health centre, if she would be his clinical supervisor. He has heard from one of Janet's supervisees that she is a good clinical supervisor.
- Nina is a school nurse who asks Mary, a speech and language therapist, to be her clinical supervisor. Mary has done a clinical supervisor training course and has had non-managerial clinical supervision herself for over two years. She is not fully aware of the extent of responsibilities of a school nurse but is willing to study the job description and relevant Trust policies.
- Valerie is a unit manager. She chooses Brian as her clinical supervisor. Brian is a part-time health care assistant in another hospital. He has recently retired from a job as a senior human resources manager in a large retail business: he is working as a health care assistant to gain insight into health care as he is now a non-executive member of a hospital Trust board. He used to train managers in mentoring skills (which is where Valerie met him) and is used to giving and receiving the equivalent of clinical supervision in a management setting.
- Feroza is new to her NHS Trust and knows nobody. She takes pot luck with someone who is on the list of people who have attended a clinical supervisor skills course and asks for a three-session trial of clinical supervision. It works out better than expected and they continue the arrangement.

---

3. *Same minority or not?* Some supervisees seek someone who is the same gender, sexuality or ethnic background. If you are in a minority, it might be helpful to have someone who really knows what it is like to struggle with your own confidence or with external prejudice. For instance, a gentle, heterosexual male nurse working with mainly female colleagues may wish to have a male supervisor who understands what it feels like to be in the minority and to cope with frequent assumptions and jibes from colleagues about being gay. A black African nurse working in a predominately white team in southern England who is finding it difficult to adapt to what she experiences as a ridiculously 'polite' and dishonest culture, may wish to

have a clinical supervisor who understands what it is like to have one's directness interpreted as aggression. For others, being in a minority may not be an issue as far as choosing a clinical supervisor is concerned.

4. *Style of facilitating in-depth reflection.* If you have experience of facilitated in-depth reflection, you will have an idea of the style of facilitation that you currently need. You might be able to judge whether a particular clinical supervisor's style is likely to be more supportive or more challenging. For instance, if you are new to a job or are going through some difficulties which affect your self-esteem, you may wish to choose someone who is especially supportive. At a more experienced or confident stage in your career, you may need someone who is more challenging. Alternatively, you might wish to consider the intuitive or logical dimension. For example, a senior nurse who spends most of her work time being very structured and logical may need some space to reflect more intuitively in an unstructured way with a clinical supervisor who has a free-flowing intuitive style. Another nurse who is strong on intuition and empathy may need to develop her ability to analyse and plan and may need a clinical supervisor with a more structured and logical style. As you become more experienced at in-depth reflection in a clinical supervision setting, you will become more aware of your changing development needs and therefore of the need to change your clinical supervisor to one with a different style or background every few years or so. We recommend that you raise this possibility right at the beginning of your supervision in order to make it easier eventually to move on, without feeling you are being disloyal or unappreciative of your clinical supervisor.

5. *In-house or external clinical supervisor?* The usual expectation is that someone will be found from within your own organization, but having clinical supervision with someone outside your organization may be preferable in a number of cases. These include the situation when you currently need to have someone from your specialty but there is no one available within your organization. Another reason may be that you work near the border of another organization which has an available clinical supervisor who is much nearer than one in your own organization. Hence it might be more appropriate to have an external clinical supervisor, provided that travelling is not a problem. However, this arrangement raises three issues:

i) *Payment.* You or your employers may need to make a payment to the clinical supervisor or their employer. Alternatively, you may be able to arrange reciprocity, either through reciprocal peer supervision in which you and your clinical supervisor take turns to supervise each other or by someone else from your organization providing clinical supervision to someone in the other organization. Hence money does not have to move between the organizations. We have seen this work very well.

ii) *Reporting back to your manager.* Your manager may be concerned that someone outside your organization may be less likely to give details of

Table 3.4 Inappropriate choices of clinical supervisor: some examples

Example	Authors' comments
Dina chooses her best friend Maggie, who is also a nurse. They plan to do 'clinical supervision' in the pub after work.	The friendship would blur the clinical supervision boundaries and the pub is a totally inappropriate setting for confidential discussions.
Kerry chooses her line manager because this is the 'done thing' locally and she does not want to offend her manager.	This is unlikely to work because she is not likely to be able reflect in depth with someone who has managerial authority over her. It is difficult to step out of the local norm, but she has a right to do so.
Sadie is a senior staff nurse and chooses someone who is junior to her on the same ward, who happened to be on the same clinical supervisor course.	This will interfere with the authority that Sadie will have to use when she is in charge.
Millie chose Yasmin who is in the same team. They work closely together and indeed their whole team is very close with a great team atmosphere. Millie does not want to have a clinical supervisor outside the team, as they have become very special to each other and other teams appear dysfunctional in comparison and they don't want to be 'infected' by any of that.	Millie's clinical supervisor will lack the objectivity needed to enable her to reflect in a different way upon her work. It's good to hear of a happy team, but there are already signs that this team is becoming collusive in their cosiness, exclusivity and viewpoint that other local teams are bad.
Bob is a newly qualified staff nurse and chooses Jodie who is an experienced health care assistant on a different ward within the same unit. Jodie is easy to chat to, Bob values her experience and they have become friends.	This relationship is already too complicated as regards his authority when Bob helps out on Jodie's ward, and their friendship would also get in the way of effective clinical supervision.

attendance and less likely to report any unsafe practice. The external contract we suggest in Chapter 9 can reassure your manager.

iii) *Organizational confidentiality.* Your manager may be concerned about confidentiality in terms of the goings-on within your organization, and an organizational confidentiality clause in a contract with an external clinical supervisor may address this concern.

Some examples of appropriate choices of clinical supervision are shown in Table 3.3. So, the choice is yours: same profession or not; more experienced or not; same minority or not; style of facilitation; in-house or external.

Where to find a clinical supervisor

You may be able to find a clinical supervisor from a list, from asking around for recommendations or taking a gamble with whoever is available. Consider the following options:

1. *A list of clinical supervisors.* There may be a well-maintained, up-to-date list of available clinical supervisors in your organization, which provides you with information covering the criteria outlined above. In which case, you can contact those who have spaces to take supervisees and ask them to consider being your clinical supervisor. This sounds simple enough, but some nurses find it daunting to risk receiving a 'no' and having to try others on the list. If this is the case for you, get some help from a colleague to call or email around until you find someone. Unfortunately, a good list of clinical supervisors is rare as it takes a lot of time and commitment to keep it up to date.

2. *Seeking recommendations.* People often find someone by personal recommendation, so try asking around.

3. *Someone you meet at a course or conference.* This is also a frequent method of finding a clinical supervisor. People who attend our supervision courses often make arrangements before the course is finished, in order to get started straightaway. Alternatively, when attending other courses or conferences, listen to others' contributions, pinpoint someone whose professionalism you respect, choose that person as a partner for any paired or small group exercises and notice their listening and facilitation skills, and then ask them before the course is over. If you leave it until after the course you are less likely to have the resolve to make the request.

4. *Existing workplace confidante.* There may be someone who you already use as a workplace confidante: you could formalize the relationship into structured clinical supervision.

5. *Take 'pot luck'.* If you are new to the organization or have tried and failed to find the 'perfect' clinical supervisor, then just try 'pot luck' with whoever is available, and agree a short-term contract of three sessions, to be mutually reviewed and subsequently either brought to an end or renewed.

Pitfalls in choosing a clinical supervisor

1. *Passivity.* Just waiting for your clinical supervision to be organized for you will probably result in your being allocated to someone unsuitable, or nothing happening at all. Likewise lack of persistence will have the same result: do not give up at the first hurdle, keep trying and seek help from your colleagues and manager if you cannot find a clinical supervisor. There will be someone in a senior position in your organization who takes the lead on clinical supervision: they should be able to help you to find a clinical supervisor.

2. *Searching for perfection.* Expecting to find the perfect clinical supervisor who ticks all your boxes is probably aiming too high. Instead, focus on the essential criteria and give it a try with someone for a three-session trial of clinical supervision.
3. *Inappropriate choice.* Make an inappropriate choice of clinical supervisor and you are setting yourself up to fail. We strongly urge you to avoid choosing your line manager, however approachable she is: either your opportunity for in-depth reflection will be impaired or the line management supervision you receive will be less effective. Also, avoid choosing someone over whom you already have, or are likely to have, line management authority. And lastly, avoid choosing a personal friend or relative as your clinical supervisor. Table 3.4 lists some examples of inappropriate choices.

Rights of the clinical supervisor

While we find that workshop participants are more concerned with the rights of the supervisee, we feel it is important for the equality of the relationship to explore the rights of the clinical supervisor as well. Taking a facilitative, empowering role such as clinical supervisor does not mean that you have to abdicate your own personal power and professional authority (see Table 3.5).

1. *Respect.* You have the right to be treated with respect as an equal partner in the clinical supervision relationship, and not be blamed for the supervisee's own errors or failings, or for the organization's shortcomings. If the supervisee acts upon any advice or information you give, those actions are still the responsibility of the supervisee.
2. *Break confidentiality in extremis.* You are entitled to break confidentiality in exceptional circumstances, which would normally have been pre-agreed with the supervisee. Suggestions about what these exceptions might be are made elsewhere in this chapter, under 'Rights of the supervisee' and 'Negotiating a clinical supervision contract'. You have the right to challenge any behaviour or values which the supervisee displays or talks about that give you concern about their practice, development or use of clinical supervision. Some guidance is provided in Chapter 6 on how to challenge the supervisee in a supportive way. You are also entitled to challenge any behaviour which is insulting or personally hurtful to you.
3. *Say no to inappropriate demands.* You have the right to refuse requests which make inappropriate demands on you in your role as clinical supervisor. This includes outside interference, whereby you receive requests from the supervisee's colleagues or manager to raise an issue which is their responsibility to deal with. It also includes requests from the supervisee which you consider inappropriate, such as giving practical help outside the clinical supervision sessions, providing ongoing personal counselling or becoming a personal friend and socializing.

Table 3.5   Rights and responsibilities of the clinical supervisor

Rights	Responsibilities
As clinical supervisor, you have the right to: • Be treated with respect as an equal partner in the clinical supervision relationship, not blamed for the supervisee's or the organization's shortcomings • Break confidentiality in exceptional circumstances • Challenge any behaviour or values which the supervisee displays or talks about which give you concern about their practice, development or use of clinical supervision • Challenge any behaviour which is insulting or personally hurtful to you • Refuse requests which make inappropriate demands on you in your role as clinical supervisor, outside interference from the supervisee's colleagues or manager or inappropriate requests from the supervisee • Set personal and professional boundaries on what issues you listen to the supervisee talking about • Choose whether to work with a person as their clinical supervisor • Take steps to withdraw from the clinical supervision relationship if you have difficulties in meeting the commitment, if the supervisee will not use the time constructively or there are relationship difficulties which cannot be resolved	**As clinical supervisor, you have the responsibility to:** • Prepare for the clinical supervision session: ensuring no interruptions; settling yourself beforehand; remembering previous sessions • Be reliable, sticking to agreed appointments, time boundaries, • Keep confidential anything the supervisee says (except for unsafe practice not being dealt with) • Avoid any line management or educational assessment role from being part of the clinical supervision session; keep the session time purely within the clinical supervision contract • Rebut inappropriate demands – e.g. outside interference from the supervisee's colleagues or manager • If you give any advice, you must always be able to justify it and you must not give advice on issues outside your own field of expertise (i.e. negligent advice) • Respond humanely with 'first-aid counselling' (not psychotherapy) for distressing issues but eventually focus on how quality professional practice can be sustained • Encourage the supervisee to seek specialist help for personal problems when necessary and have access to sources of such help • Challenge any behaviour or values which the supervisee displays or talks about which give you concern about their practice, development or use of clinical supervision • Ensure that you yourself have the necessary backup support – e.g. your own clinical supervision and support systems • Keep records of attendance, not content of sessions (unless unsafe practice)

4. *Choose to be a clinical supervisor to a particular person.* You are entitled to have some choice about whether or not to be the clinical supervisor of any particular supervisee. If, from knowing the supervisee previously or as you get to know her during the first session, you realize that you thoroughly dislike her or that she thoroughly dislikes you, you have the right to choose not to work with her. Having embarked on the clinical supervision relationship, you have the right to take steps to withdraw from it if there are relationship difficulties which cannot be resolved or you have difficulties in meeting the commitment.

5. *Personal and professional boundaries.* You also have the right to set personal and professional boundaries on what issues you listen to the supervisee talking about. As nurses and human beings we all have limits and occasionally your boundaries may need to be asserted. There may be areas of work which are totally outside your professional expertise that you would wish to refer on to others who have the knowledge. For example:

> Ursula urgently needs guidance on child safeguarding procedures but this is not Jan's field. She makes some suggestions about contacting experts in the organization but has to draw the line at giving any practical guidance about it, though she is more than willing to listen to Ursula reflecting on the stress of the situation.

There may also be personal vulnerabilities which mean you are temporarily unable to listen to certain topics. For example:

> George has recently returned to work after compassionate leave for a bereavement, his partner having been suddenly killed in an accident. He leaves a message to warn his supervisee Natalie, who works on a cardiac unit: 'I think you've heard what happened: well, I'm still pretty wobbly about it and I just need to say that I don't think I could manage dealing with topics directly related to bereavement: anything else, fine. If this gets in the way of any burning issues you may have, perhaps we could fix you a clinical supervision session with someone else? Let me know.'

Responsibilities of the clinical supervisor

1. *Settle yourself first.* It is your responsibility to prepare for the clinical supervision session by ensuring that you will not be called or interrupted and by settling yourself before the supervisee arrives. Answering the phone and knocks at the door gives the supervisee a sense of being devalued and trust cannot develop. Giving yourself space and time to remember previous sessions is important, so that you can tune in quickly to being with the supervisee as a person.

2. *Reliability.* This is very important, such as sticking to agreed appointments and time boundaries and to the agreements made in the clinical supervision contract.

3. *Confidentiality.* You need to keep all personal information confidential, except for unsafe, unethical or illegal practice that the supervisee reveals (see point 4).

4. *Accountability.* In the event of unsafe practice being disclosed, as clinical supervisor you have no more or less responsibility than any other professional colleague who becomes aware of unsafe practice: you must disclose information to the appropriate person in authority if the supervisee reveals unsafe practice that is not being dealt with *and* the supervisee is unable or unwilling to proceed with appropriate haste to deal with it themselves having discussed it with you. You must keep a record in such a situation and reveal it when/if required.

5. *Boundaries.* Maintaining the boundaries of clinical supervision is your responsibility. You also need to refuse requests that make inappropriate demands on you in your role as clinical supervisor, whether outside interference from the supervisee's colleagues or manager or the supervisee attempting to step over the boundaries of the working alliance. You need to be definite about avoiding any line management or educational assessment role being part of the clinical supervision relationship or sessions.

6. *Emotional first aid, not counselling.* As part of the support role in clinical supervision, it is your responsibility to respond humanely, giving 'emotional first aid' (not ongoing psychotherapy) if necessary when the supervisee is distressed for whatever reason, but eventually you must focus the discussion back onto how quality professional practice can be sustained in spite of the workplace distress or the personal difficulties. There is an example of this in Chapter 5 when a supervisee becomes distressed after a mild challenge.

7. *Refer on if necessary.* It is your responsibility to encourage the supervisee to seek specialist professional or personal help or advice when their personal or professional problems are outside the boundaries of clinical supervision or about clinical topics outside your field of expertise. It is also your responsibility to have access to some information about people and services available to the supervisee.

8. *Challenge the supervisee.* It is not only your right but your responsibility to challenge any behaviour or values which the supervisee displays or talks about which give you concern about their practice, development or use of clinical supervision.

9. *Have clinical supervision yourself.* It is your responsibility to ensure that you yourself have the necessary backup support to enable you to deal with the strains involved in being a clinical supervisor. This includes having your own clinical supervision and developing and using your own support systems.

10. *Records of attendance not content.* Equally with the supervisee, you both have the responsibility to keep a record of attendance at clinical supervision, showing dates, times and who was present, and be willing to share this for monitoring and audit purposes. Also, if requested for monitoring and audit purposes, you must keep a record of this clinical supervision's value to yourself and your practice and professional development, as well as the supervisee keeping a parallel record. You and the supervisee may wish to provide each other with references regarding the other's commitment to and development of skills in your respective roles in this clinical supervision: these could be part of your professional portfolios or to share at staff appraisal sessions with your own line managers. However, no records should show the details of what the supervisee disclosed to you, unless it was about unsafe or unethical practice.

Negotiating a clinical supervision contract

The clinical supervision contract involves exploration of supervisee and clinical supervisor's expectations of each other and agreeing to boundaries.

Every relationship between people is based on their expectations of each other. The relationship goes well when expectations are met and goes badly when they are not, leading to disappointment, disruption and possibly to a sense of betrayal and even breakdown of the relationship in extreme cases. These expectations may be explicit, such as those laid out in an employment contract, but the majority are implicit. Open discussion of expectations can help establish and maintain a relationship and go towards healing one that is going wrong. In many informal relationships it would be stilted and unnatural to negotiate a contract at the outset ('I'd like to be your friend and draw up a friendship contract'!). However, clinical supervision is a formalized type of professional support, in which the people involved meet fairly infrequently – therefore it is important that the supervisee and clinical supervisor make an agreement about how they work together in clinical supervision (see Table 3.6 for an example). This helps to clarify expectations of each other, gives you both the same view of where you are going, builds trust when the supervisee and clinical supervisor come to see the agreement enacted in practice and provides a common language for talking about and reviewing the working relationship.

With regard to boundaries, we can draw on the experience of supervisors in the counselling and therapy professions and their strong emphasis on boundaries. For instance, Woods (2007) highlights the importance of boundaries in supervision: they offer a secure frame and may enhance the supervisee's sense of safety and containment, and this allows the exploration of sensitive, anxiety-provoking material. The supervisee may sometimes need to take the risk of disclosing feelings of workplace incompetence, inadequacy, ignorance, guilt and shame. The boundary-setting contract as well as regularity, privacy and reliability, contribute to the necessary sense of safety.

Table 3.6 One example of a clinical supervision contract

As supervisee and clinical supervisor, we both agree to the following:
- That the aims of our session together are to enable (supervisee's name) to reflect in depth on issues affecting practice in order to develop personally and professionally towards achieving, sustaining and creatively developing a high quality of practice.
- Meeting on average once per calendar month for one hour, minimum 10 sessions per year.
- Protecting the time and space for (supervisee's name) to reflect in depth by sticking to agreed appointments and time boundaries, being punctual, ensuring privacy and no interruptions.
- Providing a record for our managers showing the dates and times of the clinical supervision sessions only. Any other notes made about the sessions during or after the sessions will be kept by (supervisee's name).
- Working primarily to (supervisee's name)'s agenda.
- Working in the spirit of learning about how to use clinical supervision, both of us being open to feedback about how we handle the clinical supervision sessions.
- Putting on the table any sensitivities and tensions we have between us arising from diversity issues between us and discussing them constructively.
- Challenge any breach of this clinical supervision agreement which the other does not already acknowledge or does not take seriously enough.

As supervisee I agree to:
- Prepare for the sessions and be responsible for having an agenda.
- Take responsibility for making effective use of the time, for the outcomes and any actions I take as a result of clinical supervision.
- Be willing to learn and change and to be open to receiving support and challenge to help me do so.

As clinical supervisor, I agree to:
- Keep all personal information you reveal in the clinical supervision sessions confidential, except for these exceptions: (A) you reveal any unsafe, unethical or illegal practice and you yourself are unwilling to go through the appropriate organizational procedures to deal with it; (B) you repeatedly don't turn up for sessions or do not use the time constructively. In the event of an exception arising, I will (1) attempt to persuade and support you to deal with the issue directly yourself through the appropriate channels; (2) check that this has been done; and (3) if not, only reveal the information as a last resort after informing you that I am going to do so.
- Not allow any management supervision or educational assessment role to be part of the clinical supervision session.
- Offer you mostly support, catalytic help and supportive challenge, occasionally sharing information or advice, to enable you to reflect in depth on issues affecting your clinical practice.
- Use my own clinical supervision to support and develop my own abilities in working with you, without breaking confidentiality.

Signed _____ Supervisee   _____ Clinical supervisor

Phases of negotiating a clinical supervision contract

We suggest four phases in negotiating your own agreement about how to work together.

1. *Open discussion.* Both of you talk about what you want from each other in clinical supervision, your understanding of the aims, your hopes and fears, why you chose each other and how you view the boundaries to clinical supervision. Notes you take from this discussion can form the beginning of a draft agreement.
2. *Clarify your contract.* You write out an agreement and agree which points to include and how to word them so that both your understandings are reflected. After your initial discussion you could consult the sample draft given in Table 3.6 or any guidelines produced in your organization and incorporate any points that are important to you.
3. *Indicate your commitment.* Your agreement is signed, with both having a copy: preferably the supervisee keeping the original, and the clinical supervisor keeping the duplicate.
4. *Review and revise.* The contract is reviewed at regular intervals and if necessary revised.

The beginning of the process is illustrated by the following example:

Liam and Sandra spend the first clinical supervision session together talking through and agreeing the contract. Liam has had clinical supervision before in a previous job, and Sandra is a clinical supervisor for the first time, and has only recently begun to receive clinical supervision herself.

Sandra: Shall we start with our hopes and fears? (Liam agrees) What do you hope to get from clinical supervision with me, Liam?

Liam: Well, I got a lot out of it with my last clinical supervisor, not particularly the first one I had, but the second one worked out well, so I hope I'll get the same. (Pause)

Sandra: And that was . . . ?

Liam: He helped a lot, listened, was a sort of sounding board, and when he criticized, it was constructive criticism, it was all right. And especially with him, he was there: he turned up on time and never cancelled sessions, except once when there was a family bereavement, but otherwise I knew I could count on him.

Sandra: So, you'd like from me: listening, sounding board, constructive criticism, punctuality, reliability – not cancelling sessions. Anything else come to mind?

Liam: Thinking about fears: what I dread is having the same set-up as the first time. We'd fix dates and she hardly ever kept to them, I know she was off sick quite a bit and she had to keep going to emergency management meetings because her unit was going to be closed at one stage, but when we did manage to have a session she was usually late. It was a waste of time.

Sandra: I can't forecast being sick and having emergencies but suppose something like that kept happening and I kept needing to change the appointment times, would it be better if we suggested another clinical supervisor is found for you?

Liam: Yes, that's what happened eventually, I had to find someone else and it turned out OK then, but I'd wasted a lot of time and I didn't think much of clinical supervision for a while.

Sandra: So we'll keep our fingers crossed, but do something about it quickly if it looks as if it's going that way. Actually, that ties in with what I was thinking about wanting from you: I'd hope you would turn up when we said and be on time, because I can't run late with sessions. So we're both concerned about punctuality. Another one of mine is feedback: as you know, I have less experience of clinical supervision than you do and I'd like feedback about what is and isn't helpful, so I can learn. What do think about those?

(Liam agrees and they go on to discuss a point Liam raises about confidentiality and what it means to them in this context.)

Pitfalls in negotiating a clinical supervision contract

1. *Copying a contract.* One common pitfall for people new to clinical super-vision is blindly adopting a pre-written contract, such as that in Table 3.6 or those produced in some organizations policy documents. This can result in lack of ownership of the agreement: the individual supervisee and clinical supervisor not fully understanding what each other means by each point and feeling less committed to the agreement than would be the case if they devised it together. To avoid this, we suggest you have the initial discussion as suggested earlier, and draft some of your own ground rules together as a result of this discussion, before you refer to any other guidelines.

2. *Making heavy weather of it.* Sometimes nurses go over the top in writing such contracts, expecting that this written agreement has to be beautifully pre-sented, typed and written in complicated language as if it were some legal or policy document. Some try to standardize such agreements, spending precious time in liaising across units, localities or throughout the Trust. However, we maintain that the agreement needs to be a record of what you as a working partnership understood and agreed between you and has to be neither comprehensible to anyone else nor standardized along with any other clinical supervision pairs or groups.

3. *Forgetting about it.* Another pitfall is to make the contract, then file it away without referring to any of the agreements again. This can result in either or both parties being more likely to break it. It may result in a growing suspicion in the supervisee that the agreement was just a paper exercise and had no lasting meaning. Suggestions made earlier about using the agreement as part of 'here-and-now' awareness, regular reviews and having it on display during sessions can help keep the agreement alive. As Wood (2007: 42) states: 'A contract might be useful in that it draws attention to the importance of boundary issues; it can be unhelpful if it fosters the illusion that boundary issues have thereby been dealt with'.

4. *Not making a contract.* Not preparing a clear contract at all may be tempting to nurses who have had some experience in clinical supervision or who know each other already. Your relationship or your general communication style may tend to be informal, but Wood (2007: 42) suggests that it is better in supervisory relationships to err on the side of caution, to dispense with informality rather than formality: 'if as a supervisor you commence with informality and excessive flexibility, it is very hard subsequently to introduce formality and restraint'. The lack of a contract can lead eventually to misunderstandings of each other and some unnecessary conflicts. The process of working together on a written agreement is an important step in establishing the structure, boundaries and mutual understanding necessary for such a specific type of helping relationship as clinical supervision.

5. *Vague comments.* Writing points such as 'trust' and 'respect' as specific ground rules is too vague to be particularly helpful. Trust and respect are the aims of such a contract, but in agreeing the details it is more helpful to be specific about the kinds of behaviour and attitudes that would help build trust and gain or demonstrate respect.

Discussing the working alliance

We recommend that the clinical supervisor and supervisee together review the way the clinical supervision relationship is developing. This is especially important in the first year and if either or both are new to clinical supervision, in order to assist mutual learning. Longer established clinical supervision relationships can be much enhanced by reviews, preventing unhelpful habits becoming established or clearing up possible points for resentment that otherwise might gradually sour the relationship. These reviews can be structured or ad hoc.

A structured review can be built into the clinical supervision contract as an agreement to review the relationship at regular intervals. The format of the review could proceed as follows:

1. *Review of contract.* The supervisee states which of the ground rules in the contract she feels that she has upheld and which she has not. The clinical supervisor gives feedback to the supervisee about this, sharing any concerns and appreciations. The clinical supervisor then states which of the ground rules she has upheld and which she has not, and the supervisee gives feedback. Any necessary revision to the contract is made in the light of this sharing.

2. *Review of the clinical supervisor's facilitation.* The clinical supervisor gives a brief self-assessment under these two headings: 'How I think I have been most effective as a clinical supervisor' and 'What I would like to do differently in the future'. The supervisee responds to this self-assessment, or gives feedback along the same lines: 'What I appreciate most about the way you carry out your role as my clinical supervisor' and 'What I would like to be different in the future from you'. One important principle is that the supervisee comments only on behaviour, not the personality of

the clinical supervisor. A second is that there should be a balance between positives and negatives, otherwise the review is likely to be experienced by the clinical supervisor as an attack or as too cosy.

3. *Review of the supervisee's use of the clinical supervision sessions.* The supervisee first makes a self-assessment, covering the following two points: 'Some ways in which I think I'm making effective use of the clinical supervision sessions' and 'Some ways in which I could make more effective use of the sessions in the future'. The clinical supervisor reacts to the self-assessment or shares points under similar headings, again with comments only on behaviour, not personality, giving a balance between positives and 'do differentlies'. For example:

> Liam and Sandra are having a review of their first three clinical supervision sessions.
>
> *Liam:* I feel that I have kept to the ground rules, though I think I could have probably given you some more feedback on the spot, as I'd agreed to do.
>
> Sandra agrees but reminds him of one occasion when he stopped her when she was giving some unwanted advice: she found it helpful to be reminded to check if advice is wanted. She also suggests that Liam need not be so wary in telling her about difficulties with a particular colleague, that she would definitely keep it confidential. Sandra then assesses herself as having met the ground rules as agreed but wants to clarify the confidentiality ground rule a bit more. When they made the contract, she had not specified that she herself would be using her own clinical supervision to reflect on her role as clinical supervisor, and while this meant disclosing a little of the content of the sessions, she wants to assure Liam that this was done without identifying him or anyone he talked about and was more focused on her own issues and development.
>
> *Liam:* That's OK with me but I'm glad we got it clear: I was wondering about it. What I'd like to say is that I've really appreciated you being reliable about the appointments and being a sounding board, plus you've given me some good ideas, especially that problem last time. The 'do differently' is what we said earlier, perhaps wait until I'm ready before you give advice.

4. *Ad hoc feedback.* This can be given at any time. As supervisee, you may feel that a certain part of a clinical supervision session has been especially helpful: you could say so at the time and specify exactly what the clinical supervisor did that was so helpful. You may be struggling with an issue and finding that the clinical supervisor's interventions are not useful to you: saying so at the time gives the clinical supervisor a chance to adapt the approach so that it is more effective. As clinical supervisor, you may be impressed with some aspects of the way the supervisee works in clinical supervision and it can be very encouraging to say this at the time. You

may notice some way in which the supervisee is hampering herself, not making best use of the time: it can be facilitative to share this at the time. More guidance on giving encouragement is given in Chapter 5, and on challenging in Chapter 6. While these pointers are focused on the clinical supervisor's facilitative role, the supervisee may also find the guidelines helpful when considering giving feedback to the clinical supervisor.

5. *Using structured evaluation tools.* Some examples of these are shown in Chapter 9. These give detailed lists of criteria to consider in assessing yourself as a supervisee and as a clinical supervisor.

Dealing with criticism in clinical supervision

We find that most nurses receiving training in supervisee skills request some help with learning how to deal with criticism. Often there is some anxiety behind the request, based on the misapprehension that clinical supervision will involve a lot of criticism. On the contrary, the major part of the work of the clinical supervisor is support and catalytic help (see Chapter 5). However, at times, the clinical supervisor will challenge the supervisee to increase awareness of, for instance, the part she herself might play in some of the problems under discussion or any blocks the supervisee seems to be having in using the session effectively (see Chapter 6).

Your clinical supervisor's intention and manner should be supportive and aimed at enabling you to learn and develop. However carefully and skilfully the clinical supervisor makes these challenges, it is likely that at times, as supervisee, you will feel some discomfort. Most people do when challenged, however constructively it is done. As compared to other professions with which we work, we find nurses especially sensitive to criticism, except those who work in settings with much robust dialogue, such as substance abuse treatment centres, prisons and forensic mental health units.

Participants on clinical supervisor training courses often request help with dealing with criticism from supervisees who are encouraged to give feedback about what is helpful and not helpful. Clinical supervisors realize that they are not going to be perfect in their clinical supervisor role and also feel nervous about the prospect of being challenged.

Whether as supervisee or supervisor, your emotional reaction to the experience of being challenged is likely to be affected by your past experiences. Most nurses have been on the receiving end of criticism which has been badly given, unjust, badly timed or humiliating, whether during their working time or elsewhere. Fear of being demolished by destructive criticism leads to many of the defensive practices explored in Chapter 2. In Clulow's (1994) study of supervisory relationships, he found there was a great deal of anxiety on both sides about their own competence and whether it was safe for either of them to reveal any lack of confidence, however transitory; there was a deep fear that disclosure would be criticized. Even the most constructive, well-timed, supportive criticism can make you feel terrible if you have been humiliated a lot in the past. As a result, it can be easy to over-react to even the most skilled, sensitive clinical supervisor or perhaps to under-react to someone who is mistaken or being unjust. The guidelines offered here suggest a few ways of dealing with criticism which might help you to cope with the discomfort and to learn something from the situation.

Steps in dealing with criticism

Consider the steps shown in Figure 3.2.

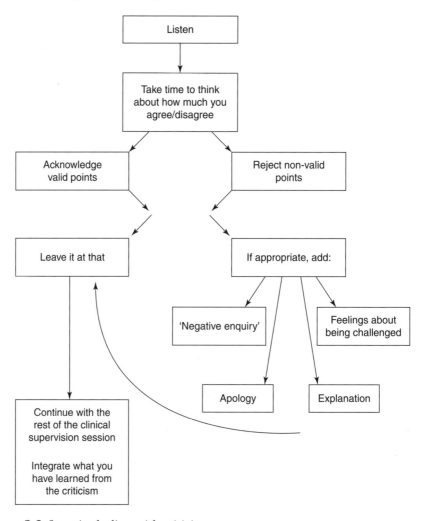

Figure 3.2 Steps in dealing with criticism

1. *Take time.* First of all, when you are challenged, listen and take time to collect yourself and think about what has been said. If your clinical supervisor does not spontaneously give you space to reflect, then ask for it.

Carol describes to David, her clinical supervisor, how an elderly patient was discharged home too early because the bed was needed for an emergency admission, and subsequently had to be readmitted after a serious fall. She describes trying to stand up to the consultant, before the original discharge, and how she was rebuffed by a rude response.

David: It sounds as if you gave up at the first hurdle and didn't try to persist to show how important your viewpoint was.

Carol: Well, I need to think about that.

Carol takes a few moments to cast her mind back over the situation.

2. *Agree/disagree?* Next, decide how much truth there is in the criticism, if any? Categorize it as either 'I totally agree', or 'I totally disagree', or 'I partially agree' (i.e. 'I agree with part of it, but disagree with the rest').

Malcolm is a practice development nurse whose role includes providing clinical supervision along with other development tasks within that sector of the Trust. His Trust has instigated a new training initiative and Malcolm is under pressure to enlist participants. During Nora's clinical supervision session with him, he gives quite a lot of information about this initiative and tries to persuade Nora to sign up for it.

Nora: Malcolm, look, this is quite interesting but this is not meeting my needs at the moment. I'm really worried about the problem I tried to discuss with you but this training initiative is your agenda. I thought this was supposed to be my time.

Malcolm realizes straight away that she is right.

3. *Acknowledge valid points.* If you think the challenge is accurate, then try to accept the valid criticism, however embarrassing it feels to admit to it. State that you agree with the criticism: a plain, direct, honest answer deals positively with the criticism and helps you to let it sink in and learn from it. Accept valid criticism without defensive justifications, excuses, passing the buck and so on. If you talk or sidle your way out of it, you are likely to learn less from it.

Carol: (continues) Yes you're right, I didn't persist. It might have got across the importance of what I was saying to him if I had.

Malcolm: (responds to Nora) That's quite true, I made a mistake pushing my agenda so much.

4. *Reject non-valid points.* If you think the criticism is inaccurate, then state that you disagree with it and contradict it with a positive statement about yourself. You need to reject criticism with which you disagree, without retaliating. The clinical supervisor is unlikely to put you down for the sake of it – they may just be mistaken. So, just respond by saying that you

disagree and contradict the critical statement with a positive statement about yourself.

> Veronica is telling her clinical supervisor Margaret about a complicated situation in which two of her staff nurses were in conflict with each other and refusing to cooperate. She had asked a particular third-year student nurse to go and work with them and had briefed her about the conflict.
>
> *Margaret:* I wonder if you were a bit rash to delegate to a student the job of sorting out the staff nurses?
> *Veronica:* Well, actually, I disagree. I think I made a very good choice in this case.

If the challenge has some truth in it but is overstated or slightly off beam, then specify exactly what you agree with and what exactly you disagree with, as Annette does to her supervisor in this example:

> *Patrick:* I'm concerned that you're always late for our sessions together.
> *Annette:* Granted I was today and a bit last time but I disagree with your saying 'always' because I've been punctual every other time.

5. *Leave it at that.* At times, it is sufficient to show agreement or disagreement and drop the issue in order to move on. You can then go on with the clinical supervision session and build into it what you have learned from the criticism. As supervisee, you might be able to use it in your reflection on the issue that you have brought to clinical supervision. As clinical supervisor, you might be able to use what you learned by adapting your approach during the rest of the session.

6. *'Negative enquiry'.* At other times, additional responses to criticism may be appropriate, though beware of saying too much out of anxiety. 'Negative enquiry' involves asking questions to elicit more useful details from a clinical supervisor who is challenging you or who you think might be feeling critical of you, but not expressing it. The word 'negative' may seem confusing here, but this is the term you will find used in the classic books about assertive communication, such as Dickson (1982). It is actually 'positive' in the sense that you are enabling your critic to give constructive rather than destructive criticism. This is based on the belief that constructive criticism is helpful and, applied to clinical supervision, that the supervisee wants to learn from being usefully challenged.

   Situations in which 'negative inquiry' may be helpful include: when you disagree with the other person when they have not given you enough information so that you can understand what they mean; when you think the other person is concerned or critical but has not expressed it; when they have used a generalization such as 'always' or have commented on your personality rather than your behaviour or manner.

   'Negative inquiry' can help you to find out exactly what actions you've done or what type of approach has bothered them. It can also help you to discover the emotional effects of your actions. So, you can use this knowledge by taking it into account next time you act. Alternatively it can open up a useful discussion about viewpoints and values.

> *Annette:* What was it that concerned you about my being late?
> This went on to become a useful discussion about Annette's commitment to clinical supervision.
> Veronica: What made you think that it was a bad decision?

7. *Explain or not.* Giving a reason may be appropriate, especially if it is about the clinical supervision session itself or about your professional practice. Explaining what happened may clear up misunderstandings, but beware of using reasons as excuses or justifications to deflect a useful challenge.

> Annette explained that today and last time there were crises on the ward just before she was due to leave for the clinical supervision session and she felt that she had to complete what she was doing rather than try to hand over to someone else. This led to a discussion about the timing of clinical supervision sessions and she and Patrick agreed in future to hold the sessions at a different time of day, when Annette was less likely to get embroiled.

> In Carol's case, there was no need to explain why she found it difficult to persist, as she had already described the difficulties of the situation and a repetition would only have been a defensive justification. Instead, they went on to explore how Carol could persist with getting her points across with this particular consultant the next time she disagreed with him.

> It seemed appropriate for Veronica to explain that the student was a mature student, older than both the staff nurses, and used to be a schoolteacher. She was really good at laughing off this type of nonsense and, as it turned out, she managed to get them both laughing about how stupid it was. As a result that team did really good work during that shift.

8. *Apology.* The person making the challenge may be entitled to an apology for something that affects her, and it might help to say what you are prepared to do about it in future.

> *Annette:* I really am sorry I kept you waiting and made you wonder if I'm not bothered about clinical supervision. Now we've changed the times I'll move heaven and earth to get here on time.

> *Malcolm:* And I'm sorry I pushed my agenda. OK Nora, let's go back to what you were saying about the problem with so-and-so.

There may be a place for sharing how you feel emotionally about being challenged or about the way the other person has challenged you.

Annette: I feel disappointed that you questioned my commitment to clinical supervision. I've put a lot into getting here and working with you and I've done a lot to get some colleagues thinking more positively about it too.

9. *Move on.* If either of you are anxious about the challenge, there can sometimes be a tendency to repeat yourself. Remember why you are meeting and move on with the clinical supervision session and try to build in what you have learned from the challenging dialogue – not only what was said, but the process. Consider what relevance it has had to your workplace.

These methods and examples may sound uncomfortable and some may fear that such methods would damage the working alliance. We maintain that it is not appropriate to strive to feel comfortable all the time in clinical supervision: getting things into the open, surfacing hidden tensions and clearing up misunderstandings are essential for an effective working alliance.

Pitfalls in dealing with criticism

The almost inevitable discomfort of being on the receiving end of a challenge can lead to non-assertive approaches; that is, being aggressive, manipulative or submissive (see Table 3.7).

Table 3.7 Pitfalls in dealing with criticism

Aggressive approach
  Retaliating by pointing out the faults of the person doing the criticizing
  Retaliating by automatically accusing the person of discrimination
  Not listening, interrupting a lot
  Walking out of the session
  Refusing to rectify a mistake out of spite

Submissive approach
  Allowing people to get away with unjust or badly given criticism
  Allowing the other person to label your personality without asking them to be more specific about your actions
  Accepting criticism second-hand instead of going to face the critic in person
  Being over-apologetic
  Absorbing all criticism, whether valid or not, and using it to feed a negative self-image

Indirect approach
  Blaming someone else
  Trying to talk the other person into changing their mind
  Throwing in red herrings
  'Poor me': trying to get the person doing the criticizing to feel sorry for you
  Criticizing the manner of the criticism, while ignoring valid content
  Insincerely appearing to agree with valid criticism

---

1. *Aggressiveness*. An aggressive approach to dealing with criticism includes various ways of attacking in retaliation. These might include dragging up some real or imagined mistake or fault on the part of the person doing the criticizing, and using it to attack them. For instance, if Annette had retaliated with 'What about you? You can talk! You were late for the very first meeting', then the discussion might have degenerated into an argument, instead of leading to some useful discussion. Retaliation might be in the form of automatically accusing the person of gender or racial discrimination, without first considering if there might be some truth in the criticism. Other aggressive responses include not listening, interrupting a lot, walking out of the session, blaming the person doing the criticizing or refusing to rectify a mistake out of spite.

2. *Submissiveness*. A submissive approach to dealing with criticism involves not setting limits or not standing up for yourself. You might be allowing people to get away with unjust or badly given criticism. It would be submissive to allow the other person to label your personality without asking them to be more specific about which of your actions they are concerned about. Submission might include accepting criticism second-hand instead of going to face the critic in person. Accepting too much of the criticism is submissive; perhaps being over-apologetic or, at the extreme, absorbing all criticism (whether valid or not) and using it to feed a negative self-image. For instance, Veronica would have been submissive if she had responded to the inaccurate criticism with, 'OK, yes, I've been told I'm hopeless at delegating, I always have been.'

3. *Indirect approach*. The manipulative or indirect approach to dealing with criticism involves deflecting the criticism in a manner which is not explicitly aggressive. Some ways of talking your way out of facing up to the criticism might include blaming someone else, trying to talk the other person into changing their mind or throwing in red herrings. The indirect approach might include trying to get the person doing the criticizing to feel sorry for you or criticizing the way they gave the criticism, while refusing to acknowledge any validity in the content of what was said. Lastly, it might involve appearing to agree with valid criticism, but just doing it to smooth things over. Annette would have been indirect if she had given excuses at length, blaming a colleague for incompetence and management for not providing cover (without being asked) and so on.

It is the aggressive, submissive and indirect approaches which can cause lasting damage to a working relationship, rather than the assertive approaches suggested earlier. Dickson (2006) and Back and Back (2005) take these basic assertiveness methods further in their books on handling difficult conversations without ruining the relationship. Chapter 9 also includes some tools for self-assessment and feedback and these can be useful for discussing expectations and how you are working together.

In response to the anxieties many nurses have expressed to us about dealing with criticism, we have given over quite a lot of space in this chapter to offering practical guidelines on this, but we wish to emphasize that this forms a very small part of an effective clinical supervision relationship. You might ask, 'How do you know if the relationship is effective?'

Features of an effective clinical supervision relationship

Imagine that you could be a fly on the wall of some clinical supervision sessions which are going well, and consider what your criteria would be for describing a clinical supervision relationship as effective. Identifying your criteria might be a useful joint exercise to add to the review structure suggested earlier in this chapter, with some exploration of what issues are emerging between you which are blocking the potential effectiveness of your working alliance. We have been lucky enough to observe many actual and practice clinical supervision sessions during consultancy work and training sessions, and will try to paint a picture here of an effective working alliance.

Seeing the relationship in action over a number of sessions, we note that the atmosphere is fundamentally one of support and advocacy for the supervisee, with the focus on the supervisee leading the session with their agenda. The clinical supervisor shows a genuine interest in the supervisee as a person, in her clients and key colleagues and in the context in which the supervisee works: it is almost as if some of the significant people with whom the supervisee works are in the room. There is a fairly relaxed beginning to each session, with short periods of general chat and there has obviously been some good communication about expectations and about the process of working together because they have a sort of shorthand language about what is wanted from the session and about how they will proceed.

In spite of the relaxed beginning there is still a slight air of formality with a certain amount of tension as complex issues are grappled with and, at times, the supervisee is obviously feeling challenged to examine their awareness of self, their own behaviour in, strengths, weaknesses, feelings and values. From time to time, there is some attempt to clarify what type of help the supervisee requires: the supervisee pauses and asks for some specific type of help from the clinical supervisor, such as helping to find a direction through the complexity, or sharing some ideas. The clinical supervisor checks occasionally if the supervisee is getting what is needed. At times, there is some humour, expressing enjoyment at achieving something or a sense of the ridiculous, or as a tension release, but it is not at anyone's expense, and not diverting from the task. Often they creatively play with ideas. The energy seems to go in waves, settling at the beginning of the session, winding down towards the end and in between punctuated by periods of intense, sometimes playful dialogue, with reflective silences and pauses to recap and complete each phase or topic.

However, not everything goes smoothly. There are times when the supervisee seems to be in a complete muddle and times when either or both the supervisee and the clinical supervisor seem at a loss to know how to sort it out, perhaps with one or other or both of them saying so. Eventually they both come out of the confusion with the supervisee developing some new insights about the complex issue under discussion. Occasionally there is disagreement or resentment between them, which causes a little tension, but they explore it, accept it, recover and move on. There is openness in the relationship: for instance, occasionally, there are disclosures of some uncertainties or personal vulnerabilities in their respective roles, either or both confessing to finding the process difficult. Sometimes one or the other draws attention to the way the here-and-now situation may have parallels with the workplace issue being discussed. At times the supervisee needs some 'emotional first aid' (allowing emotional release and enabling recovery) when she is feeling vulnerable. The supervisee has enough trust in herself and the clinical supervisor to reveal some of the personal difficulties and mistakes that they experience in whatever aspects of their work they are addressing in the sessions, and to explore the embarrassment or shame that accompanies these errors. There is also an interest in exploring what has gone well and what can be learned from that experience about the supervisee's taken-for-granted expertise and knowledge.

There is a sense of mutual enquiry. The supervisee brings complex issues which have no single answers and they explore them together. The clinical supervisor is obviously equally curious as to where the discussion will lead them and how things will turn out in reality. There is an atmosphere of joint endeavour: supervisee and clinical supervisor seem tuned into and paying attention to one another. The work that is done in the sessions involves the supervisee doing in-depth reflection on practice situations and issues affecting that practice, in dialogue with the clinical supervisor who also ponders on the issue with the supervisee. There is no sense that the clinical supervisor feels obliged to come up with solutions, instead there is more of a partnership in enquiry.

The beginning of each session usually includes a report by the supervisee of how she has put into practice the learning from the last session. Each session usually ends on time with some clarity about what has been achieved and how it will be put into practice, and both parties are clear about the date and time of the next session.

Summary

This chapter has offered some practical guidelines for clarifying rights and responsibilities, negotiating the clinical supervision contract and reviewing the relationship with the intention of equipping you to develop an appropriate symmetry of power and to build a secure psychological base for the supervisee within the organization. Linking back to the structural discrimination issues and blocking factors highlighted in Chapter 2, we urge you to be alert to and honest about your own prejudices, negative attitudes towards each other, any sensitivities that the other may trigger for you and your fears about clinical supervision itself; and that you seek to minimize their destructive influences on the clinical supervision relationship. While the work in this chapter has aimed towards providing appropriate boundaries and taking responsibility for the quality of the relationship, other conditions for developing effective working alliances depend on committed management sponsorship, choice of delivery framework, allocation of appropriate amount of protected time, skills training and continuity: these are explored in Chapter 9.

The next four chapters focus in turn on the reflective skills of the supervisee, the enabling skills of the clinical supervisor and the skills of group clinical supervision. While we have had to separate these out of necessity, we would like you consider all within the context of the clinical supervision relationship. This working alliance between supervisee and clinical supervisor aims towards providing a secure psychological base for the supervisee within which to feel safe enough to grasp the nettle of accepting support for vulnerabilities, consider challenges to actions, values and attitudes, and reflect in depth on their own clinical practice and their own part in it.

4 Supervisee skills of in-depth reflection

This chapter aims to paint a picture of the experience of reflection in effective clinical supervision and to provide some practical frameworks to stimulate your reflective processes, with the long-term aim of enabling you to maintain and deepen the process of reflection in your everyday practice. It highlights the need for balance between analytical thinking skills and those of intuitive and emotional understanding and expression. All three of these areas of skills are needed to foster creative reflective practice through the qualities of thoughtfulness and emotional depth.

The nature of reflection in clinical supervision

Pondering on the nature of reflection, we are reminded of a particular painting: *The Rokeby Venus* in the National Gallery, London. It is a painting by Velázquez in which a naked woman reclines on a couch with her back to the viewer. A mirror is held up to her by a child/nymph. She is not looking at herself but is looking at us, the viewer, looking at her. At least it seems that way as the face is fairly blurred. All manner of interpretations have been put on this picture of reflection, and interpretations can shift depending on where you 'place' yourself mentally and in the gallery room and on what you think is going on. When you know more about what the artist had in mind, and the political context in which he painted the picture, it adds greater layers of complexity still, but as in all art, it is the external interpretations of the person outside of the picture that enables even more in-depth reflection.

Similarly a process of reflection within clinical supervision, shared with another, enables both sides of the supervisory relationship to occupy different positions. When the supervisee is 'in' the picture with another (patient or colleague), engaging in the complexities of health care, they will see and think about things differently from a thoughtful person on the outside looking in. The clinical supervisor needs to imagine what it is like to be within the situation, but also needs to occupy a separate place. The supervisee needs to be open to this benevolent scrutiny from another perspective. Together they can move about in the discussions and engagement with the problem, to occupy different reflective angles until more clarity is gained.

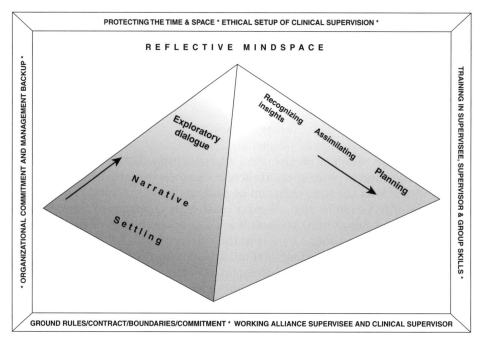

Figure 4.1 Pyramid of reflection in clinical supervision, showing phases of in-depth reflection

The dynamics of reflection in clinical supervision

We observe that this collaborative process of reflection in an effective clinical supervision session tends to go in phases, provided that the 'frame', the (conditions conducive to in-depth reflection), is firmly in place to provide a secure boundary. (see Figure 4.1). The phases are:

1. *Settling.* The clinical supervisor has arrived early and settled, in order to be able to welcome the supervisee and enable her to make the transition into the session (as outlined under 'Support skills of the clinical supervisor' in the next chapter.) After some preliminary discussion, including reporting back on action plans from the previous session, the supervisee moves on to the next phase.

2. *Narrative.* The supervisee outlines the experience which she has brought to reflect upon. The supervisee recounts the experience at her own pace and in her own sequence. The clinical supervisor listens actively, saying little, but supports and encourages.

3. *Exploratory dialogue.* The clinical supervisor becomes more actively involved and there is more two-way dialogue as they explore what was said in the narrative further, while the supervisee expands on certain aspects.

4. *Reflective mindspace.* The dialogue becomes increasingly reflective and the supervisee enters a state of mind in which reason, emotion and intuition seem to be to working together, a combined state of analysing, feeling and

pondering, often with a sense of playing with ideas. The clinical supervisor also enters this reflective mind-space, but with an eye to the process and her role in facilitating it within the clinical supervision framework.

5. *Working with insights.* Neuroscientists Jung-Beeman et al (2004) suggest that it is possible to notice when insights occur and emphasize the importance of capturing them before they are forgotten. Their studies indicate that the moment of insight has two brief phases. Firstly, the supervisee's focus moves inwards and there is a momentary change of posture, facial expression (often eyes closing) and/or breathing, such as holding breath or a deep breath. Tests show an increase in alpha waves in the brain and an increase in serotonin. The second phase is the moment that a new idea crosses the supervisee's mind, and can be observed by another slight change in posture or facial expression, such as the eyes opening again. Tests show an increase in gamma waves from many different parts of the brain as information is put together in a new way to form an insight, and there is increased adrenaline, dopamine and serotonin release. The supervisee may experience an emotional 'buzz'. Then there is a return to normal brain waves and levels of brain chemicals. The studies carried out by Jung-Beeman et al (2004) also demonstrate that unless the insights are captured, acknowledged and integrates, they were forgotten within one hour. The implications for clinical supervision lie in the supervisee being aware of their own process and the clinical supervisor allowing the space for this crucial part of the reflective process to occur, being aware of subtle and quick changes in body language when insights, verbalise them and integrate them into their action plans.

While this might often appear to be the process, there are some background issues which need to be held in mind: self-disclosure and the unknown (see Figure 4.2).

Self-disclosure

In-depth reflection involves a degree of self-disclosure on the part of the supervisee, and to some extent the clinical supervisor, when entering into an exploratory dialogue and reflective mind-space from which insights, decisions and the unexpected might emerge. Many nurses have serious concerns about self-disclosure and while there may be intrinsic psychological defences against it (as explored in Chapter 2), there may also be just cause for the concern: 'Can I trust my clinical supervisor?'. While we may be taking the metaphor of *The Rokeby Venus* a bit too far to refer to her nakedness at this point, course participants and supervisees do speak about fears of feeling 'exposed' and 'revealing too much of themselves'.

So first we need to define 'self-disclosure' in this context. Self-disclosure is the process of revealing more about ourselves to others. We each have our own levels of privacy, from the public to the professional, personal, private, intimate and finally, secret. Typically, when we meet someone for the first time, we reveal information about ourselves which we are comfortable about being public. As we get to know

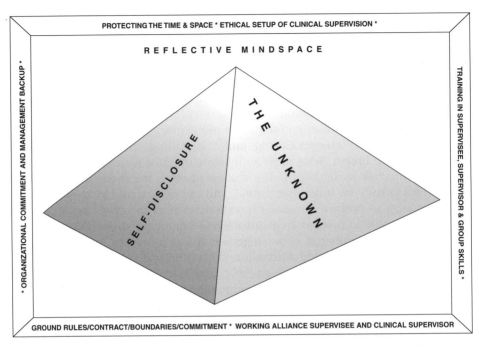

Figure 4.2 The other sides of the pyramid of reflection in clinical supervision

one other, we disclose more professional and personal information. In close personal relationships we reveal personal, intimate and sometimes secret information. The progression is usually gradual and may be conscious or unconscious.

Part of Gregory's (1996) definition is 'disclosing is showing others who you are' (p. 119) and she contrasts this with 'the professional shield' (p. 252), which emerged strongly in her study of nursing students who reported that the shield was modelled by (and corroborated in her study by) the senior staff working with them.

Given that the assessment of nurses in training now includes a significant element of assessment of reflective journals, case studies and critical incident analyses, we have seen evidence in our postgraduate courses that this scrutiny is leading some nurses to develop extended versions of the 'professional shield'. Not only are they learning to hide behind a façade of doing the right practical procedure and shutting up about their feelings, some seem to be building a façade of appearing to be a 'reflective practitioner'. In recent years, the following example has been a common occurrence on our courses for trained nurses: although the topic was a real-life complex issue brought by the supervisee, she said after 10 minutes: 'I've done a "Gibbs" on this one and I'm finished: this is what happens in my clinical supervision sessions, I don't need an hour.' She was referring to a classic and valuable model by Gibbs (1988) which is taught on many nursing degree courses but she had applied it in a superficial and mechanistic manner. This tendency is supported by Saltiel's (2010: 139) critique of current reflective practice which includes the assertion that in both social work and nursing 'there is a strong tendency for reflection to become something superficial, conformist and . . . a technical exercise to fulfil certain study or employment requirements'.

We consider that at the heart of this diminution of reflection in clinical supervision is fear of self-disclosure, some of which may be justified. This is the reason we have put so much emphasis in this book on creating the conditions for reflection to happen safely: by establishing the 'frame'; in the way clinical supervision is set up (Chapter 9), in the building of the working alliance (Chapter 3), in both supervisee and clinical supervisor receiving training in the appropriate skills, and in the way the clinical supervisor facilitates reflection (Chapters 5 and 6). These factors are central to the instances when we have observed clinical supervision working well.

The unknown

The process of reflection is an open-ended exploration and neither the supervisee nor the clinical supervisor knows where it might lead. In addition to relevant insights, creative ideas and inspired decisions, issues may arise which are outside the bounds of clinical supervision. This is another reason for our emphasizing the need for clarity and ethics in setting up clinical supervision. If you can feel secure enough with the boundaries, you can relax into the reflective mindspace and should anything come up which is outside the frame, both the supervisee and clinical supervisor will know when to take it outside appropriately.

Existing skills of reflection

How you as supervisee use the clinical supervision time to think, select, describe, analyze, disclose and so on, will also draw upon the skills you have developed in your personal life. Earlier attachment and educational histories may affect the range of thinking and emotional skills immediately at your disposal. The frameworks offered in this chapter must be seen in the context of the clinical supervision relationship: time must be allowed for enough feelings of trust and self-confidence to develop before the frameworks can be used effectively as part of the working alliance. Not all of this chapter will be relevant to every reader, but some of the guidelines may enable you to identify some of the gaps in your skills and to reflect on them with reference to the blocks and attachment implications explored in Chapter 2.

Reflection on/in practice, and from/through practice

We also wish to distinguish between reflection *on* practice and reflection *in* practice. This distinction relates to Fish *et al.*'s (1989) terms 'learning *from* practice' and 'learning *through* practice'. Learning from practice suggests that there is an ideal way to practise, sanctioned by theory and the 'way it is done around here'. Learning through practice suggests more of a dynamic process 'through which to learn something wider and of more significance' (Fish *et al.* 1989: 32). This more sophisticated absorption and integration of a range of skills allows for on-the-spot processing, reflection, prioritizing and action as appropriate, so that you

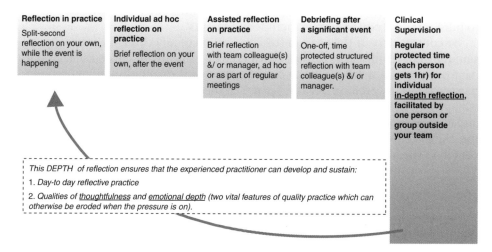

Figure 4.3 Where clinical supervision sits in reflective practice

both 'do' and refine practice at the same time. In clinical supervision, a similar developmental process can happen, moving from being in supervision with
a clinical supervisor or group where reflection on practice can take place, to
developing your own 'internal supervisor'. This is the part of you that inter-
nalizes the composite mixture of skills developed with the help of the clinical supervisor, to use 'on the job' as reflection *in* practice. Implicit in 'internal
supervision' is the processing of the relationship and communication elements of
your work with the client, as well as the more technical aspects of clinical practice.

Where clinical supervision sits in reflective practice

In everyday work, an experienced practitioner reflects in practice, taking seconds
or minutes, and at times stopping for a short period to consciously reflect on
what has just happened, and then at times consulting with colleagues or a line
manager. Regular meetings with colleagues and line managers will explicitly have
periods of reflection, especially after critical or distressing incidents. These periods
of reflection in day-to-day working life are of necessity short as there are many
immediate and competing factors to be addressed. Complex, long-term issues are
put to the back of the mind because stopping to reflect on them requires time and
a different mindset: the reflective mind-space.

Clinical supervision provides protected time for the transition into this state of
mind, for deeper reflection, an opportunity which does not occur in the rest of
a nurse's working life. The regular experience of clinical supervision supports the
maintenance and development of the qualities of thoughtfulness and emotional
depth, two vital features of quality practice which can otherwise be eroded when
a nurse is under continuous pressure.

Choosing a topic to take to clinical supervision

As supervisee, it is important that you give some thought to your agenda for the clinical supervision session, and make a start on reflecting on those topics. Preparation will help you to make the transition from action-oriented work to in-depth reflection during clinical supervision. The opportunity for you to be empowered to use the session as your time for reflection will be lost if you are unable to initiate the work. Sometimes the choice of topic will be straightforward, since you may have a burning issue on your mind that you have already tried to think through on your own and for which you have a pressing need for support and guidance. At other times, you may find it difficult to think of something to bring to the session.

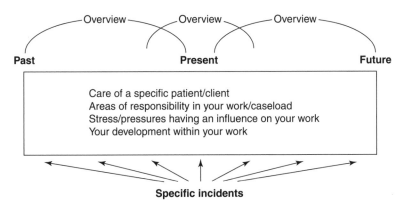

Figure 4.4 Pinpointing topics for reflection in clinical supervision sessions

Figure 4.4 and the following suggestions may help you plan your agenda. To find a relevant issue for reflection, you could scan through each of the four main areas shown in centre of the diagram.

1. *Particular patient/client/family.* Consider your care of a specific patient or client, including establishing the relationship, care assessment and planning, technical nursing procedures, communication about care plans and progress, emotional support, health education, work with their family or carers, delegation to and monitoring of other nurses, evaluation of care, preparation for transfer and finishing the relationship.
2. *Other responsibilities apart from direct patient care.* You could focus on one area of responsibility in your role, such as caseload management, being a team member, time management, management of junior staff, training of staff and students, liaison with other professionals, record-keeping, specialties within your role and so on.
3. *Stress of work or affecting work.* Your need may be more to explore some of the stresses or pressures arising from the job. You could consider the

stresses that arise from the nature of your work with clients or their families, from communicating with other nurses and professionals or from working within the organization. Alternatively, you could look at stresses from elsewhere in your life which have an influence on your work: it can be relevant to look at personal stresses provided you relate your reflection to finding ways of maintaining your standards at work in spite of those difficulties.

4. *Your development.* You could consider your personal and professional development and ask yourself which personal qualities and types of professional expertise are being utilized and developed within your work, or which you would like to develop more in the future. You could tackle any one of these from two perspectives: taking an overview or focusing on specific incidents. You could think in terms of scanning a particular span of time, choosing perhaps to review the past or the recent past/present/near future, or to consider the long-term future. Alternatively, you could focus on specific complicated events, whether in the past, recently, in the present or anticipated in the near or long-term future.

Still can't think of anything? Mental block?

If considering these options does not help you clarify something significant to reflect upon during clinical supervision then you probably have a mental block about it. Whatever you do, we urge you *not to cancel the session.* Take the mental block as your topic to clinical supervision: we have often found that these sessions turn out to be the most fruitful. We find there are usually two main reasons for the mental block:

1. *The dormant 'Big Issue'.* The pressures of dealing with many tasks and achieving specific targets can lead you to mentally park the complex issues which are not within your immediate focus. The issue becomes bigger and more daunting to tackle the longer you leave it, and unconsciously you bury it even further. Sometimes arriving at your clinical supervision session without an agenda, being welcomed and having the chance to settle, will create the space in your mind for the dormant topic to come forward.

> Heather arrived cheerfully at her session without a topic. She settled and just started talking and found herself going over a multidisciplinary team decision which seemed to have been dealt with. As she spoke, the clinical supervisor, Raj, picked up that Heather was not happy about the decision. They explored it and it seemed to Raj that it was a potentially serious case of team collusion: the decision was possibly unsafe because one crucial factor had not been clarified, and Heather agreed, with relief. Heather went back after the session and immediately checked out some crucial information that had not been taken seriously, and when she highlighted that fact, the team realized their mistake and changed the decision. Raj did not have to break confidentiality to report the situation as he trusted Heather's account

of dealing with the unsafe decision (she telephoned him as agreed to tell of the outcome), but he kept a record of that session and informed Heather that he had done so.

2. *Unacknowledged feelings.* The contributing factors to such a block may be your unacknowledged emotional feelings about the clinical supervision. When you arrive at your session, ask yourself 'How do I really feel about being here?' Perhaps you have some resentment about doing clinical supervision or specifically about your clinical supervisor or clinical supervision group. You may have unacknowledged fears to do with being criticized, or about lack of confidentiality and organizational links. Your feelings may be of unacknowledged sadness leading to your perhaps not wanting to let go of the past, such as a previous clinical supervisor or a previous job, or nursing-as-it-used-to-be. Realization of any of these feelings might enable you to work through the block and become more able to prepare for and use the time available in clinical supervision. Clinical supervision is an ideal time and place to talk about your emotions and this is considered a sign of emotional competence, not a failing.

> Geordie went to his clinical supervision group without a topic, in spite of racking his brains for one. He felt reluctant to attend, but went anyway. When it was his turn to speak and he still had no topic, one of the group members asked, 'How do you feel about being here right now?' He found himself looking at Tony and realized that he felt uncomfortable in the group today with him. Geordie had recently had a heated disagreement with a colleague that he knew shared a house with Tony. He didn't know if they were partners, but either way, he wasn't sure that confidentiality would be kept if he revealed the nature of the disagreement in the group, which he had just realized was the topic he really needed to talk about.

Intuitive methods of reflection

We offer some structures that may be helpful for making the transition between activity and reflection, and you can use these before, during and after your clinical supervision sessions. They can be applied to any personal notes or reflective diary you might want to keep, to face-to-face work with your clinical supervisor or clinical supervision group or to any reflection you do as part of your professional practice.

Many of the methods for reflection identified in the nursing literature are based on frameworks for *logical* thinking, and have been developed by their authors to a level of complicated cognitive mapping which many nurses find daunting and dissonant. We find that workshop participants are relieved and feel validated when we suggest that *intuitive* thinking skills are equally important. Experienced nurses internalize their knowledge and expertise and their work is based to a large extent on this *informed intuition*. Benner's (1984) seminal work emphasizes the part intuition plays in expert nursing, and this has been developed by many authors including Gobet and Chassy (2008).

Some issues require mainly one or other of the types of thinking skills; most demand a combination. Intuitive thinking can be useful when the issue you have to reflect upon is not clear-cut: you may have incomplete information and cannot realistically get any more. In this type of situation, you are not clear what your goals are and it is not certain whether or not you will be able to achieve anything. The options open to you are not precise and you cannot easily predict the outcomes of any course of action. You can see from this that intuitive thinking can be especially useful when reflecting on complex and unpredictable issues involving emotions and human relationships.

Logical thinking on its own can be useful when the issue upon which you wish to reflect is fairly straightforward: when you have enough information about the problem, you can clarify what you are aiming at and it seems likely that you can at least in part achieve that aim. In this type of situation, the options open to you can be identified and you can more easily predict the outcomes of each option.

We find that some of the most frequent issues of concern that are brought to clinical supervision involve relationships with colleagues, managers, the client or their relatives. Applying a purely logical framework to trying to think these through would be a non-satisfying and ineffective process. Therefore we first suggest some intuitive methods of reflection which can be used on their own or combined with the more logical, sequential methods which follow. These intuitive methods are summarized in Table 4.1.

Table 4.1 Intuitive methods of reflection

- TOP-OF-THE-HEAD REFLECTION – Start talking or writing, without censoring; look back and pick out themes, significant points, gaps, steps in reflection so far
- FREE-FALL WRITING – Write a 'stem' phrase at the top of a blank sheet; write anything, that comes into your mind, without censoring; stop at the end of time limit and look back; highlight one especially loaded phrase and write that at the top of another sheet as a new 'stem' phrase; continue; look back over your sheets and pick out any themes
- BRAINSTORMING – Write a specific question; within a time limit, list any ideas without censoring; rest; continue brainstorming for a further, shorter time limit; look back over all the ideas and cross out those which are totally out of the question; consider the others
- SLEEPING ON IT – Go to sleep at night thinking 'I wonder such and such' and note any insights when you wake
- SHORT RELAXATION BREAK – Use physical relaxation techniques, 'time out' break to walk around or daydream or silence during the clinical supervision session, in order to allow intuitive thoughts to pop up
- DRAWING THE ISSUE – Ponder silently about the issue that you have identified; begin to draw freely in an abstract way, covering the paper; sit back and reflect on what you have drawn
- MIND MAPPING – Write a main heading; write the thoughts this heading stimulates, in a circle around the central point, linking each to the central heading with a line; expand on each of the thoughts by adding key words related to each one, in a little cluster around it; sit back and look at the overall map, noticing links

---

1. *'Top-of-the-head reflection'*. This is the most commonly used intuitive method in clinical supervision. You start talking or writing about the issue and say whatever comes into your head about it, without censoring and without any deliberate order or structure. Then when you have run out of steam, you look back over what you have said and try to pick out any themes, significant points that came out and surprised you or any gaps in your account that, in retrospect, you can see you omitted. You might notice that you covered some of the steps in one or other of the logical reflection cycles. Your clinical supervisor or clinical supervision group can be helpful in assisting you to identify the themes and logical steps you have already covered and the gaps in your thinking so far. Sometimes, the clinical supervisor may feel obliged to try to get you to organize your thoughts before you are ready, so it can be useful to warn her that you just want space to talk about it in your own words first before you marshal your thoughts.

2. *'Free-fall writing'*. This technique was pioneered by Goldberg (1986) and developed subsequently (Goldberg 2001). You write a 'stem' phrase at the top of a blank sheet of paper, for example, 'It all started when...' or 'I remember...'. Then, for seven minutes you write absolutely anything that comes into your mind, without censoring. You should keep writing for the whole time without lifting your pen from the paper, without thinking, correcting or crossing out. At the end of the seven minutes, look back over what you have written and highlight one particularly loaded phrase. Write this at the top of a fresh sheet as your new 'stem' phrase. Then repeat the process for another seven minutes. Then look back over both sheets and see if you can identify any common themes. This technique is rather like bungee-jumping on paper: it is a leap into thin air and can be very productive. However, it is important to keep the contents of your writing private, and only discuss the emerging themes with your clinical supervisor or supervision group if appropriate.

3. *Brainstorming*. This is probably the best known intuitive method. Write a specific question at the top of a sheet of paper, or agree with your clinical supervisor to consider a question, such as 'What are the factors which contribute to the problem?' or 'What are the options for dealing with the problem?' Set a time limit, say, five minutes. Within that time limit, make a list as quickly as you can of any idea at all that comes into your head: do not censor, but instead include any extreme, rude, dangerous, silly or ridiculous ideas that occur to you. After the time limit, take a few deep breaths and briefly scan the ideas, then continue brainstorming for a further, shorter, time limit – say, two minutes. Look back over all the ideas and cross out those which are totally out of the question. Then consider the others. The aim of brainstorming is to loosen up your thinking, away from your usual train of thought towards more creativity. Although many of your ideas will need to be crossed out, these may have served the purpose of stimulating some useful ones that you otherwise may not have considered. You can do this on your own or with your clinical supervisor: either of you

could do the writing or both of you could call out the brainstormed points. Brainstorming is a useful method to use in clinical supervision groups to collect ideas and stimulate some mental energy.

4. *Sleeping on it.* Plan your topic to bring to your clinical supervision session at least 24 hours beforehand. This gives you the chance to sleep on it. 'Sleeping on it' is an intuitive skill which you can enhance by asking yourself a question, just before you go to sleep, beginning with 'I wonder ...', such as 'I wonder what I'll say about that problem during clinical supervision tomorrow'. Then let your mind wander away from the topic, forget about it and go to sleep. When you wake or when you get to that issue in clinical supervision, sometimes some surprising insights can come to you without trying.

5. *Short relaxation.* Letting yourself just relax sometimes allows intuitive thoughts to pop up. You can do this before the clinical supervision session, whether using relaxation techniques per se, or just having a 'time out' break to walk around or daydream. Don't strain to think about the problem, just let your mind drift. Sometimes an insight or a solution spontaneously emerges if you let it. You can use silence during the clinical supervision session to allow ideas to emerge in this way.

6. *Drawing the topic.* Drawing the issue utilizes and develops your capacity to think in pictures. Again, you can do this before the clinical supervision session and take your drawing along to discuss with your clinical supervisor or clinical supervision group, or you can take some pens and paper and do the drawing there. There are three steps: first of all ponder silently about the issue that you have identified. Begin to draw while you ponder and let your hand flow freely in an abstract way. Let the drawing develop until it covers the sheet of paper. Do not think about the drawing, or about whether or not you are producing a work of art. Just draw shapes and use colours while you think about the issue. You might want to include symbols or key words that mean something to you. Then sit back and look at what you have drawn. Ask yourself what any of the parts of the drawing might symbolize about the issue or about yourself. Then discuss this with your clinical supervisor or clinical supervision group. Anyone can use this method: even if you think you cannot draw, you will be able to doodle something about the issue in hand.

7. *Mind map.* Using a mind map, a technique devised by Buzan (2006), is another effective intuitive method. It is based on the idea that thoughts arise out of the network of interconnections between the brain cells, not sequentially as if in a list. The electrical activity of the brain occurs so quickly that we cannot be conscious of every thought. You can slow down and capture some of these thoughts by recording them in a sort of map which takes into account how thoughts occur in the brain. Using a mind map to lay out your thoughts about an issue helps you to capture the range of thoughts you have, and then step back and look for themes and further connections. Making a mind map has four stages. The first is to

write a word or phrase by way of a main heading in the centre of a sheet of paper, summarizing the issue you want to think through. Then write the thoughts this heading stimulates, in a circle around the central point, linking each to the central heading with a line. Third, expand on each of the thoughts by adding key words related to each one, in a little cluster around it. Then sit back and look at the overall map. Notice if any of the thoughts under separate sections link together, and draw a line across the page to link them. Add any further thoughts that arise from each link. Emphasize any solutions or learning points, either in a different colour or with a bolder border. You can use this method as part of your preparation for clinical supervision and take the map to discuss with your clinical supervisor or clinical supervision group, or you can map it out during the clinical supervision session.

Intuitive methods on their own can be inspirationally effective or spectacularly unreliable because some crucial elements can be omitted. Using logical structures for reflection can help you to check that your intuitive thinking has taken everything into account.

Logical frameworks for reflection

Part of the alienation which many nurses feel when trying to get to grips with published models for reflection may be due to what Davies (1995: 51) describes as 'masculine logic', which she suggests 'fears, denies and contains the world of bodily needs and emotions and interdependencies'. Much of the nursing literature on reflective practice makes dry reading, focusing on mainly analytic approaches to reflection, and the sheer plethora of models drives many nurses to 'analysis-paralysis': they cannot get started at all. Others try to cope by fixing on just one framework and trying to apply it, with inevitable difficulty, to every topic they wish to explore. To avoid being overwhelmed by the choice and complexity of models of reflection we recommend that as supervisee you first become acquainted with at least two different frameworks, one problem-solving framework and one experiential learning cycle, and use a simplified version of each to begin with. Then you can apply or combine them according to the issue in hand. As a rule of thumb, we suggest that you use a problem-solving framework when further action is going to be required from you with regard to dealing with a current problem. When the issue is past and gone and you are wishing to reflect on your learning from it, then choose an experiential cycle. When you are adept at using both, you will be able to combine them for maximum effectiveness. Then you can expand your repertoire of frameworks for reflection by using a second problem-solving framework and a second experiential learning cycle and so on. As you become more familiar with your options, you could use the map in Figure 4.5 to help you choose a framework for each issue you want to explore.

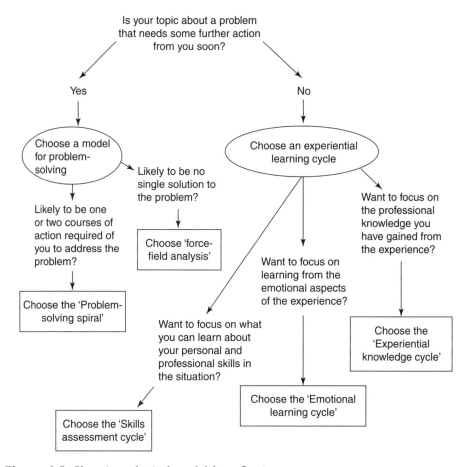

Figure 4.5 Choosing a logical model for reflection

We have come across some organizational rigidity with regard to logical models of reflection, in that policies may insist that a particular model is used. We consider this oppressive and this view is supported by Bradbury *et al*.'s (2010) suggestion that such efforts at 'mind control' miss the point. Hence the supervisee should have the autonomy to choose their own models for reflection.

Problem-solving frameworks

There are many structures for problem-solving available to you, especially in books on management skills. We have adapted two which are of most interest to nurses attending our courses.

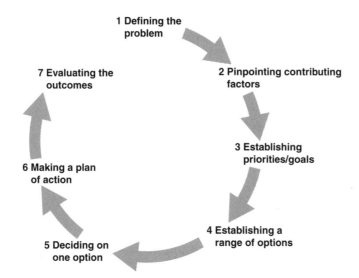

Figure 4.6 A problem-solving spiral

A problem-solving spiral

This spiral is useful when there are likely to be one or just a few courses of action required.

Figure 4.6 shows one step-by-step process of working through a problem to enable you to come to a clear decision. Although it is expressed in a certain sequence, you may have to take it in a slightly different order, or go back and forth until you are ready for the next step. For instance, having defined the problem and looked at contributing factors, you might realize that one of the contributing factors is the main problem that needs to be tackled first. In that case, you redefine that as the problem and then analyse the factors that contribute to it and move on through the cycle.

You can amalgamate some of the intuitive methods of reflection into this cycle. For instance, drawing the issue or mind mapping may be a good way of starting to define the problem and its contributing factors. Brainstorming is useful for considering options for action. This framework may highlight the steps you go through automatically when using intuitive methods such as 'top-of-the-head' reflection. However, we find that the most common pitfall for nurses is to go to the 'deciding on one option' stage too quickly, being anxious to answer the question 'What am I going to do about it?' without thinking in depth first (see Figure 4.7). This framework can remind you not to skip important stages in reflection on a problem that you are keen to solve.

The questions in Table 4.2 may help you to work your way through the spiral. A number of questions is offered for each stage and it is important that you are very selective, perhaps using just one per stage in the cycle.

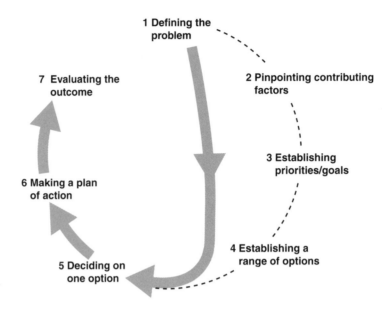

Figure 4.7 A common pitfall in problem-solving

Force-field analysis

The method was first described by Lewin (1951), and is a classic which has been tried and tested over the years and is now very widely used, for example by Nash and Young (2009). It is a framework for dealing with a many-faceted problem for which there is no single solution. It is a useful structure for reflecting on many of the complex issues that you can bring to clinical supervision, especially when you feel stuck in trying to solve the problem. Figure 4.8 suggests a format for writing in each step.

1. *Describe present position.* The first step is to describe the present situation – the 'frozen' or stuck position. Again, you might wish to use some intuitive methods such as mind mapping or drawing the issue to enable you to describe the complexity of the present situation.
2. *Vision or hope.* Then you need to take a leap of imagination and try to describe how you would really like the situation to be – the 'vision'. (If you are writing or drawing this, use a different sheet of paper.) Try to include in your description the emotional tone and the relationship aspects of your vision, as well as any factual circumstances.
3. *Restraining forces.* Next make a list of all the present factors which get in the way of your moving towards the vision: the restraining forces.
4. *Driving forces.* Ask yourself, 'What are the present factors which would push the situation towards the vision if there were no restraining forces?'

Table 4.2 Select a few of these questions as prompts through the stages of the problem-solving cycle

1. **Defining the problem**
   - What's bothering you?
   - What exactly is the problem?
2. **Pinpointing contributing factors**
   - What do you think contributes to this problem or difficulty?
   - How do you think you contribute to the problem?
   - What's behind the problem?
   - Think of a time when this problem did not exist. What was different about the situation then?
   - Which of these factors do you think should be tackled first?
   - Do you need to redefine the problem or are you clear about what exactly the problem is?
3. **Establishing priorities/goals**
   - What are you hoping to achieve?
   - What are you hoping for/aiming at in the long run?
   - Imagine that it is now, say, six months later and this problem has been dealt with. What's different now?
   - What are your ultimate goals?
   - What short-term goals would help towards that end?
   - Are your goals realistic? If not, what would be more realistic?
4. **Establishing a range of options**
   - What solutions have you tried already?
   - What options have you thought of so far?
   - Allowing your ideas to flow freely, what ways can you think of to achieve your goals? Brainstorm and don't censor, just let anything, however crazy, come into your mind

   - What's the most outrageous or extreme course of action that comes to mind? What's the most extreme form of inaction? Putting these two extremes at each end of a continuum, what options are there in between? Cross out anything which you are definitely not prepared to do under any circumstances whatsoever
5. **Deciding on one option**
   - Which is likely to be the most effective course of action, bearing in mind your goals?
   - Given that all your options are going to be difficult, which is the least worst?
6. **Making a plan of action**
   - What's your plan?
   - What is your very first step?
   - Then what next?
   - Whose help do you need?
   - When exactly are you going to do these things?
   - How will you keep up your courage and resolve to carry out this plan?
   - How will you know if you have been successful?
   - When exactly will you evaluate the outcome?
7. **(Later) Evaluating your decision**
   - How far were your goals achieved?
   - In the light of further information or events, what, if anything, needs to be done next?
   - Looking back at the factors contributing to the initial problem, is there anything else which could usefully be tackled?

Alternatively, if it is hard to think so positively, ask yourself, 'What factors prevent this situation being even worse?' These are the driving forces.

5. *Reduce each restraint a little.* Next consider how you can reduce the power of some of the restraining forces. Again, brainstorming can be an effective

Step 4 Driving forces	Step 1 Frozen position	Step 3 Restraining forces		Step 2 Vision
List here	Describe here	List here		Describe here
1		1		
2		2		
3		3		
4		4		
5		5		
6		6		
7		7		
8		8		
Step 6 Plan steps to enhance the power of each driving force		**Step 5** Plan steps to reduce the power of each restraining force		

Figure 4.8 Force-field analysis chart

method of coming up with some creative ways of tackling these restraining forces. Write next to each one a small thing you can do to reduce its power.

6. *Enhance each driving force a little.* Then think about how you might enhance the power of the driving forces and write one small plan next to each point. You now have a detailed plan of a number of actions which will improve the situation: the incremental things you do add up to moving you from the present situation in the direction of what you hope to achieve.

Experiential learning cycles

Kolb (1984) first described a process of learning from experience: the experiential learning cycle. This has been much adapted since (e.g. see Atherton 2009). Here we outline some adaptations which focus on different elements of the learning experience: self-assessment of skills, personal professional knowledge and emotional learning. All experiential learning cycles have three fundamental stages of reflection as their core, which can be summarized under the headings: 'What?', 'So what?' and 'Now what?' (see Figure 4.9).

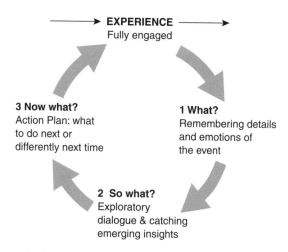

Figure 4.9 Stages of a basic experiential learning cycle

The starting point for maximum learning from experience is to be fully engaged in the experience: to be involved with your concentration, emotions and active participation. Taking an observer role results in a relatively shallow experience and, correspondingly, a relatively superficial level of experiential learning. While there is a place for observing another experienced nurse at work in order to pick up tips about procedures or how to handle difficult situations, the deepest learning comes from the occasions when you yourself are fully involved in a situation. You can maximize your learning from experience by taking regular time to step back and reflect on significant experiences. Doing this with an experiential learning cycle to guide your thinking, and a clinical supervisor or clinical supervision group to help you deepen it, can enable you to continue building up your professional knowledge, expertise and realistic confidence as you deepen your knowledge of your clients and yourself. Being able to monitor your practice by using an experiential learning cycle while you work, rather than only waiting for your clinical supervision sessions, is the ultimate aim in building these reflective skills.

Experiential learning cycles are frameworks to enable you to step back and look under the experience, have an exploratory dialogue with your clinical supervisor,

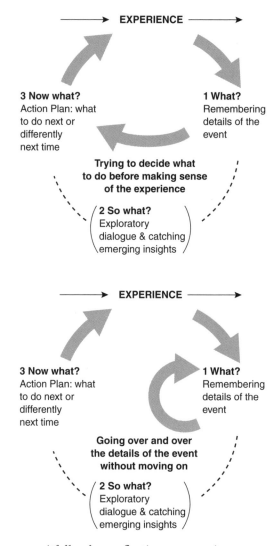

Figure 4.10 Common pitfalls when reflecting on experience

catch your emerging insights analyse it and consider your learning from the experience and how you can apply that learning. During workshops, practice exercises and observations of real-life clinical supervision sessions, we see some common pitfalls which ensnare the supervisee into superficial reflection (see Figure 4.10). One is to stay preoccupied with recalling the event, going over and over the details without moving on to include the emotional dimension and analysing it in more detail to find its meaning and learning points. A second pitfall is to jump straight from the recall stage to the action planning stage, bypassing the in-depth reflection that is needed in order to discover the significance of the experience and your learning points. Both pitfalls are examples of avoidant, superficial reflection.

Since the first edition of this book, we have become aware of interest from some nursing students about the provenance of the 'What?', 'So what?', 'Now what?' framework. This framework has existed in education for many decades, handed down from teachers of teachers to their students. Our version here was adapted from that taught by Kilty (1977). The earliest reference we could find is Borton (1970), who was involved in the area of T-groups and encounter groups applied to outward-bound courses.

Some of the frameworks which follow may help you to deepen your reflection in each of the various stages of the experiential learning cycle. Each framework takes a slightly different focus.

A skills-assessment cycle (see Figure 4.11.) may help you to make a self-assessment of the skills and abilities you used in the situation and how you can develop them in the future. It is especially useful for enabling you to practise taking a balanced view of the part you play in the complex situations you experience in your work. You are encouraged to balance acknowledgement of your strengths with that of your weaknesses, and to consider how to use your strengths to greater effect as well as develop your areas of weakness. We find that nurses have a tendency to understate their strengths and overstate their weaknesses, although those who have been in a particular post for a long time can often go to the opposite extreme. Using this skills assessment cycle in dialogue with your clinical supervisor or group can enable you to achieve and sustain a confidence about your expertise alongside an openness to learn.

The following is a list of some pointers which might help you to reflect on the experience, taking the focus of personal and professional skills. Again, the

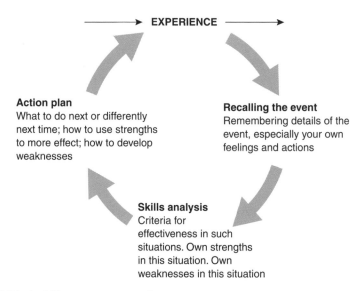

Figure 4.11 A skills-assessment cycle

framework offers a selection of pointers for each stage: just pick the ones which seem most helpful in enabling you to deepen or move your thinking on.

1. *Recalling the experience.* Describe the experience in your own words, in whatever sequence comes to you, putting the emphasis wherever you wish.
    - If you haven't already, describe your own actions, thoughts and feelings at significant points.
    - If you haven't already, pinpoint the reasons why you acted in the ways you did or why you failed to act.
2. *Skills analysis.*
    - Make a list of the professional and personal skills which would contribute to high quality practice in this type of situation. Put as many as you can into your list of criteria for excellence (minimum number: 15). Ensure that you write a phrase or sentence about each one, because single-word criteria are usually too general.
    - Include a wide range of professional skills, such as those which come within the categories of technical, interpersonal, care planning, team work, health education, support, staff education and so on.
    - Include a wide range of personal skills, such as those which come within the categories of time management, stress management, self-assessment, reflection, problem-solving, decision-making, emotional skills and so on.
    - Looking at this list, pick out one which was one of your strengths in this situation. If you cannot think of anything positive, if perhaps your confidence is having a bad day, pick one at which you think you were least hopeless! You could also ask your clinical supervisor or group for prompts.
    - Then select one criterion from the list which was one of your weaknesses in this situation. If you cannot think of anything in terms of a weakness, perhaps because your humility is having a bad day, then select one at which you were least perfect! Or ask for prompts.
    - Repeat the last two steps until you have three of each type of criterion: three strengths and three weaknesses. Ensure that you have an equal number of strengths and weaknesses.
3. *Action plan.* Make a step-by-step plan of how you are going to develop one of your strengths and one of your weaknesses.
    - Make a similar plan for the other strengths and weaknesses.
    - Outline how you hope to apply this development should you ever be in a similar situation again: what would you do differently?

A personal/professional knowledge cycle of experiential learning

Johns (1994) has utilized some of Carper's (1978) work on four ways of knowing, and incorporated it into this experiential learning cycle. Johns' classic cycle is especially useful for building your awareness of and confidence in the professional knowledge that you develop from personal involvement in the experience of working with a client. He suggests that the emphasis on research-based practice has become too extreme. This has devalued the knowledge nurses gain from their own experience and those areas of nursing practice which cannot be easily measured, such as compassion, caring, motivation, intuition, personal and interpersonal skills and so on. Johns takes a 'new paradigm' stance on research: that using any of the experiential learning cycles in order to enquire into one's own personal professional knowledge is a valid method of research – see Reason and Rowan (1981) for an account of this.

Figure 4.12 shows our adaptation of Johns' cycle. We follow his cue questions to lead you through the process. Again, the list gives a selection of questions for each stage: you would not be expected to try to answer them all. Use them to identify how far you have got already in your thinking, then pick out only the ones which help you to think more deeply or move on.

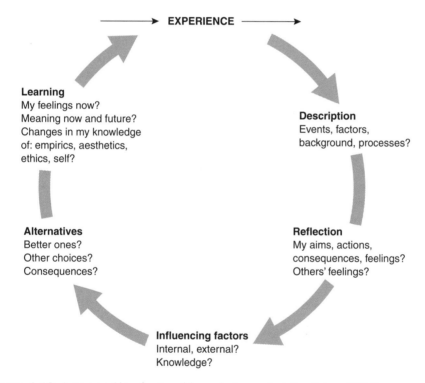

EXPERIENCE

Learning
My feelings now?
Meaning now and future?
Changes in my knowledge
of: empirics, aesthetics,
ethics, self?

Description
Events, factors,
background, processes?

Alternatives
Better ones?
Other choices?
Consequences?

Reflection
My aims, actions,
consequences, feelings?
Others' feelings?

Influencing factors
Internal, external?
Knowledge?

Figure 4.12 A personal/professional knowledge cycle (after Johns 1994)

Questions to guide you through the personal-professional knowledge cycle are taken from Johns (1994: 112):

Core question: *'What information do I need access to in order to learn through this experience?'*

1. *Description of the experience.*
   • Phenomenon: describe the 'here and now' experience.

- Causal: what essential factors contributed to this experience?
- Context: what are the significant background factors to this experience?
- Clarifying: what are the key processes (for reflection) in this experience?

2. *Reflection.*
   - What was I trying to achieve?
   - Why did I intervene as I did?
   - What were the consequences of my actions for:
     – myself?
     – the client/family?
     – the people I work with?
   - How did I feel about this experience when it was happening?
   - How did the patient feel about it?
   - How do I know how the patient felt about it?

3. *Influencing factors.*
   - What internal factors influenced my decision-making?
   - What external factors influenced my decision-making?
   - What sources of knowledge did influence/should have influenced my decision-making?

4. *Could I have dealt better with the situation?*
   - What other choices did I have?
   - What would have been the consequences of these choices?

5. *Learning.*
   - How do I feel now about this experience?
   - How can I make sense of this experience in the light of past experiences and future practice?
   - How has this experience changed my ways of knowing: empirics (the science of nursing); aesthetics (the art of nursing); ethics (the moral component of nursing); personal (self-knowledge)?

An emotional skills learning cycle

We aim to demystify the emotional element of clinical supervision and ensure that it has its place alongside professional knowledge and skills as worthy of examination. This emotional skills development framework may help you to reflect on what can be learned about your abilities in using your emotional energy (see Figure 4.13). It includes some adapted elements from Boud *et al.*'s (1985) framework of reflection in learning. It provides a structure for thinking about your emotions.

We suggest some pointers which might help you to reflect on the experience with the focus on emotional skills. Again, use the framework to augment your existing thinking about the experience and to highlight any stages you have left out in your reflection so far or that you need to explore in more depth. Pick the pointers which seem most helpful to you.

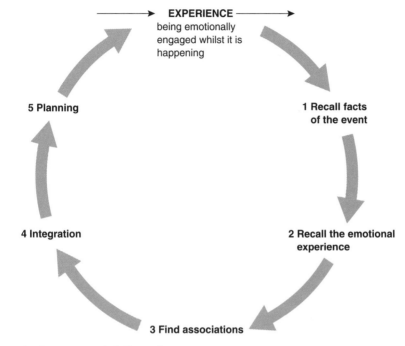

Figure 4.13 Emotional skills cycle

Questions and prompts to guide you through the emotional skills cycle:

1. *Recall the facts of the event.*
   - Describe the sequence of events as factually as you can without interpreting or analysing them at this point and without describing your feelings.
2. *Recall the emotional experience.*
   - Describe the whole experience, or the most important part of the experience, again, but this time in the present tense.
   - What kind of atmosphere do you pick up?
   - What colours, tone, sounds, sensations do you notice in particular?
   - What are you thinking?
   - How are you feeling?
   - What do your feelings lead you to do?
   - How do your emotional feelings help or hinder you in this situation?
   - What emotional skills did you use?
3. *Find associations.* Use any of the intuitive methods shown earlier in the chapter to discover associations: 'top-of-the-head' reflection; free-fall writing; drawing the issue; mind mapping, brainstorming. Do not censor. While you are doing this, consider these questions and include your answers in the account:

- What does this situation remind you of?
- When have you felt like this before?
- Taking each of the emotions you identified in Stage 2, brainstorm associations using the seed phrase 'Times I've felt ...'.

4. *Integration.*
   - What themes or linking patterns can you see?
   - How did your emotion positively and negatively affect your actions?
   - What conclusions do you draw from reviewing the emotional content of the experience like this?

5. *Planning.*
   - Make a step-by-step plan that is possible and realistic.
   - How will you apply these conclusions now?
   - How might you apply these conclusions in future?
   - With whose help?
   - What emotional skills will you use?
   - Rehearse how you will apply them: either by talking through the sequence of action, writing it down, setting up a role play with your clinical supervisor or clinical supervision group, or a colleague.
   - When and how will you review your plan?

Emotional skills

Concepts such as 'emotional competence' (Heron 1983) and 'emotional skills' (Bond 1986) have been used for some time and are gaining ground, along with 'positive emotional processes' (Heron 1999), 'emotional literacy' and 'emotional intelligence' (Cherniss and Goleman 2001). As we outlined in Chapter 2, evidence is emerging from neuroscience of the centrality of emotions in the networking of the brain and the necessity to value their place alongside rationality in cognitive functioning. Therefore, for effective professional decision-making within clinical supervision and in professional practice, as much attention needs to be paid to the development of emotional competence as to logical thinking abilities.

Emotional skills can be summarized as shown in Figure 4.14, a framework adapted from Heron's (2001) 'positive emotional processes'. Emotional skills can be described as the two central skills of awareness and self-acceptance, from which emerge the skills of being able to calm and settle oneself (containment, switching, contemplation) and the skills of emotional expression (communication, redirection, release). The key to emotional balance is to have a repertoire of skills from both sides of the scale and to use both types equally, each in their appropriate setting. Over- or under-use of either side leads to emotional imbalance and has a negative impact on practice. The nurse who spends an inordinate amount of time in the workplace communicating to anyone nearby how stressed she is, fascinated with her own misery, exhausts all support which is available from colleagues, and is a burden on clients who are too unwell to bear the strain of hearing it. On the other hand, the nurse who is so contained that she appears unconcerned about anything at all is callous in the face of others' vulnerabilities, including those of

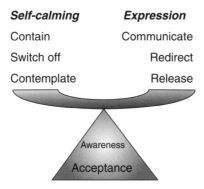

Figure 4.14 Emotional skills used in balance

clients. The alternative to these imbalances is to learn and use a balanced range of emotional skills in order to fuel the professional qualities of good decision-making, thoughtfulness and emotional depth which underpin effective professional practice.

Looking at each of the skills in turn, we start at the fulcrum of the balancing scale.

1. *Awareness.* This involves noticing your own emotions, being able to identify them and noting the extent to which they can positively and negatively influence your behaviour. This is essential for being able to selectively control emotional impulses rather than put a blanket repression on all of them. This leaves room for choice about expressing emotions and using them as a resource as well as containing them. One way of becoming more aware of your emotions is to notice their physical effects: a sensation of energy, tingling or alertness can tell you that you are interested, motivated, excited, pleased or delighted. Warmness in the chest and arms may indicate liking and affection while heaviness in the chest may be sadness, grief or despair. Tensions in the jaw, neck and shoulders may indicate irritation, resentment or anger. Stomach churning, lower back tensions, unpleasant tingling, tightness in the chest or fidgety legs may tell you that you are worried, anxious or fearful.

2. *Acceptance.* Non-critical acceptance of the existence of your emotions is important, though difficult in the culture of the health service. It involves not blaming or crediting the feelings on someone else, and not being critical with yourself for having them. Awareness and acceptance go hand in hand. The more you can come to accept your feelings non-judgementally, the easier it will become to be increasingly aware of your emotions and the energy that goes with them. Repression and suppression take up a lot of energy and can leave you feeling exhausted, whereas awareness and acceptance of emotions liberates energy which you can use

positively. Using clinical supervision to put your feelings into words can help to develop your self-acceptance provided your clinical supervisor can listen non-judgementally.

3. *Communication.* Communicating your emotions helps to reduce superficiality and build trust in relationships. It includes taking the risk of sharing positive feelings, revealing emotional vulnerability and giving constructive criticism. Verbal communication about emotions requires you to be emotionally articulate, to have a vocabulary of words that you can draw on to describe the feelings you experience. Communication may also be in a creative form such as poetry, dance, painting, drawing, music, etc.

4. *Redirection.* This is about channelling the energy of emotions into constructive thought or action. For instance, if your ability to do your work is hindered by a certain policy and you are in danger of blowing your top if you try to challenge the system, you could temporarily divert the energy of the frustration away from the problem and channel it into getting a lot of office or household chores done quickly. Then when you have calmed down a little, you could use the energy to tackle the problem constructively, perhaps by getting together with colleagues to collect evidence and go through the correct channels to suggest a change of policy.

5. *Emotional release.* As a skill, this is a controlled process of letting go: you are aware of what you are doing and choosing to do it safely at the appropriate time and place. It may involve yelling, bashing cushions, crying, laughing or putting a lot of strength of feeling into verbal communication about emotions. You need to choose times of privacy or times with non-judgemental family, friends or colleagues with whom you can release feelings from time to time. Clinical supervision may be an appropriate place for short periods of letting off steam. We have found that nurses often feel ashamed at crying in clinical supervision sessions but are relieved, if not amused, when it is pointed out that they are actually using an emotional skill by choosing an appropriate time and place to do this. We find that the more senior our supervisees are in the hierarchy, the more likely they are to need to have a cry in clinical supervision as there are fewer colleagues with whom they would feel safe to do this.

6. *Containment.* This is about holding back or holding onto emotions. There are many occasions when you need to hold back, perhaps to avoid hurting someone or when people are depending on you to act efficiently, or to restrain yourself from spilling out your stresses inappropriately to a client. The usually accepted concept of control is a sort of grit-your-teeth-holding-back-the-reins, which is ultimately exhausting. Containment is about expanding your sense of your own personal strength so that you can contain the feelings, psychologically 'holding' that part of you which is feeling emotional and postponing expressing the feelings until a more appropriate time. Earlier in this book we referred to the containing function of clinical supervision where we can name and acknowledge anxieties and the inner conflicts they can produce. Nurses who have good clinical

supervision speak of the containing effect of just knowing they can rely on getting their clinical supervision and how much this helps them to contain some of the difficult feelings triggered by day-to-day work.

7. *Switching off.* Nurses can have a variety of ways of switching off. You get yourself into a more settled emotional state by positive self-talk, doing something neutral like making a cup of tea, taking the proper breaks you are entitled to and using these to get a change of environment by going for a walk or some other physical exercise.

8. *Contemplation.* Emotional contemplation is a meditative process of staying still with the emotions and their accompanying physical feelings. There is a range of levels, from daydreaming, to physical relaxation, to using mental images or repetitive phrases or tunes, to transformation through feeling emotions intensely until your experience takes you to an altered state of consciousness. Most religions have prayers or meditations which can enable calming or transformation of emotions and there are secular techniques of relaxation and meditation which also have this effect.

For further guidance about practical ways of building emotional skills, you may wish to refer to guidelines we have provided elsewhere, such as in Bond (1986, 1989) and Holland (1987). Some stress management books address this issue, though not all view emotions as such potentially positive resources.

Here is an example of using emotional skills in clinical supervision:

Matt almost fell through the door at the start of the clinical supervision session. He blurted out that he'd never needed clinical supervision more in his life as he'd had to contain himself for the last three days. He burst into tears and cried for some time. Graham, the clinical supervisor, gave him space and reminded him it was OK to let go. He did not ask him to explain at this point. After about 10 minutes Matt collected himself enough to be able to speak and spoke tearfully about the sudden death of his colleague Mike, who was also a senior staff nurse on the same oncology ward. Mike had been a young man who had become a personal friend and he had a young family who were distraught. Because the ward manager was on annual leave, Matt had taken charge of the ward and had spent the last three days consoling the staff and patients. Most of his time off was spent with Mike's family. Having recounted this much, he sat back, resting his head and closed his eyes, sighing a lot. His breathing settled and he stayed still. Graham was very moved by the situation, and his mind was racing, firstly wondering if Matt was too exhausted to be safe at work: Matt obviously needed to stop and rest, which was exactly what he was doing at that point. They both stayed silent for some time. Matt eventually spoke about how welcome those peaceful minutes were. He spoke more about what he had done to support patients and staff and Mike's family. Prompted by Graham, he explored how he could get more support for himself at work, and he also considered his main supporters out of work. As he spoke he realized how exhausted he was. Without needing any prompting, he soon decided it would be safer if he went home early and got some sleep. He rang his manager and explained how exhausted he was and she was more than willing to arrange cover. He was concerned that the junior staff would feel abandoned so said he should go to the ward and explain that he would be back tomorrow, but the manager offered to do that for him, and she arranged to see him the next day. By this time it was near the end of the session and Graham offered an extra clinical supervision session in a week's time, which was agreed. Matt recovered well and there were many professional aspects of this situation which were picked up and explored during subsequent sessions (which reverted to monthly after the extra session) as well as Matt needing to revisit the trauma of the situation. Graham was struck by how emotionally skilled Matt was, how much he learned from the experience about team leadership and self-care and how thoughtful and empathic he seemed with his clients and staff.

In Chapter 2 we suggested that although clinical supervision provides an important space for feelings to surface, uncomfortable or painful emotions cannot always be magically removed or made better, however much we may unconsciously want to rescue and repair. For example, feelings of grief and loss need to be replayed and relived over and over before the intensity can lessen. Developing your emotional skills enables you to use clinical supervision and any other appropriate setting for giving air time to both celebratory and uncomfortable feelings and releasing the positive energy that they generate, in order to be effective back in the workplace.

Developmental stages in using clinical supervision skills

As with any other set of skills, as supervisee you will learn from the experience of using the time offered in clinical supervision. As your skills, confidence in yourself and trust in your clinical supervisor develop, you will be able increasingly to deepen your reflective process during clinical supervision sessions. The 'So what?' phase of the experiential learning cycle will become deeper and your ability to put into practice what you have learned from reflection will be increasingly effective. You will find yourself being more and more able to use the support and guidance of the clinical supervisor or clinical supervision group and to give yourself this type of support and guidance while you are working in practice.

Stages in developing in-depth reflection skills

You will notice your development in the way you reflect about your care of specific clients. Figure 4.15 suggests some phases through which you may progress.

This framework is adapted from an idea by Hawkins and Shohet (1989) and is based on our observations of clinical supervision practice sessions during courses and some real-life clinical supervision sessions, but is suggested tentatively. Although we have tended to see these stages according to the length of time the supervisee has been receiving clinical supervision, some individuals may start at a different point. For some, the focus of Level 4 may be the easier starting point, yet they may not have highly developed problem-solving skills. A danger that we see in using such a developmental framework is that some nurses

Level 1	Level 2	Level 3	Level 4
Focus: Problem-centred	(Includes Level 1)	(Includes Level 1)	(Includes Level 1)
Key question: 'Am I doing the right thing?' 'What do I do next?'	*Focus:* Client/patient centred	(Includes Level 2)	(Includes Level 2)
Level 1	*Key question:* 'How is the client/patient developing?'	*Focus:* Relationship with client/patient	(Includes Level 3)
	Level 2	*Key question:* 'How am I and the client/patient relating and what's my part in that?'	*Focus:* Developing the 'internal supervisor'
		Level 3	*Key question:* 'What's happening now in this situation that parallels what happens in my practice while I'm working with the client?'
			Level 4

Figure 4.15 Developmental stages in using clinical supervision as supervisee

can apply a hierarchy of value to the stages: diminishing the importance of, say, problem-solving, when they have achieved the dizzy heights of Level 4: a competitive 'I'm-more-self-aware-therefore-a-better-person-than-my-practically-oriented-colleagues' approach. We maintain that all stages in the framework are important and no early stage should be abandoned in favour of the later stages.

The internal supervisor

The term 'internal supervisor' was coined by Patrick Casement with reference to the needs of trainees in counselling and psychotherapy, but it is also relevant and applicable to the process of clinical supervision in nursing. This is a fairly advanced part of the reflective process and needs to be developed slowly over a period of time, moving from an initial focus on specific incidents or problems to a continuous internalized reflection and supervision by you as supervisee about your own skills, perceptions, understanding of and relationship with your client. This mirrors the concept of 'learning through practice' as described by Fish *et al.* (1989). Casement describes the developmental process well; we change the words slightly to adapt it to clinical supervision in nursing:

> At the outset, [supervisees] may rely a good deal upon the advice and comments offered by the supervisor. . . . During the course of being supervised, [supervisees] need to acquire their own capacity for spontaneous reflection within the session . . . they can learn to watch themselves as well as the [client], now using this island of intellectual contemplation and mental space within which their internal supervisor [the skills acquired and absorbed in supervision] can begin to operate.
>
> (Casement 1985: 32)

The time you spend reflecting on practice during your clinical supervision sessions enables you to build and deepen your skills of reflecting *in* practice. Implicit in these skills is your capacity as supervisee to be in two places at once: in the shoes of your client, and at the same time having your feet firmly embedded in your own footwear. This is what makes such skills different from more cognitive self-analysis because the ability to empathize, feel and respond using your intuitive skills is vital to this interactive process which includes rather than excludes the client. It can prevent what Davies (1995) continues to see as a problem in Schön's (1983) framework of reflective practice, namely the continued professional emotional distance from the client. Although 'internal supervision' is about the ability to stand apart, from both yourself and from your client, you are still engaged in the process of interacting with the client while monitoring the relationship between you. Swain (1995) reminds us that it is not the same as standing aloof or disengaging, as this would severely damage our clinical and human responsiveness. But you can use this heightened awareness of your own inner responses to develop and improve your attentiveness and effectiveness at the same time as being attentive to the client.

This awareness can be manifest in your clinical supervision sessions when you reflect on the here and now dynamics of what is happening in the session and considering the extent to which this parallels what has been happening back in the workplace.

Summary

We hope this chapter has been a helpful resource from which to select some frameworks to aid your reflection during clinical supervision sessions. Your taking the initiative in selecting from these frameworks will give you intellectual freedom and the the power you require to make full use of the clinical supervision relationship, to lead the sessions and ensure your time is spent on your own in-depth reflection on your practice and the part you play as an individual in the complexity and quality of your practice. We hope also that it has been useful to highlight the longer-term, ongoing development of your skills of reflection-in-practice as a result of your experiences as a supervisee. The next two chapters are addressed to clinical supervisors and members of clinical supervision groups, but even if you do not fall into either category, they may yet cover some useful ground to illustrate what you might expect from your clinical supervisor.

5 Support and catalytic skills of the clinical supervisor

The clinical supervisor is expected to emphasize the 'power to' aspects of the power relationship, seeking to empower the supervisee and use enabling skills in which are embraced all the main principles of clinical supervision. The supportive and formative elements are the main means by which the normative function is carried out. This chapter will focus on these supportive and formative elements but these need to be balanced with normative elements as well, seen within the context of the working alliance between supervisee and clinical supervisor and within the organizational setting. Chapter 6 addresses the more authoritative aspects of the clinical supervisor's role more specifically, but in looking in this chapter in more depth at the support and catalytic skills of the supervisor, we need to bear in mind that the aim of clinical supervision is the development and maintenance of quality practice.

We are aware that the chapters of a book such as this are rarely read sequentially. However, in tune with our view that the clinical supervisor needs to have her own clinical supervision, we recommend that you read Chapter 4 fully before you proceed with this or the next chapter. It will clarify where we are coming from and what it is that we are expecting the clinical supervisor to facilitate.

Building on those concepts in Chapter 3, we suggest that the clinical supervisor's role is to encourage exploratory dialogue and a reflective mind-space in which the supervisee can engage and build some or all of the following: their own professional and personal knowledge; their logical and analytical thinking abilities; their emotional awareness, expression and energy; realistic self-esteem; intuition and inspiration; advocacy for themselves, their clients and colleagues; their beliefs about what is important; and their personal and professional ethics, and through this exploration capture insights and inspiration and make their own decisions. The results of this sort of facilitation enables the supervisee to own their own plans and to have the energy and commitment to act on them.

In this and the next chapter, we refer to the clinical supervisor mainly in the context of one-to-one clinical supervision. However, we wish to emphasize that these skills are also necessary for all members of a clinical supervision group. Chapter 7 places this in context.

A framework for exploring the enabling skills of the clinical supervisor

Through using support, catalytic, challenging and informative skills, the clinical supervisor can provide the opportunity for mutual enquiry into the many complex aspects of practice for which there are no straightforward answers.

This chapter and Chapter 6 focus on the specific helping skills of the clinical supervisor which, when applied well, enable the supervisee to settle, lead the exploratory dialogue and reach a reflective mind-space. Together you will be able to explore and process whatever comes out of that reflective mind-space and move towards assimilating the emergent insights and planning to apply them in future reflection or action.

Much of what we have written about these skills will look familiar to you since they are already an intrinsic part of your work in any helping relationship, whether with clients, colleagues, students, your own friends or family. We find that workshop participants gain from identifying these helping skills and applying them in this very specific way to clinical supervision: we seek to give you the chance to identify your own strengths and weaknesses and to focus on and develop both Fig. 5.1.

We looked at the concepts and skills of reflection in Chapter 4 and in these chapters we focus on the facilitation skills of the clinical supervisor and clinical supervision group member. Before we identify the nature of these skills, it might be useful to clarify the meaning of 'facilitation'. This has come to mean, in many areas of professional communication, to supportively enable another person or group of people to decide, do or learn something for themselves. Tosey and Gregory's (2002)

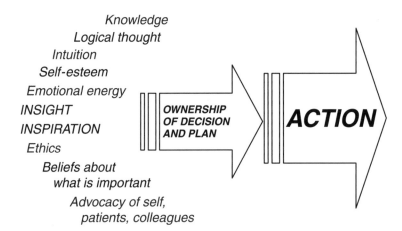

Figure 5.1 Exploratory dialogue enables the supervisee to have ownership of their own action plan and the commitment to put it into practice

definition is: 'Facilitation literally means "easing". A facilitator helps to create the conditions within which other human beings can, so far as possible, select and direct their own learning and development'. Underpinning this is the belief that enabling the other to engage their own knowledge, intellect, intuition, ethics and so on, increases their sense of ownership of the outcome, and provides a motivating learning experience which can contribute positively to increased personal and professional effectiveness in the future (see Figure 5.1).

Jacques (2000: 124) describes facilitation in this way: 'It involves careful listening and eliciting rather than giving one's own knowledge ... there is a sense of shared or developed responsibility for learning'. In our framework, we identify four main types of facilitation skills: supportive, catalytic, challenging and informative (see Figure 5.2). These have similarities to those identified in Heron's (2001) six-category intervention analysis (supportive and cathartic, catalytic, confronting, prescriptive and informative) and the intervention styles described by Cockman et al. (1998) (acceptant, catalytic, confrontational and prescriptive). Each of these four types of skills depends on your intention: that is, what you intend as far as your communication with the supervisee is concerned. This framework does not indicate that any one of these is 'better' than another. Any helping relationship will need to include a mixture of these four skills of communication, and the relative balance between the four types of communication is defined by the type of relationship, its purpose and any agreed contract between the people involved.

As a clinical supervisor, your aim is to achieve an appropriate balance by using mainly the non-directive (supportive and catalytic) interventions: these are the heart of your communication in clinical supervision. The more directive (informative and challenging) interventions very occasionally arise from and quickly return to your non-directive communication base. This might be in contrast to, say, a preceptor who is working with a newly qualified nurse taking up her first post in a unit new to her, when the preceptor may need to define more of the agenda and pass on a body of information because she has more knowledge of what needs to be covered. As another contrasting example, a team manager who is meeting

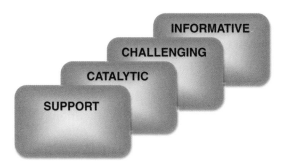

Figure 5.2 Four main types of facilitation skills of the clinical supervisor

with a team member to apply a management-by-objectives approach would use more directive skills in outlining organizational and team objectives and challenging any lack of achieving them, in addition to drawing out the team member's own objectives within that framework. The clinical supervisor's approach should be focused on the supervisee's agenda and on mostly non-directive facilitation of the exploration of those topics.

Many of the pitfalls in facilitating the supervisee arise from:

- a genuine desire to show that you are listening and that you are wanting to help, but the type of support turns out to be inappropriate advice;
- lack of knowledge of ways of showing explicit support;
- lack of skill;
- lack of awareness of your own uncontained feelings of anxiety, helplessness, embarrassment or frustration;
- lack of skill in containing or expressing your own feelings when you become aware of them.

This chapter highlights some aspects of support and catalytic facilitation that especially apply to the clinical supervision situation. These non-directive skills of the clinical supervisor are the bedrock of the relationship. There are some similarities between this aspect of clinical supervision and counselling, but also some crucial differences.

Distinguishing between clinical supervision and counselling

Many of the skills outlined in this section will be familiar to you, possibly reminiscent of counselling skills training sessions. It is important, however, to be clear about the difference between clinical supervision and counselling. Table 5.1 highlights some of these differences.

Following through your intention to take a non-directive or directive approach requires conscious and intuitive use of specific skills. Many clinical supervisors assess themselves as being strongest at supporting and giving information, and less strong at challenging. So, perhaps starting with one of your strengths, we'll start looking at the supportive skills of clinical supervision.

The rest of this chapter aims to help you to:

- give names to the skills of support and catalytic facilitation that you already use;
- relate them to your role as clinical supervisor;
- clarify your supportive and catalytic intentions and your options for putting those intentions into practice;
- pinpoint some of the pitfalls that you might encounter when intending to be supportive and catalytic, and clarify some ways of avoiding these pitfalls.

Table 5.1   Distinguishing between counselling and clinical supervision

	Counselling	Clinical supervision
Agenda	Agenda defined by the supervisee and is based on a personal problem	Agenda defined by the supervisee, and does not necessarily have to have a problem. Topics are work related. Clinical supervisor may add items arising during previous sessions or refocus on how any personal issues discussed affect practice
Confidentiality	Total, with legal exceptions. Counsellor may keep own records that are absolutely confidential	Almost total, with exceptions of legal or professional ethics. Record may be made to pass on within the organization of attendance dates and times. Record of content may be negotiated between practitioner and clinical supervisor, for their eyes only
Information from facilitator	Information, advice or guidance very rarely given, and then usually focused on emotional issues	Some information, advice, guidance offered to supplement the supervisee's own professional expertise, to help the supervisee see options available and make own informed decision
Challenge from facilitator	Non-judgemental about the person's emotional issues. Challenges about defences against emotional expression and growth	Occasionally challenging any technical mistakes, inadequate clinical standards, contribution to problems with teamwork, unhelpful or self-defeating behaviour or attitude, blind spots, broken contracts. Based on evidence gained during the clinical supervision session only
Support from facilitator	Support for the client as a person, especially for emotional awareness and expression. Disclosure of personal issues expected	Support for the supervisee as a person and encouragement given to help supervisee recognize and use own expertise and personal abilities towards developing their professional expertise. Disclosure of personal issues not required, but any which are disclosed are acknowledged and eventually related back to how these affect practice
Catalytic help from facilitator	Enabling reflection and problem-solving of deeper exploration into the personal and relationship aspects of the problem, including the transference relationship between client and counsellor	Enabling reflection on issues ultimately affecting practice (including some consideration of issues involved in the clinical supervision relationship), learning from experience, problem-solving, pinpointing ways of dealing with difficult emotions, decision making and planning. With the ultimate emphasis on reviewing application to practice

Support skills of the clinical supervisor

As Swain (1995: 29) points out, there is a need for staff support, peer support and 'courteous, sensitive, consultative organisational management': clinical supervision should not replace any of these. She goes on to say: 'That said, a support element is intrinsic to the clinical supervision process. This, while not "cosy", should be holding; while not counselling in a formal sense, will be listening to the individual's "feeling state", as she carries out her work, and will use counselling skills; while not occupational health, will take note of the supervisee's "health" state'.

Be explicitly supportive

As a clinical supervisor, your approach to the supervisee needs to be fundamentally supportive at all times. The time available in clinical supervision is short and it is important to find ways of showing support openly and explicitly so that the supervisee can quickly recognize the support that is available. However, one common pitfall in setting out intentionally to be supportive is to lack genuineness. The key to being genuine is to listen carefully to what the supervisee says and to express your support as a reaction to what you hear.

Ways of showing support

In this chapter, we will give illustrations of ways of showing support that might apply to the following example so, to set the scene, it is introduced here and we will return to it later.

> Aileen is telling her clinical supervisor, Chandra, about a traumatic incident in her ward, of which she is the new manager. The son of a very ill patient had been physically violent with another relative, causing a severe injury, and had also been verbally violent and threatening towards staff. The details of the incident are shocking and Aileen recounts everything she did to deal with the situation at the time. She is anxiously asking Chandra to tell her where she went wrong, what else she could have done or should be doing now.

We suggest 10 distinct ways of showing support explicitly through your actions, your manner and what you say (see Table 5.2).

1. *Reliability and punctuality.* It is important to make appointments with your supervisee a priority, only postponing or cancelling them in dire emergencies. The planned, regular protected time gives a regular structure to the support the supervisee experiences from clinical supervision. This psychological 'holding' is almost as important as the process of the session itself and meets some of the human need for security in the workplace which we discussed in Chapter 2. A practitioner who knows she can rely

Table 5.2 Ways of showing support in clinical supervision

- RELIABILITY AND PUNCTUALITY – Making appointments with supervisee a priority; being punctual and sticking to time boundaries
- SETTLING – Enabling the supervisee to settle, relax and put their journey to the session behind them (you need to be composed, settled and relaxed yourself first!)
- SHOWING YOU ARE LISTENING WITH ACCEPTANCE – Paying attention to the supervisee as a human being and seeking to understand the supervisee's perception of the situation they are describing; showing you are listening by your non-verbal responses and by summarizing their viewpoint, respecting it as their perspective
- ENCOURAGEMENT – Showing interest, pointing out strengths or achievements that the supervisee has shown, encourage the supervisee to talk positively about herself
- TUNING IN – Tuning in to the emotions being expressed or which are implicit and tuning in to their level of intensity; putting into words and acknowledging the level of emotion that underlies what supervisee is saying; tentatively to allow supervisee to find their own words for their feelings; accepting of the emotion, non-critical
- ADVOCACY – Indicating when the supervisee deserves better, perhaps more consideration, information, respect for personal or professional rights, support, etc.
- SUPPORTIVE SILENCE – Space to reflect
- EMOTIONAL FIRST AID – Supporting emotional release without making a fuss; showing your acceptance; enabling emotional recovery
- SELF-DISCLOSURE – Sharing a little of your own experience or feelings; expressing any caring and concerned feelings you have about the supervisee
- APOLOGIZING – For any of your mistakes, without defensiveness

---

on the regular sessions is more able to contain the stresses and distresses of her work. Punctuality in starting and finishing the session is part of this structure of support. By repeatedly sticking to the agreed time boundaries you are building the supervisee's responsibility and ability to use the time effectively. If you find there are other pressures in your own work that might lead you to postpone, cancel or be late for sessions, then you need to consider whether being a clinical supervisor is appropriate to your role in the organization. Many managers attending our workshops find that they are so often called to emergency management meetings or to deal with management crises that the clinical supervision they can offer is only a haphazard, low priority affair.

2. *Settling.* Your first supportive task in a clinical supervision session is to enable the supervisee to settle into the session, to make the often difficult transition from the busy-ness of action-oriented work to sitting and reflecting. Your relaxed, thoughtful manner at the beginning of a session can be very supportive in enabling this transition. In practical terms, this means you need to settle yourself, taking a few minutes of undisturbed time before the session to put aside your other preoccupations, and to focus your thoughts on the individual with whom you are about to work. When the supervisee arrives, you need to be explicitly welcoming and to use the

usual settling conversation about, say, the journey, and perhaps offer a cold or hot drink, to enable the supervisee to 'arrive' and make the transition into the space for the session. If the supervisee does not do this spontaneously, you should mark the start of the session, perhaps by asking what the supervisee hopes to get from the session or what they would like to talk about.

3. *Showing you are listening with acceptance.* A clinical supervisor needs to be able to listen with acceptance, paying attention to the supervisee as a human being, giving space for them to find their own words. Showing that you are listening by your non-verbal responses is important, not only giving good eye contact, but reacting with your facial and body expression and with non-verbal sounds such as 'hm' to the supervisee's emphatic points. You listen not only to the words but also to the tone, the 'real' meanings and emotions, the supervisee's own perception of the situation they are describing. Your listening needs to be active, proving that you are listening by your occasional attempts to summarize what the supervisee is saying. This summary can be experienced as supportive if it shows an attempt on your part really to try to understand the supervisee's perspective, without adding your interpretation or challenging them to look at it another way. Of course, there is a place for challenging, but here we are focusing on times when your intention is to get across your support for the person.

4. *Encouragement.* You can encourage the supervisee by listening particularly for anything which tells you about this person's strengths (e.g. abilities or qualities) in surviving and dealing with the situation, or something that they have achieved or obviously could achieve with the right help. Your summary of this observation can feel especially supportive.

> Chandra listens attentively and when Aileen stops and seems to be looking to her supervisor for a response, Chandra finds herself mute, unable to think of anything to say in the face of such a traumatic event. However, she pulls herself out of it and suggests that before they think about what else could be done, they recap together the strengths and achievements that Aileen displayed in dealing with the situation so far, and Chandra reflects back some examples: her quick thinking in acting appropriately to secure the safety of the patient, the injured relative and her colleagues; her resilience in leading her staff through what became a long, drawn-out problem.

5. *Tuning in.* Tuning in to the emotions which are being expressed or are implicit in what the supervisee is saying can be supportive. To do this, listen particularly to the supervisee's tone, to emotive words or metaphors, so as to imagine yourself in the supervisee's shoes, and to notice the emotional feelings which are stirred up in yourself when you listen. Notice not only which emotions are being expressed or are implicit in what the supervisee

is saying, but also the level of intensity of those emotions. You can show that you are tuning in by your non-verbal responses. Occasionally you might say a few words summarizing as best you can the emotions and their level of intensity. Put into words and acknowledge the emotion that underlies what the supervisee is saying and its level of intensity, as shown by the cues the supervisee is giving off (e.g. 'So, it seems you are feeling a bit worried about dealing with X?'). It is essential to be tentative and allow the supervisee to correct you, to find their own words for their feelings. Your tone needs to be accepting of the emotion, and non-critical. This kind of explicit support can be very helpful in enabling the supervisee to develop the central emotional skills of self-awareness and acceptance of their own emotions.

> For instance, Chandra suggests: 'Naturally enough, you seem to be feeling quite shocked and very anxious about this incident. Is that right?'

6. *Advocacy.* You can show support by making *advocacy statements.* By advocacy statements we mean listening to what the supervisee has to say about an experience, and formulating some explicitly supportive responses about the supervisee's rights. While you are listening, you could ask yourself, 'Which of the supervisee's individual rights were not respected? What intrusion, humiliation, oppression, deprivation was experienced? What do they deserve as a human being in terms of respect, care, concern, acceptance, protection, information, opportunity, etc.?' Then you could indicate that the supervisee deserves better, perhaps more consideration, information, respect for personal or professional rights, support, etc.

> For instance, Aileen berates herself for somehow not preventing this incident and she feels a failure for having to involve the police. Chandra reminds her that the violent visitor was responsible for his own behaviour and was committing a serious offence and that she, staff and patients had the right to have police protection.

7. *Supportive silence.* Become used to spotting when the supervisee is thinking something over, and stay silent when she is moving into the reflective mindspace, without interruption or prompting.
8. *Emotional first-aid.* Allowing emotional release without making a big fuss about it can be supportive. We find that it is not uncommon for nurses (especially senior nurses and managers) to burst into tears with the relief of having protected time and support for themselves, after competently and effectively giving out intensive support and leadership to others. Being able to accept this as normal without bleeping the duty psychiatrist is important. The supervisee who can express feelings, release tensions (without taking them out by attacking you), and eventually refocus on reflection and problem-solving is emotionally competent: they are using an appropriate time and place let off steam. However, this may not be the prevailing

attitude in the organization. The supervisee may berate themselves for expressing feelings or feel embarrassed afterwards.

> For instance, when Aileen bursts into tears and then struggles to stop them straight away, saying she shouldn't be crying, Chandra says: 'You've been through a lot. Anyone in your position would need a place to let the tears out and it's OK to do that here'.

The supervisee may need some help to recover from releasing feelings. You can gently help them to refocus on the issue or problem at hand, or, if they are too distracted to think straight, to take a mini-break, perhaps making tea or talking about neutral things for a while.

> For instance, after Aileen has had a good sob and is blowing her nose, she comments on her smeared make up, Chandra asks if she'd like a another tissue. Aileen ends up laughing about her make-up and they chat about brands of mascara that are waterproof enough to survive a weep. After a while, Aileen gets back to the topic in question herself and is able to think a little more clearly.

9. *Self-disclosure.* Some self-disclosure on your part can be supportive, when you share a little of your own feelings. For instance, you might explicitly let the supervisee know when you care about them as a person and care about what happens to them. You might share that you also find a certain type of situation difficult, or that you went through a similar difficulty yourself in the past (this needs to be said with humility, otherwise it may sound patronizing).

> For instance, Chandra discloses: 'I felt quite shocked when you told me what you'd been through. I've always found physical violence scary and I respect the way you handled it.'

10. *Apologizing for any mistakes.* As the 'pitfalls' sections of this and the next chapter highlight, there is a lot of scope for making mistakes as a clinical supervisor and it can be supportive to admit to it when you have done so and to apologize, without being defensive.

Pitfalls in giving support in clinical supervision

1. *Premature focus on facts or solutions.* One of the most common pitfalls (see Table 5.3) is to focus prematurely on facts, interrupting the supervisee's flow with factual questions and not letting them explain the situation in their own words and sequence. You rush in with factual questions too quickly.

Table 5.3 Pitfalls in giving support in clinical supervision

- PREMATURE FOCUS ON FACTS OR SOLUTIONS – Interrupting the supervisee's flow with factual questions, not letting them explain the situation in their own words and sequence; focusing on solutions too quickly, interrupting reflection
- LACK OF SUPPORTIVE RESPONSE – No non-verbal response to what the supervisee is saying; lack of explicit verbal support
- PATRONIZING – Talking down to the person as though they are going through a difficult phase that you conquered long ago; speaking in over-simplified manner
- MISPLACED SUPPORT – Colluding, giving encouragement about something you know is not in the supervisee's or their client's best interests
- MOUNTAINS OUT OF MOLEHILLS – Being too earnest, over-dramatizing a natural bit of emotional release
- TONE JUDGEMENTAL OR FALSE – Tone comes across as critical, non-accepting or false, using support techniques without genuineness, such as in a back-handed compliment
- TOO DEEP, TOO SOON – You actively delve into supervisee's personal feelings too much (rather than following the supervisee's own pace), thereby increasing vulnerability
- OVERDONE – Being over the top with compliments which are too general to be useful, or sickly
- ABSORBING STRESS – Taking too much responsibility on yourself for making the supervisee feel better if they are upset; rescuing, trying to take away their emotional discomfort at all costs (but really making yourself feel better), thereby diminishing the person
- SUPPRESSIVE SYMPATHIZING – You overdo the sympathy by swamping them with 'there, theres' or pats on the back

For instance, Aileen is articulate and can describe the situation very well, though her emotional turmoil may have led her to relate the incident a bit out of sequence. Chandra would have interrupted and possibly missed the main point if she had fired factual questions such as, 'Was he the client's son or brother?', 'What did you say to him then?', 'Did the visitor lose consciousness after he was knocked down?', 'What did you do next?', 'How long did the police take to arrive?', 'What did the police say were his previous convictions?', 'Who did he attack that time?', 'How long was he in prison before?', and so on.

You can avoid this pitfall by mentally tagging any information-seeking questions you want to ask and postponing using them till later. Often you will find that the supervisee covers most of the information you seek if they are given space to explain the situation in their own way. You can also avoid this pitfall by reminding yourself that you need to hear the supervisee describe the situation in their own way in order to understand their perception of the situation and their priorities: the way the supervisee describes the experience can tell you as much about her as the facts she is recounting. If you have factual queries, make a mental note to come back to them when the supervisee has finished their explanation.

Similarly, you may prematurely focus on solutions. This is when you jump in with questions which focus on action or when you give advice before the supervisee has had the chance to finish explaining the situation and to reflect upon it in some depth. You can avoid this pitfall by channelling your urge to support into making explicit supportive statements, as outlined earlier in this chapter. You could also remind yourself that the purpose of clinical supervision includes in-depth reflection, which requires some patience on your part.

2. *Lack of supportive responses.* However, there are pitfalls in staying silent too. A deadpan expression, with no non-verbal response to what the supervisee is saying, is inappropriate for a clinical supervisor. The supervisee is likely to feel unnecessarily disconcerted and unsupported. There are schools of psychoanalysis which advocate striving to eliminate personal reactions to the client, to allow for deeper transference to be established, but it is not the role of the clinical supervisor to deliberately attract more transference. We have found that some mental health nurses who work with such psychoanalyst colleagues, or who work with highly provocative patients, can sometimes use the blank approach inappropriately in clinical supervision.

Another common pitfall is to assume that by your staying silent, looking at the person and nodding, the supervisee will know that you are listening and supporting. In counselling, the counsellor has more time to show support silently, by their presence and supportive attention during sessions held once, twice or more times a week. The clinical supervisor has less time and needs to be more explicit. The situation that the supervisee talks about may be so traumatic that the clinical supervisor may be mute in response. Saying nothing explicitly supportive may come from inappropriate inhibition: you may not be able to prevent your shock or embarrassment from getting in the way. To avoid this pitfall, try to be aware of your emotions, accept that's how you feel, but go ahead and say something explicitly supportive anyway.

> In Chandra's case, Aileen was looking for something from her and it would have been unnerving to have had a blank response.

3. *Patronizing.* You might overdo your attempts at explicit support by coming across as patronizing. This is easy to do if you are disclosing that you have also had a similar experience, and hint that it was a less mature phase and now you are through it. This can make you sound superior. You can sound patronizing if you state the obvious (commonly done when advice-giving) or speak in an over-simplified manner or sing-song voice. You might go over the top with compliments which are too general to be useful, such as complimenting the supervisee's personality, rather than their actions. Your tone might sound too sickly. So, keep your support statements low-key and make any reference to your past experience with a tone of humility.

4. *Misplaced support.* Your support might be inappropriate. For instance, by continuing to support the supervisee who is going round in circles, you

may be colluding in a blaming state of mind or in avoiding tackling the real problem. You might give encouragement about something you know is not in the supervisee's or their client's best interests, such as a self-destructive course of action. You can avoid this by clarifying what exactly you are supporting and what you are not supporting.

5. *Mountains out of molehills*. A common pitfall is to over-react by being too earnest and reacting over-dramatically to something that the supervisee can, given time, handle quite well. A supervisee bursting into tears can sometimes trigger this over-reaction from a clinical supervisor, whereas to the supervisee it may be a natural, short-lived bit of emotional release. You can avoid this by looking at your own anxieties when listening to supervisees, accepting that is how you feel and considering ways of containing the anxiety when with your supervisee. This highlights the importance of having your own supervision sessions to deal with such issues.

6. *Tone judgemental or false*. The clinical supervisor's unaware and uncontained anxiety can lead to an inappropriate tone or manner, perhaps coming across as the opposite of what is intended. Your being tense can result in your sounding judgemental, perhaps your tone coming across as critical, or non-accepting. Deliberately relaxing your body, especially your throat, can help your tone to come out as you intend. Trying too hard might lead you to sound false, as if you are using support as a technique. A common example is to use a back-handed compliment to soften the blow of criticism; the positive comment has a sting in the tail, ending with a 'but ...'.

7. *Too deep, too soon*. Clinical supervisors who have skills in counselling, mental health nursing or co-counselling may be tempted to use techniques which push someone towards releasing feelings. This may be because you are used to working with people intensively in this area and are using the skills automatically, without considering the different boundaries which should operate in clinical supervision. Sometimes the perspective that 'it will do them good to let it out' makes the clinical supervisor too pushy in this respect. Remembering the following rule of thumb might help here: in clinical supervision, cathartic release of emotions through short periods of crying, storming, shaking and so on are appropriate if the supervisee spontaneously does this or gives definite cues that they wish to do so. Your role is to offer 'emotional first-aid' and allow and support their release of emotion in order eventually to help the supervisee refocus on reflecting on the issues involved. Manipulating or pushing the supervisee into cathartic release is not appropriate: it will only increase their need to protect themselves by resorting to defensive action – and they would be quite right to do so.

8. *Absorbing stress*. Support may be overdone by the clinical supervisor absorbing the supervisee's stress. You take too much responsibility on yourself for making the supervisee feel better if they are upset. In your role as clinical supervisor, it would be inappropriate to agree to take action yourself,

outside the clinical supervision sessions, rather than enabling the supervisee to do it for themselves (although of course the exception is unsafe practice that the supervisee is unable or unwilling to address herself). You might try to rescue the supervisee from the inevitable emotional discomfort of reflecting on difficult issues: rescuing comes from the clinical supervisor being unaware of or unable to contain their own feelings of anxiety and helplessness when hearing about the supervisee's difficulties. Rescuing is really about trying to make yourself feel better, and diminishes the supervisee. Again, finding ways of becoming more aware and accepting of your own anxieties can pave the way to your being more able to contain them when you are a clinical supervisor.

> For example, Chandra would have been interfering and undermining Aileen if she had offered to facilitate a staff debriefing session on her ward. However, Chandra was aware that Aileen's topic was hitting a raw nerve in herself and she knew she could take this to her own clinical supervision. This helped her to contain her anxieties and avoid acting from them inappropriately.

9. *Suppressive sympathizing.* Another pitfall may be over-sympathizing, encouraging the supervisee to be repetitively preoccupied with misery, perhaps swamping them with 'Yes, isn't it awful' comments. This seems especially common in dealing with the despair many nurses feel about the NHS: if this is your feeling too, try not to disappear down the plughole along with your supervisee. Avoid this pitfall by giving some space for expressing feelings, then encouraging the supervisee to move on to reflecting more logically on the issues involved, and practical ways of dealing with the feelings. Use your own supervision to explore emotions that have been triggered by your supervisee.

If you find yourself sliding into one of these pitfalls, all is not lost: you can usually retrieve the situation by recalling that you have many options open to you to show explicit support and choosing the one that feels right.

In summary, the most important principles in supporting supervisee are:

- giving space, listening and showing that you are listening;
- being explicit about your support;
- following cues, acknowledging emotions non-judgementally;
- using your own supervision for support in dealing with emotions which are stirred up by the supervisee.

The 'being supportive' category needs to be involved in *all* your communication with the supervisee, whether explicitly in your words, or implicitly in your tone and manner.

Catalytic skills of the clinical supervisor

When you use catalytic interventions, you are showing that you are listening and trying to understand, and enabling the supervisee to tell her story, think aloud, reflect on learning from an experience, surface her own insights, assimilate them and make her own decision for herself. In chemistry, a catalyst is a substance which speeds up a chemical reaction without itself becoming part of it. In clinical supervision, using catalytic interventions means you enable the supervisee to reflect in depth on an experience and to move towards clearer learning and decision-making outcomes, without contributing your own solutions.

All the support skills we outlined earlier in this chapter are likely also to have a catalytic function. A supervisee will be able to think more clearly and in more depth from a position of feeling supported. Sometimes the supervisee who is skilled at using supervision may require little more than support to flourish in her use of the clinical supervision time. However, any supervisee will benefit from the careful use of some specifically catalytic skills, and one way of emphasizing caution in using these skills is to consider them being used in phases (see Figure 5.3).

1 Open-ended
   encouragement

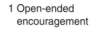2 Focusing on the most
   important elements of
   the issue

3 Exploratory dialogue

4 Working with
   emerging insights

Figure 5.3 Phases in using catalytic skills

Phases of using catalytic interventions

When using catalytic skills, you need to have some idea about why you are using them. Although it could be said that catalytic methods are comparatively non-directive, in that they do not offer information or advice or challenge, they can often channel the supervisee's thinking in a certain direction. If you use them without due consideration of the reason why you are using them, your supervisee may be led up many blind alleys or into scattered thinking. They may end up being more confused than when they started. Or you may indirectly lead the supervisee along a path of your choosing, rather than theirs.

Consider four main reasons for using catalytic skills. These would be to enable the supervisee to do the following.

Table 5.4   Catalytic skills phase 1: open-ended encouragement to speak

---

- Support skills
- Prompts to continue: non-verbal encouragement, e.g. nods, 'uh huh', 'hm'; verbal prompts, e.g. 'yes', 'really?', 'go on', 'and so . . . ?', 'and then . . . ?'
- Echoing the last word or phrase
- Very open questions, e.g. 'What would you like to talk about today?', 'What else would you like to say about that?', 'What do you think/feel about that?'

---

1. Think aloud and speak their narrative in their own words, sequence and pace, given open-ended encouragement.
2. Pick out the most important elements of the issue to explore.
3. Engage in exploratory reflective dialogue with the clinical supervisor and experience a reflective mind-space.
4. Recognize emerging insights, assimilate them and move towards planning how to apply the insights to professional practice.

This framework is an adaptation of Egan's (2009) classic three-stage helping framework.

Again, the example of Aileen and Chandra will be used to illustrate the skills and pitfalls. In a real clinical supervision session, not all the skills and pitfalls would apply to one session, but here they are referred to as illustrations to bring the text alive.

Phase 1: open-ended encouragement to speak (see Table 5.4)

All the support skills which were outlined earlier give open-ended encouragement to think aloud. Other methods include prompts to continue, last-word echoing and very open questions.

Prompts to continue include the many non-verbal encouragements that we give each other in any interaction, such as nods, 'uh huh' and 'hm'. Verbal prompts include brief encouragements such as 'Yes', 'Really?', 'Go on', 'And so . . . ?', 'And then . . . ?' You can give a prompt to continue by echoing the last word or phrase, to encourage the supervisee to go on or elaborate. Very open questions have little or no specific focus and encourage the supervisee to give more than just a brief reply. Some examples include: 'What would you like to talk about today?', 'What else would you like to say about that?', 'What do you think/feel about that?'.

Phase 2: focusing on the most important elements of the narrative
(see Table 5.5)

You could use selective echoing, selective summary, closed questions and inviting self-summary to help the supervisee to focus on the most important aspects of the experience being discussed.

Selective echoing is when you echo a specific word or phrase that seems especially significant, in order to encourage the supervisee to explore a bit further.

Table 5.5 Catalytic skills phase 2: focusing on the most important elements of the narrative

- Selective echoing: echo a significant word or phrase
- Selective summary: pick out the aspects that seem important. Express this tentatively
- Closed questions: questions that could be answered by a brief factual reply or 'yes' or 'no' to help supervisee focus on one aspect
- Invite self-summary: ask supervisee to pick out the main points for themselves

> *Aileen:* It was like I was watching myself dealing with it, I couldn't believe my hands were so steady ... (pause).
> *Chandra:* Couldn't believe it?

Any summary you make of what the supervisee is saying will have an element of selection about it: you will automatically pick out the aspects that have had an impact on you, that *seem* important. It is important to be aware of this and to be tentative in offering the summary: you may have missed the most important point as far as the supervisee is concerned. You can express this tentativeness by adding a checking-out question or by making your statement sound like a question: 'So far, you seem to be saying ... Have I missed out anything important?' or 'Do you mean that you ... ?' or 'It seems to me that the most important aspect of this situation to you is ... is that so?'

Closed questions are questions that could be answered by a brief factual reply or 'yes' or 'no', and are useful to help the supervisee focus on one aspect.

> *Chandra:* Is it that in spite of acting professionally, inside you felt in a state of shock?

You could invite a self-summary by asking the supervisee to reflect back over what they have said and pick out the main points for themselves.

> *Chandra:* Looking back over what you've told me so far about this very difficult situation, what would you like to focus on in particular in the time we have left here together?

Table 5.6 Catalytic skills phase 3: exploratory dialogue

- Logical prompts to analyse the experience, using problem-solving or reflective models and 'logical building' to point in which direction the supervisee seems to be going
- Engaging imagination, such as Socratic questioning, encouragement to draw
- Intuitive exploration, emphasizing wondering, mulling over, pondering, musing, sensing, speculating, hunches, e.g. "I wonder ... .'; 'I've been mulling over what you said about... .'
- 'Emotional barometer': aware of possibility absorbing and reflecting supervisee's suppressed feelings
- Acknowledging the unknown
- Identifying parallel processes

Phase 3: exploratory dialogue (see Table 5.6)

1. *Logical exploration.* The supervisee may be intuitively or consciously using elements of some of the reflective frameworks outlined in Chapter 4. While you are listening you may be able to spot the stages the supervisee has covered in her thinking so far and give feedback to clarify this. Then you might help the supervisee to revisit a previous stage in one of the reflective or problem-solving frameworks, to deepen their exploration of the stage they have reached, or move on to the next phase. As far as possible, without interrupting the supervisee's flow, try to be transparent about which framework you are using. This may help the supervisee to understand the reflective framework and be able to use it more in everyday practice.

   > For example, Chandra sees that Aileen might usefully go back to the beginning of the problem-solving cycle and redefine the present problem: 'I'm wondering if it would be useful to focus on what the main difficulty is for you right now?' Aileen seems confused and repeats some of the information she has shared previously. Chandra makes a quick drawing of the problem-solving cycle to remind Aileen of a framework they have discussed in the past.

   Then you could use 'logical building' (Heron 2001): summarize the content of what the supervisee is saying and point to any direction in which it seems to be leading.

   > For instance, Chandra sees the stages that Aileen has gone through in the 'learning from experience' spiral outlined in Chapter 4 and in Figure 4.7. Aileen has described the experience in terms of the events and her observations of her own and other people's actions and reactions, and looked in some depth at her feelings about the issue. She is in some confusion about the meaning of it all and is jumping towards evaluating her own and her deputy's performance in an overly negative way. Chandra shares these observations with Aileen before using 'logical building': 'And this seems to be leading towards an exploration of a leader's role in that situation and some lack of confidence about your leadership skills in an emergency. Is that right?'

2. *Engaging imagination.* This can help the supervisee to use the right brain and get into a reflective mind-space. One way of helping the supervisee to engage imagination is by using 'Socratic questioning': you encourage the supervisee to imagine that the situation had happened to someone else and they were listening to this other person recounting it.

   > *Chandra:* You've already said you can step back and observe yourself while you were dealing with all this: let's take that a bit further. Imagine that the time is now two weeks ago, before this happened.

> A colleague, let's call her Abigail, comes to you and tells you exactly what you've told me, the same details about how she had to deal with a patient's relative who had been physically violent with another relative and verbally violent and threatening towards staff. What would you think about Abigail and her situation?

Another imaginative approach is to encourage the supervisee to draw a diagram or freehand picture.

- Offer the supervisee some paper and pens and suggest they draw a diagram or picture.
- Look at the picture with interest, saying something like: 'Do you want to tell me about your picture?', 'I'm just wondering what this is', or 'I wonder what this shape/colour symbolizes.'
- Give plenty of space for the supervisee to speak about the picture and their perception of its significance.
- Do not give interpretations (that would be the province of art therapy).

3. *Intuitive exploration.* This is also about explicitly enabling a state of reflective mind-space. You yourself go into a reflective mind-space and use words such as wondering, mulling over, pondering, musing, sensing, speculating or hunches. For example, 'I wonder … ', 'I've been mulling over what you said about … ', 'I have a hunch that … '. Avoid pushing for a response, just leave your comment in the air.

4. *Emotional barometer.* This is an everyday phrase for what counsellors and therapists call using counter-transference (described in Chapter 2). At times, you may find that you have a strong emotional reaction to what the supervisee is saying or to her manner. It is possible that as the clinical supervisor you pick up the supervisee's unacknowledged strength of feeling. Helping the supervisee to acknowledge and accept her emotions can be an important step in deepening her reflection and enabling her to move on. You notice your own strong feelings and wonder if they are really your own feelings or if you have become a 'barometer' of the supervisee's feelings of which they are unaware. If you think your feelings might be the latter, you could tentatively explore this.

> For example, in a later session, Chandra says, 'Listening to you talking about all the things you've achieved since our last session, I've become more and more sleepy. Do you ever feel exhausted?' In this case Chandra was surprised that she felt so sleepy as she had slept well the night before and what the supervisee was saying was interesting, yet her eyelids became very heavy indeed. Her question elicited a relieved response and Aileen dropped her 'dynamic' façade and admitted to exhaustion. This and the imagined requirement to keep up a 'dynamic' impression in her new senior post was a fruitful issue to reflect upon as regards the development of her leadership style (the clinical supervisor's tiredness dispelled immediately).

You need to be tentative in using this catalytic method. Bear in mind a '50-50 benchmark': that 50 per cent of the time your strong reactions to the supervisee could reflect the supervisee's unacknowledged feelings; and 50 per cent of the time the feelings are nothing to do with the supervisee at all, but relate only to your own past experiences. Even if you are right, the supervisee may not be ready to explore those feelings and anything other than a tentative approach on your part can be too intrusive and cross the boundaries between clinical supervision and psychotherapy.

5. *Acknowledging 'the unknown'.* A new clinical supervisor may have a tendency to feel that she should have the answer or be aware of everything that could be happening in the session, but this is patently impossible. The more experienced and skilled you become, the more you will realize that there are more and more 'unknowns' in the clinical supervision process and it is honest to admit it and to seek to explore them together. Van Ooijen (2003) gives some useful examples:

- I get the feeling that there is something blocking us here.
- I could be wrong, but I have the sense that we are missing something.
- I don't think we have quite got to whatever is behind all this yet.

6. *Identifying parallel processes.* This is building on the 'emotional barometer' phenomenon, by exploring whether the here-and-now feelings extend as far as the people involved in the situation back in the workplace: they have unacknowledged feelings which become stirred up in the supervisee; the supervisee does not acknowledge them in herself and the clinical supervisor then feels them. Enabling the supervisee to acknowledge her feelings can in turn help her to enable the client to acknowledge theirs.

> At one stage in the discussion about the violent incident, Chandra noticed herself feeling helpless and wondering what to do to help Aileen. She asked Aileen if she had felt particularly helpless at any point during this incident. Aileen agreed that that feeling was very strong at the time and she had to fight it to take charge of the situation. Chandra suggested perhaps that violent relative also felt helpless in the face of his father's impending death and that he felt he had to fight the feeling and ended up fighting his brother. Aileen was immediately energized by this idea and reflected on how she might have shown the son more understanding, which might have calmed him sooner. Or even possibly prevented the outburst by spending some time with the brothers to show them how to make contact with their semi-comatose father.

Phase 4: Working with emerging insights (see Table 5.7)

1. *Enable recognition of insights.* As you engage with the supervisee in exploratory dialogue, and she enters a reflective mind-space, your role is to

listen carefully and notice any new ideas, insights, options, learning points and decisions which emerge while the supervisee is talking. If the supervisee does not stop and recognize them herself, your role is to remember them and remind the supervisee when there is a pause.

> Aileen's thinking rushed on to planning a debriefing session with her team, which was a very useful train of thought for her and she planned it very clearly with Chandra listening but not needing to prompt. But Chandra thought that she had also missed the significance of another insight. At the next pause, Chandra said: 'That's an excellent plan and it's really important for the staff to have the chance to offload and reflect on what they have learned from the situation (pause). I wonder if there's also some mileage in exploring your idea about demonstrating understanding to an angry person and showing relatives how to relate to a very sick patient?'

In this example, the clinical supervisor invited the supervisee to explore the significance of one important insight that she seemed to have left unnoticed, but she also needed to remember the plan about the debriefing session, as this was also important.

2. *Assimilation of insights*. The supervisee needs time to think over the insights which have emerged and to explore what they mean to her and the implications for practice. A plan of action often emerges from this assimilation without the need for prompting.

3. *Enable planning*. When the supervisee has reached a state of reflective mindspace and insights have emerged, there is often a rush of energy and their plan becomes clear and falls into place without the need for any further prompts (as in the example above). Then the clinical supervisor's task is to validate the plan (unless you think it will lead to disaster) and hold the supervisee to it at the next session. Sometimes the supervisee's plan may be too vague and they may need some prompting to come up with a specific plan of action, with the occasional focused questions about specifics: 'What?', 'How?', 'With whose help?', 'When?' etc. However, bear in mind that not all insights can be assimilated and an action plan completed within the time boundary of the session. The supervisee can continue with the process after the session and report back next time.

Table 5.7 Catalytic skills phase 4: working with emerging insights

---

- Enable recognition of insights – listen, remember, remind
- Time to assimilate insights – invite supervisee to explore their significance
- Allow the emerging plan to flow. Enable movement towards planning how to apply the insights to professional practice, focussed questions about specifics of the plan, 'what?, how?, with whose help?. when?' etc.

> Aileen's clinical supervision session was coming to an end and she needed more time to mull over her insight about responding to angry relatives and possibly preventing outbursts. Her plan in this respect was to think it over more and to explore this in an 'I wonder . . . ' sort of way with her team at the debriefing session.

You will have noticed that in this example, the process of facilitated reflection has moved Aileen from a negatively critical examination of her performance and that of her colleague, to a blame-free enquiry into constructively learning from the experience. She is also beginning to develop a more reflective approach as part of her leadership style.

Pitfalls in using catalytic skills

1. *Interrogating.* One of the most common pitfalls (see also Table 5.7) is interrogating: when you machine-gun the supervisee with questions or prompts, going through your own checklist rather than giving the supervisee the chance to explain in her own words. This links to the first of the pitfalls in supporting.
2. *Prematurely action-oriented.* Coming in with advice about solutions or inviting the supervisee to plan what they are going to do before they have reflected more deeply on the issue. You would be encouraging shallow thinking by doing this and perhaps insulting the supervisee's intelligence by covering options she had already considered or dealt with.

   > In Aileen's case, she had dealt conscientiously with all practical aspects of the situation and Chandra would have demeaned her by coming in with action-oriented advice before Aileen had a chance to tell the whole story.

   One way to avoid this pitfall is to remind yourself that your role is to enable in-depth reflection, not instant advice-giving.
3. *Mechanical processing.* You might become too attached to one of the models for reflection or problem-solving and try to control the supervisee's thinking process. In this case you have one fixed framework in mind and relentlessly question the supervisee to hound them to think sequentially through the framework. We consider this to be intellectual oppression and the common reaction from any supervisee is passive resistance, by going through the motions superficially. We have also highlighted this common pitfall in other parts of the book. These frameworks should be used as mere tools to pick up and put down when needed. Given the appropriate intellectual freedom, many supervisees will move between frameworks or back and forth between stages of one framework rather than follow a pre-programmed thought pathway. One way to avoid this pitfall is to be transparent about which model you have in mind and give the supervisee

Table 5.8 Pitfalls in being catalytic in clinical supervision

- INTERROGATING – Machine-gunning the supervisee with factual questions
- PREMATURELY ACTION-ORIENTED – Advice about solutions or inviting the supervisee to plan what they are going to do before they have reflected more deeply on the issue
- MECHANICAL PROCESSING – Being too attached to one of the models for reflection or problem-solving and relentlessly questioning the supervisee to hound them to think sequentially through the model
- ANSWERING YOUR OWN QUESTIONS – Following an open question with a closed one which indicates your answer
- CURIOSITY-QUESTIONING – Questions to satisfy your own interest and curiosity may lead the supervisee off on a tangent, away from the issue that is most concerning her at this time
- FOLLOWING THE RED HERRING – Diversion as a result of your directing the topic towards your focus of interest, but can also be as a result of the supervisee diverting away from an uncomfortable issue onto something more comfortable but less relevant
- PROJECTING OWN FEELINGS ONTO SUPERVISEE –
- COMPULSIVELY CATALYTIC – Relentlessly putting everything back to the supervisee to work out or find out for themselves rather than giving appropriate advice or information
- COMPULSIVE SEARCH FOR ORDER – Pushing supervisee to be more coherent than they are ready to be
- DULL ANTENNA – Miss important cues and instead blunder on to something less important to the supervisee
- INTERVIEW RAPE – Probe into private aspects of the person's life or feelings without invitation
- SCRAPING THE BOWL – Going over ground which supervisee has discussed, decided and finished with
- PREMATURE CLOSURE – Pushing the supervisee to reach a neat conclusion so you yourself have a sense of completion
- FEAR OF THE UNKNOWN – making assumptions about what the supervisee is going to say next.

a genuine choice about whether to use it or not. In addition, you could ensure that you have enough understanding of more than one framework for reflection and for problem-solving and use a mixture in your own reflection during your own clinical supervision. This will help you to stand back and observe which elements of which frameworks the supervisee is using and summarize and validate what thinking she has done herself.

4. *Answering your own questions*. This is when you follow an open question with a closed one which indicates your answer. For instance:

> *Chandra:* What do you think about your staff nurse's reactions? Don't you think she has a right to feel upset?

If this is one of your tendencies, imagine a large full stop hanging in the air after you have asked an open question. Give the supervisee space to pause and reply in her own time. 'Don't you think she has a right to feel upset?' is also an example of a leading question. Leading questions are a common pitfall: these are questions phrased in a way which indicates what answer you expect the supervisee to give.

5. *Curiosity-questioning.* This is when you ask factual questions to satisfy your own interest and curiosity. This can lead the supervisee off on a tangent, away from the issue that is most concerning her at this time. Some of the examples under 'interrogating' could be curiosity-led questions. One way of avoiding this pitfall is to stop yourself by thinking 'This is *her* time' and focusing back on what the supervisee is saying.

6. *Following the red herring.* This may be a diversion as a result of your directing the topic towards your focus of interest, but can also be a result of the supervisee diverting away from an uncomfortable issue onto something more comfortable but less relevant, which diverts from the decision to be made.

7. *Projecting own feelings onto supervisee.* Over-confident use of the 'emotional barometer' and 'parallel processes' might lead you to being pushy about what you think the supervisee *ought* to be feeling, when you may be mistaken about the emotional issues. Your reading of the emotional issues involved may be more about you and your past experiences than about the supervisee's present feeling state. Even if your view might have an element of truth, you can be mistaken about the supervisee being ready to understand these complex interventions.

8. *Compulsively catalytic.* Being compulsively catalytic can be a pitfall for someone who is a recent convert to non-directive approaches to facilitating reflection in clinical supervision. There will be times when giving advice or information would be more appropriate than relentlessly putting everything back to the supervisee to work out or find out for themselves.

> For instance, Chandra had information about a helpful pamphlet outlining a suggested process for debriefing after traumatic situations that had been produced by staff at the mental health unit of the same Trust. If Aileen had been struggling to plan the debriefing sessions, it might have been more helpful for her to offer Aileen a copy than to let her struggle on without it.

Heron (2001) highlights some pitfalls to bear in mind: compulsive search for order, dull antenna, interview rape, scraping the bowl and premature closure.

9. *Compulsive search for order.* You try to push the supervisee into being more coherent than they are ready to be.

> For instance, at the beginning, Aileen needed to blurt out the story to Chandra, and did it in a fairly illogical way, getting the sequence out of order. If Chandra had interrupted and demanded that she get her thoughts more organized in the early stages of the session, she would have been falling into this pitfall.

10. *Dull antenna*. This is when you miss important cues and instead blunder onto something less important to the supervisee.

> For example, if Chandra had pursued the facts of the violent man's past history, she might have missed the important issue, which was the feeling of helplessness that Aileen and her team were experiencing.

11. *Interview rape*. You probe into private aspects of the person's life or feelings without invitation. Delving into the personal or childhood origins of workplace feelings is the province *only* of counsellors and psychotherapists. The clinical supervisor's focus is on past workplace experiences, the recent past, the present and the future, and your role is to enable expression of emotions and then clarification of how the supervisee can find practical ways of dealing with them, whatever their origins.

> For instance, if Chandra had asked: 'Is feeling responsible for other people's violence a pattern from childhood?', this would have definitely been overstepping the boundaries of clinical supervision. She would have been falling into 'interview rape': attempting to open up a private topic when she had no contract to do so in the clinical supervision relationship.

12. *Scraping the bowl*. Going over ground which the supervisee has discussed, digested, decided and finished with.
13. *Premature closure*. Pushing the supervisee to reach a neat conclusion to reflecting on a topic so you yourself have a sense of completion. Working in a facilitative role such as clinical supervisor can leave you with some frustration when the supervisee does not achieve a neat solution or plan by the end of the discussion. This frustration goes with the role and you will need to learn to sit with it. The supervisee is capable of continuing to reflect on the issue after the session, and may need some more time to assimilate insights or seek more information in order to come to an appropriate conclusion.

Many of the above pitfalls can arise from a fear of the unknown. When a supervisee is in a reflective mind-space, anything can emerge unexpectedly. As a new clinical supervisor, this fear may lead you to assume the supervisee's train of thought is going to leave the station on the same track as yours, and your comments manipulate the supervisee in that direction. An experienced clinical supervisor may feel they have heard it all before. If you start to feel that you know what the supervisee is going to say next, it is important to have the humility to check yourself and give the supervisee the opportunity to surprise you.

Summary

The focus in this chapter has been on the clinical supervisor but this must be placed in the context of the working alliance between supervisee and supervisor. Effective use of these skills requires an underlying care and concern for the supervisee and her clients and staff, and a desire to see them flourish. Any tendency to want to use a slick array of techniques needs to be privately acknowledged and contained, otherwise the supervisee will sense a lack of genuineness and respect. You may have to modify your own defensive reactions, and be alert to any tendency towards being over-critical or a desire to take over and try to dazzle with your own experience. Bear in mind that the purpose of support and catalytic skills is to provide a secure enough psychological base within which the supervisee can feel sufficiently supported to take on the challenge of learning and developing their clinical practice, and their part in the complexity and quality of that practice that they play as a person. The opportunity that the supervisee gets in thinking these issues through for herself, exploring the reflective mind-space, builds the skill of the supervisee's 'internal supervisor' that will be used in everyday practice.

The next chapter examines the more authoritative skills used by the clinical supervisor.

6 Informative and challenging skills of the clinical supervisor

Most of the help that you as clinical supervisor give to the supervisee is in the form of support and catalytic facilitation of the supervisee's own reflection on issues affecting practice. However, while you will need to be relatively sparing in giving information, advice or challenging, this authoritative dimension of the role of the clinical supervisor or supervision group member is an essential element of the process.

Some readers may look in dismay at the emphasis that we place in this chapter on the authoritative aspects of the clinical supervisor's role, especially regarding challenging the supervisee, and consider that it contradicts what we have written in the last chapter. This dismay is sometimes expressed on our courses when we cover clinical supervisor skills in this sequence. However, support and challenge are not either/or elements: they sit together. This is consistent with both the concern nurses and managers have about professional accountability and standards and with the support and growth principles of clinical supervision.

The authoritative dimension of being a clinical supervisor

In Chapter 2 we asked you to think about the use of power within the clinical supervision relationship, and suggested that there was a great deal of confusion and ambivalence about its use in all professional relationships, both with clients and colleagues. On the one hand, nurses can have a tendency to give too much information and advice: this is shown in numerous communication studies in nursing (see the literature review in Kendall 1991). On the other, there is a tendency to avoid using challenging, illustrated by Burnard and Morrison's study (1988), obviously not considered out of date as it is frequently quoted as still being relevant.

We find that once nurses learn the effectiveness of support and catalytic skills, they can sometimes become excessively non-directive, withholding information, advice or challenge inappropriately as far as the clinical supervision relationship is concerned. In Chapter 2 we suggested that some practitioners shy away from or minimize the authoritative dimension of their professional relationships and can be quick to feel anxious or resistant to perceived authority themselves and in others. In this chapter you are urged to remember the distinction we drew in Chapter 2 between authoritative and authoritarian, when we suggested that authoritative skills were based on valid experience, knowledge and skills, which can be used non-abusively to enable and support others. Therefore most of the guidance offered in this chapter applies to all professional relationships. The clinical supervisor has no more or less responsibility and authority for dealing with inadequate professional standards than any other nurse who discovers such causes for concern, but it might be the case that the clinical supervisor becomes privy to more information about poor standards than her non-clinical supervisor colleagues.

To elaborate on the authority dimension: imagine a continuum with 'very authoritative' at one end and 'very facilitative' at the other. You could place a number of options between those two poles, in varying degrees of either along the continuum. Table 6.1 illustrates the range of leadership characteristics between those two poles, applicable to any leadership role. If we take one task involved in clinical supervision, that of decision-making, Table 6.1 also highlights that in clinical supervision the emphasis is firmly towards the facilitative end of the continuum, where the supervisee is responsible for making their own decision, facilitated by the clinical supervisor, while being prepared to move to the authoritative end of the scale if necessary. Likewise with the leadership task of initiating action, the clinical supervisor role is concentrated at the facilitative end, while again being prepared to move to the authoritative end if the issue is an ethical one, perhaps concerning dangerous practice that is not being dealt with. You could contrast this with the version of this matrix shown in Chapter 9, highlighting a different emphasis in line management supervision (Table 9.3).

This chapter focuses on the skills necessary to achieve an appropriately authoritative approach within a clinical supervision context. It will also be useful to those seeking guidance about forms of supervision in which there is a greater emphasis on the supervisor's authority, such as line management, safeguarding supervision and day-to-day feedback to colleagues, whether peers, junior or senior staff.

Our examples focus mostly on directive skills in the 'average' clinical supervision session, with the occasional example of more extreme situations. The skills that are the focus of this chapter can be applied to any level of concern, although their use is also often brought into sharp relief when there is specific concern about accountability and standards.

We begin by examining the skills of giving information and advice.

Informative skills

We distinguish between giving information and giving advice in that giving information is sharing facts, opinions and procedures in order that the supervisee can extrapolate and make her own informed decision about what course of action to take. Giving advice is offering one or more examples of specific courses of action that the supervisee can take when considering her options. Again, the emphasis is on the supervisee making the decision about what action to take: she remains responsible for her practice whatever advice you give as clinical supervisor, although you also have a responsibility not to give negligent advice. We encourage you in most situations to give any information, advice or instructions in such a way that the supervisee can take it or leave it, use it in their decision-making or not, and, if

Table 6.1 A leadership matrix, indicating examples of the range of leadership characteristics within the authoritative/facilitative dimension, highlighting the emphasis (shaded) in clinical supervision

CONTINUUM	AUTHORITATIVE				FACILITATIVE
LEADERSHIP CHARACTERISTIC	DIRECTIVE	NEGOTIATING		CATALYTIC	SPACE-GIVING
LEADERSHIP TASK	DECISION-MAKING				
Whose responsibility is it to make the decision?	Yours / Mostly yours	Yours & supervisee(s)		Mostly supervisee(s)	supervisee(s)
Who decides?	You decide — You decide, then consult, then change decision or not — You consult, then decide	You decide then negotiate compromise — You give a few options from which supervisee(s) can decide	You explore options jointly & jointly decide	You indicate the overall boundary & enable supervisee(s) to decide within that. — You give information or possible options to enable supervisee(s) to decide	You impartially & catalytically enable supervisee(s) to decide for themselves — You do nothing, wait for supervisee(s) to decide, but stay alert to what decisions are made or not.
LEADERSHIP TASK	INITIATING ACTION BY SUPERVISEE(S)				
What do you do?	You give an unequivocal order — You direct — You persuade	You request then negotiate compromise — You give limited options, supervisee(s) choose which ones to act upon	You indicate the overall parameters & enable supervisee(s) to get things done within them.	You provide the necessary information & give supervisee(s) space to act upon it in their own way. — You enable the supervisee(s) to reflect in-depth, connect with their intuition, knowledge, feelings, & motivation & give them space to carry out the action in their own way.	You do nothing, wait for supervisee(s) to do what needs doing, but stay alert to what's happening or not happening.

you have a tendency to be too informative, to restrain yourself in using this skill and focus on developing the other three skills more.

Giving information or advice, rather than purely support and catalytic help, is appropriate when certain conditions apply. A general rule of thumb is that the more technical a problem is, the more relevant it is to offer information or advice. The more the issue concerns feelings and human relationships (the most common issues that we see brought to clinical supervision), the less appropriate it is to be informative.

However, it may be appropriate to give information or advice in the following scenarios:

- the supervisee is stuck in their thinking: support and catalytic help has not worked, so some information or advice about *how* to reflect, such as intuitive methods of reflection or frameworks for problem-solving or reflection may provide a way forward (see Chapter 4);
- the supervisee is going along the wrong track because they are genuinely unaware of or do not understand some key facts or options that would easily clarify the situation;
- the supervisee's gaps in knowledge, misunderstanding or misinformation are part of the problem that they bring to clinical supervision or are likely to experience soon;
- the supervisee is floundering because their confidence and decision-making ability is shattered and some key information or advice would start them on the road to doing something to rectify their emotional situation and begin to get their confidence back;
- the supervisee is totally unaware of some important information or options and you need to share these in order to help them to progress and make informed decisions and choices about what to do;
- the situation is critical and requires quick action;
- the problem is within your specialist field of expertise and the supervisee knows little about it;
- the supervisee has asked for information or advice and giving it would not be colluding with inappropriate dependency on the clinical supervisor;
- the supervisee has decided to take precipitate action which has not been thought through and is obviously inappropriate, too risky for them or others or is an incorrect procedure, and strong advice is required to help the supervisee get back on track;
- the supervisee seems to be stuck in a cycle of behaviour which is destructive and attempts to help supportively and with catalytic and challenging interventions have not worked, so repeated firm advice is necessary.

For example:

Kunu is a member of a clinical supervision group and is attending a session which happens to be held on the last day of her annual leave, but she has come into work just for the session. She was about to use her time in the clinical supervision session to talk through some long-term plans for managing the team on her unit that she had thought through while on holiday in West Africa. The group froze when they realized that she was unaware that there had been plans made at senior management level which would affect her unit. Laura, the group facilitator, felt she had to give her the information now otherwise Kunu's session would be a waste of time and in any case all the other group members knew about it.

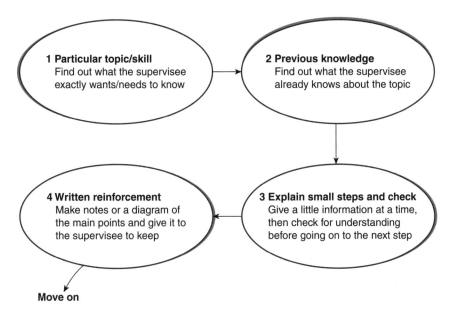

Figure 6.1 Steps in giving information

Steps in giving information

Step 1: what information is needed?

You may have a vast amount of information on a topic but the supervisee is likely only to require a small amount of it. Assessing which specific aspects of the topic are required is important, otherwise you will swamp the supervisee with information or enthusiasm. This is not a teaching session, so you need to be very sparing in your information-giving. First of all, find out exactly what the supervisee wants or needs to know.

Step 2: existing knowledge?

Then find out the supervisee's existing level of knowledge: what the supervisee already knows about the topic. You will be using your catalytic skills to elicit this information, for instance: 'What exactly would you like to know about … ?', Tell me what you know already about … ?', 'Have you ever tried to do this or seen anyone doing this before?' Here is how Laura approaches the situation with Kunu:

> *Laura:* Kunu, before you go on, am I right in thinking you don't start back until tomorrow and you haven't been to the ward yet?
> *Kunu:* That's right.
> *Laura:* So you haven't heard the bad news?'

Step 3: explain in small steps and check understanding

Give the information in small steps: give a little information at a time and try to relate it to the supervisee's situation or to her choice of words. Leave space for questions and, after each step, check for understanding before going on to the next step. Be careful to stop yourself when you have given enough and give the supervisee time to mull it over.

> *Laura:* I'm sorry to have to tell you this, Kunu. Your manager was probably going to meet you tomorrow to tell you. As far as I understand it, the plan is to close your ward and combine it with Nightingale ward in four weeks' time.

Checking for understanding involves using your catalytic skills again: use open questions such as 'What has struck you in particular about what I've just said?', 'Which parts of that are especially relevant to your situation?', 'How might you use this information?'

Closed questions like 'OK?', 'Is that clear?', 'Did you understand?', or 'Got that?' are not going to give you a good idea of what the supervisee has really understood. In Kunu's case, there is no need to check: her shocked reaction shows that she understands only too well.

Step 4: written reinforcement

Often it can be useful to make notes or draw a diagram of the main points and give it to the supervisee to keep, since much verbally given information is forgotten within an hour or so if there is no written or visual backup to reinforce it.

Ways of giving advice

Advice-giving is distinguished from information-giving in that advice is a suggestion for action. There are two types of advice: soft and firm.

Soft advice

This is appropriate for most clinical supervision situations. You give the advice as one suggestion or option, implying or explicitly pointing out that there are other courses of action that might be equally effective. You phrase the advice tentatively, for instance: 'I suggest . . . ', 'You could try . . . ', 'You might . . . ', 'Possibly . . . ', 'One thing you could try is . . . ', 'One option could be . . . ' and so on.

> Ros, one of the group members, says to Kunu: 'Kunu, I think it might be a good idea to go and speak to your manager right now. You're not going to be able to concentrate until you know where you stand. Please come back though and tell us.' The group decides to have their coffee break early and Kunu leaves the clinical supervision session to phone her manager to get more information: Ros goes with her for support. They soon rejoin the group and Kunu spends her time in the session getting 'emotional first-aid' support from them.

Firm advice

You would give firm advice when you feel strongly about the course of action you are suggesting. You still need to be conscious that the supervisee has the right to reject your advice, but that they must take responsibility for the consequences of doing so. Express your strength of conviction and spell out the consequences of not following the advice: for instance: 'I strongly advise/urge/suggest you do such and such, otherwise – will probably happen', 'It's vital/very important/essential that you – or else – will happen.'

> Ros says to Kunu at the end of the session: 'I think it's important that you go and have a break and something to eat before you drive home, you didn't have any lunch and you've said yourself you still feel a bit wobbly.'

In giving advice, it is preferable to be positive: to speak more of 'dos' rather than 'don'ts'. Of course, you may need to point out pitfalls, but emphasize the positive course of action that you are suggesting the supervisee takes, as this is clear communication. This is especially the case if someone is stressed or confused: they can easily get the wrong end of the stick if you emphasize the 'don'ts'. You can see this when, say, helping a very disorientated patient to eat: if you say 'Don't spit this out' the patient often does just what you said, spits it out, not registering the 'don't'. 'Try to chew this and swallow this food' usually gets a better response. Likewise a stressed supervisee: say what you positively advise the supervisee to do, not what you don't want them to do. Giving a positive instruction puts the positive idea in the other person's mind and reduces misunderstanding.

Pitfalls in being informative

1. *Overload.* The most common pitfall we have seen is swamping the supervisee with too much information, advice or enthusiasm for the subject, so the supervisee has no space to mull over and apply relevant information. Consciously stopping, allowing pauses and checking for understanding can help you to slow down and avoid getting carried away. We find that nurses who have a tendency to give too much information or advice may

Table 6.2 Pitfalls in being informative

---

1. OVERLOAD. Giving too much information or advice, not selecting what is really wanted
2. INFO/ADVICE NOT WANTED. Giving instructions or advice without supervisee having the chance to reflect on it
3. NEGLIGENT ADVICE. If advice outside of your area of expertise, you are liable if it turned out to be dangerous
4. PUSHY ADVICE. Being over-anxious about your advice being taken, hounding the supervisee with reminders. Annoyed that the supervisee hasn't taken your advice
5. PUT-DOWN ADVICE. Your manner implies that the supervisee is stupid for not knowing
6. PATRONIZING. Giving information which the supervisee already knows well. Using over-simplified vocabulary, a sing-song, nursery teacher tone of voice, exaggerated patience with an edge of impatience
7. DELIVERY INEFFECTIVE. Too fast, slow, indistinct, loud/soft, no written reinforcement; being too complicated, using terms not known by supervisee
8. COMPULSIVE NON-DIRECTIVENESS. Always putting it back to the supervisee when sometimes it is appropriate to give information or advice
9. WHY DON'T YOU....YES, BUT. See Figure 6.2

---

do so as a means of showing they want to explicitly support the supervisee. In this case, learning about the skills of giving explicit support, as shown in the previous chapter, can reduce this tendency.

2. *Information/advice not wanted/needed.* Related to overload is giving information or advice which is not wanted: perhaps the supervisee knows already, or is quite capable of working it out for themselves, or is giving off cues that they do not want advice at that point. This could be said to be interfering: giving information or advice about problems which are nothing to do with your expertise or your contract with the supervisee. You can avoid this pitfall by checking if some advice or information is wanted before you give it. Here you need to be sensitive to cues of hesitancy or uncertainty: nurses will often find it difficult to say no. It may be important to you as a clinical supervisor to be seen as someone who has something to offer, to be identified as the knowledgeable person who solved a difficult situation. Coping with your feelings of lack of acknowledgement and appreciation are part of the job: the more effective you are at facilitating, the more the supervisee will be pleased with herself for solving the problem, rather than pleased with you. The origins of giving too much advice may lie in a need to help by rescuing the supervisee from the discomfort of puzzling something through for herself: the clinical supervisor cannot bear her own discomfort while sitting with the supervisee. However, whatever the motives, Casement (1985) reminds us to stay with not-knowing, when the issue is one of feelings or human relationships: anything else can be either too premature or too dishonest.

3. *Negligent advice.* If you give advice that is outside of your area of expertise, then you could be liable if it turns out to be dangerous (see Jenkins 2006).

4. *Pushy advice*. You might become too attached to your advice, perhaps being overanxious about it being taken, hounding the supervisee with reminders and follow-ups. Even though other options may be equally or more effective, you may show annoyance that the supervisee hasn't taken your excellent advice.

5. *Put-down advice*. Your manner can come across as a put-down if your tone implies that the supervisee is stupid for not knowing the information or not knowing what to do. This can happen when you feel surprised that the supervisee appears not to know something basic or appears not to see the obvious solution to the problem. Sometimes the very fact that you are giving advice too early can seem like an insult to their intelligence. You may be stating the obvious course of action that anyone would think of: the supervisee has tried it unsuccessfully long ago. Remember that you do not know every single detail of the supervisee's story: there may be other factors that are unknown to you which get in the way of the obvious solutions. However, it may be the case that stress can make the supervisee forget or temporarily be blind to the obvious solution, but tread carefully in raising it.

6. *Patronizing*. The clinical supervision can come across as patronizing if information is given which the supervisee already knows well. Also, if you have had a similar experience but the way you share it implies that you are now more mature and through that phase now, this can sound patronizing; likewise using oversimplified vocabulary or showing exaggerated patience by using a sing-song, nursery teacher tone of voice. Finding out what the supervisee already knows, or helping them to remember and have confidence in their own knowledge, can help avoid this pitfall.

7. *Ineffective delivery*. The delivery of information or advice may be too fast, slow, indistinct, too enthusiastic, too flat or boring, with no written reinforcement, or too complicated, using terms not known by the supervisee. Following the guidelines suggested earlier may avoid this pitfall, especially eliciting the supervisee's specific wants and needs and their previous knowledge. You can then use some of the supervisee's vocabulary in your explanation, and relate your points to their concerns.

8. *Compulsive non-directiveness*. This may occur when the clinical supervisor continues to use support and catalytic interventions when some information or advice may be more appropriate. This seems to happen most often with nurses who are used to listening non-directively to clients for long periods of time, such as mental health nurses or nurses with a specific counselling role. Alternatively, a clinical supervisor who is a fervent recent convert to non-directive approaches may have a tendency to overdo non-direction.

9. *Why don't you . . . Yes, but*. This is the advice-defence trap, outlined by Berne (2004) (see Figure 6.2). This can happen when the clinical supervisor gives advice inappropriately, using the 'Why don't you?' phrase which can be taken as containing an element of criticism. The supervisee then replies defensively, 'Yes, but . . . ' giving a reason why it wouldn't work. The

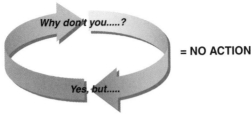

Figure 6.2 Pitfalls in giving advice: 'Why don't you ... ?', 'Yes but ... ' (adapted from Berne 2004)

clinical supervisor tries again with another piece of advice, the supervisee says she has tried it but it didn't work, and the two of them go round in circles and become irritated with each other. No plan is made and nothing is done about the problem.

Skills of challenging the supervisee

The intention in challenging the supervisee is to help them to be more aware of behaviour or values which actually or potentially contribute to the problem in question, or which block their potential for developing high quality practice, or block their ability to use clinical supervision well.

Most people on clinical supervision courses find this skill is one of their weakest. The exceptions seem to be those whose work involves the necessity of using challenging skills a lot, such as those who work in substance abuse clinics, secure units, prisons and accident and emergency departments. Williams *et al.* (2005) also found that members of a clinical supervision group felt challenging to be the most difficult skill to use. It causes anxiety for almost everyone, partly because in reality you never really know how the supervisee will react and partly because of the emotional baggage we bring from our own past experiences of being on the receiving end of destructive criticism. You may not wish to upset the supervisee, but, as Egan (2009) points out, people have enough emotional resilience to be able to manage the discomfort that can result from having behaviour and values challenged in a supportive way.

Historically there has been very little help for practitioners to learn and practise challenging skills. This framework will help to focus on ways of following through your intention to challenge, but probably nothing will completely take away the inevitable anxiety of challenging. However, the principles and step-by-step format offered here may help you to manage that anxiety.

Three conditions for challenging the supervisee

1. *Information gained during the clinical supervision sessions only*. As a clinical supervisor, you have the right and responsibility to challenge

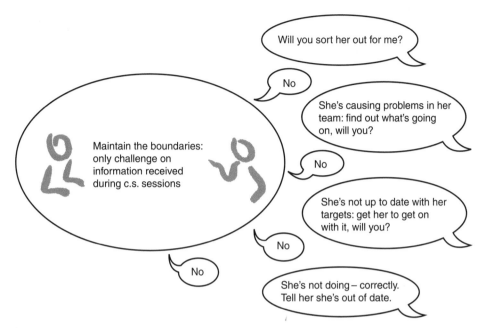

Figure 6.3 Maintaining the boundaries by rebutting outside interference

issues that concern or alarm you, provided that you have gained the information during the clinical supervision sessions. This means that if someone else asks you to challenge the supervisee about something that concerns them, it is important that you refuse and put it back to them to deal with (see Figure 6.3). Otherwise you undermine the principles of clinical supervision, collude with whoever is abdicating their responsibility and undermine their authority. This type of request is often reported by clinical supervisors attending our courses. If you also work with the supervisee outside clinical supervision and you see or discover errors elsewhere, it is important that you challenge them there and then rather than comment during the clinical supervision session. The boundaries to the clinical supervision relationship are vital and we have covered the rationale for this a number of time elsewhere in this book.

2. *Supervisee not already aware or not addressing the problem.* The second condition is that the supervisee does not appear to have insight into the negative effect of their behaviour or values, chooses to ignore it or does not take it seriously enough.

3. *Use supportive and catalytic facilitation first.* You should already have used supportive and catalytic facilitation which have not succeeded in raising awareness. The exception is if the issue is of such pressing importance, such as unsafe practice that is not being dealt with, that it would be inappropriate to spend time using these other approaches.

Table 6.3 Some topic areas for challenging the supervisee

---

a) Inconsistencies
b) Mistakes
c) Avoiding responsibility
d) Unsafe practice not being dealt with
e) Mental blocks
f) Misuse of clinical supervision time
g) Avoiding awkward topics in the clinical supervision relationship
h) Signs of an unacknowledged problem
i) Prejudices and unfounded assumptions

Bear in mind that as a professional person, the supervisee has enough emotional resilience to be able to manage the discomfort that can result from having gaps in knowledge or ability exposed, and from having inappropriate behaviour and values challenged within a safe space.

Topics for challenging the supervisee

You need to be clear about what it is exactly that you are challenging about what the person does. Table 6.3 lists some examples of topic areas and each of these are illustrated by scenario's A to I.

- *Inconsistencies.* There may be a lack of fit between the supervisee's self-image and what she actually does, or the inconsistency may be between the supervisee's espoused values and her behaviour.

  > **Scenario A.** Angela is complaining to Pete about an agency nurse who is temporarily in her team and seems to be slow in learning the ropes. She recounts some of their conversations in which it sounds as if Angela has frequently been quite harsh. The agency nurse goes to pieces when she is on duty, but apparently not when Angela's deputy is in charge. Angela maintains she is always patient with new staff but that this person is beyond the pale and she is thinking of contacting the agency to get her replaced.

- *Mistakes.* Shaw (2004: 66) defines a mistake as an 'unintended slip in good practice or a common therapeutic blunder'. We would add to this: a judgement that you consider is mistaken.

  > **Scenario B.** Brenda is a staff nurse on an accident and emergency unit, who recently returned to work after a career break. In her clinical supervision she is reflecting on another issue when, in passing, she mentions that she was about to show a student how to treat a patient with hypothermia with a space blanket, but couldn't find one.

- *Avoiding responsibility*. The supervisee might be describing an event in which she appears not to have fulfilled the expectations of a professional within her role, whether towards her patients, team members or employers. This might be an explicit organizational contract, such as working a certain number of hours or carrying out certain functions, or may be an explicit person-to-person agreement between the supervisee and a client or colleague. Implicit contracts are more about what people might reasonably expect from each other according to their roles.

    Scenario C. Charlotte is telling her clinical supervisor Pauline about a conflict with her new manager. Charlotte has always refused to sort out the holiday roster directly with her two immediate health visitor colleagues, with whom she is barely on speaking terms. The previous manager used to do it for them to keep the peace. Charlotte does not see it as her responsibility to negotiate with her colleagues.

- *Unsafe practice not being addressed*. There may appear to be unsafe practice that the supervisee or her team are not willing or able to deal with, or more subtle aspects of the NMC (2008) code that are not being addressed.

    Scenario D. David tells his clinical supervisor Hannah about having witnessed a colleague repeatedly slapping a patient with learning difficulties. David has reported this verbally to the team leader who has done nothing about it, apparently not believing him and pathologizing his concern by saying that David is having a very difficult time due to a marriage break-up and needs support. The abuse continues. He feels that he has fulfilled his responsibilities, considers that no further action is required on his part and washes his hands of the affair.

- *Mental blocks*. These are the defences, mental rigidities or emotional blind spots which lead the supervisee to avoid dealing with something difficult which needs to be addressed.

    Scenario E. Evelyn has spoken to her clinical supervisor Zara about a difficulty with a colleague who is not pulling her weight in the team. At the last two clinical supervision sessions she has gone away with an action plan to confront the colleague but keeps procrastinating.

- *Misuse of clinical supervision time*. The supervisee may be not be using the time for in-depth reflection – for example, being frequently late for sessions, answering her mobile phone, bringing inappropriate topics, being mechanistic and cursory in using reflective cycles, staying closed about anything other than technical topics, expecting the clinical supervisor to teach her or tell her what to do, and so on. Clinical supervisors often report that supervisees have difficulties in the early stages of clinical supervision with taking responsibility for their use of the time. This is especially the case if the supervisee has not been able to attend training in supervisee skills, or has chosen not to attend such courses on offer. Lack of understanding of clinical supervision, lack of skill in reflection or resentment about having to attend may contribute to this type of situation.

> **Scenario F.** Fergus tends to describe a problem to his clinical supervisor Mohammed in a manner that implies: 'There it is, now see if you can sort it out'.

- *Avoiding awkward topics in the clinical supervision relationship.* You may have a sense that something is being avoided that relates directly to the clinical supervision relationship. The clues may be to do with lack of commitment, lateness, superficiality, defensiveness or in themes within the topics that the supervisee brings to the sessions that point towards the reality of the relationship.

> **Scenario G.** At each of his first three sessions with Catherine, Gamada has brought a topic about conflicts with colleagues and his manager. Catherine notices that each example concerned a white woman who was senior to him. Although Catherine is of the same grade as Gamada, she is white and Gamada had little choice about having her as his clinical supervisor as she was the only one available at the time. She wonders to herself if there is any significance to this, or whether she is feeling awkward about having a black male supervisee.

- *Signs of an unacknowledged problem.* The supervisee may be talking negatively about her patients/clients or her colleagues in such a way that you sense there is some underlying problem which has not been acknowledged.

> **Scenario H.** In clinical supervision, Fran notices that her supervisee Holly (a nursery nurse) is complaining a lot about the parents of the patients she works with on the paediatric ward, whereas she used to speak about enjoying this aspect of her work.

- *Prejudices and unfounded assumptions.* The supervisee may exhibit some negative assumptions about certain sectors of society, such as people of a different race, class, religion, sexuality, age, level of physical or mental ability and so on. She may make unfounded assumptions about people who are different from herself.

> **Scenario I.** Iris is a practice nurse and describes to her clinical supervisor Norma how she enjoys working at the main surgery premises, her practice base, which is situated in a leafy suburb, but dislikes holding clinics in the satellite surgery situated in a large housing estate. She speaks of the residents of the estate as 'riff raff'.

Challenging: some principles

Focus on positive change: the challenge should be given in the spirit that the supervisee has the potential for development and that your role is to support them towards that. Your tone therefore should avoid sounding punitive.

It is very important that you comment only on the supervisee's actions, decisions or apparent values, not on their personality. Commenting on personality will feel more like a personal attack and is not supportive of development in the clinical supervision context. Personality change is not the remit of clinical supervision. Some principles to bear in mind are as follows.

- *Be supportive.* When you have challenged a supervisee, be prepared to let them respond and have their say: that in itself is supportive. You may wish to draw them out about any background reasons or feelings about the problem, or to offer other support. The manner in which you express the challenge needs to be supportive rather than carping or critical. Remember, your intention is to raise awareness and throw some light on and explore the situation, not to punish or take out your frustrations on the supervisee. Ensure that you follow your challenge with an offer of support towards development, such as encouraging the supervisee to explore the issue further and consider other approaches that might be more positive.
- *Keep within the boundaries of clinical supervision.* Comment on information you have gained during the clinical supervision session only.
- *Be specific.* It is important that you refer to specific actions or things the supervisee has said to you. Avoid generalities such as 'You always ... '.
- *Speak concisely.* You may not need to say it all at once, so be brief. Allow silences, so the supervisee can absorb and respond. The inevitable anxiety involved in challenging tends to lead many people to say too much or repeat themselves, not allowing the supervisee the space to have her say.

Challenging questions

These are focused on enabling the supervisee to think through what they have said and come to some insight about the issue at hand. For example, scenario A continues:

> *Pete:* (to Angela, gently) You say you are always patient with new staff. In what ways have you been patient with this agency nurse?'

> Pete's challenging question to Angela led her to realize that she had been especially hard on the agency nurse and eventually she came to the conclusion that she was feeling a bit insecure in her authority as a very young ward manager, because the nurse was much older and more experienced in the field than Angela was. Had the question not achieved this awareness-raising, Pete might have tried to take it further by asking: 'It sounds to me that you've been especially harsh with this agency nurse and that her confidence goes to pieces when she works with you. What triggers your irritation in particular?'

Steps in challenging: Level 1

Often it is clearer to get to the point. The steps shown in Figure 6.4 can help to make the challenge constructive. Scenario I will be used here to illustrate the steps.

- Step 1. *Introduce the topic.* Sometimes you may need to pinpoint the topic upon which you want to comment, especially if the discussion has gone off the point towards something else.

    Norma: (to Iris, gently) I'd like to say something about the way you referred earlier to the residents of the estate.

- Step 2. *Specify behaviour.* Come to the point as quickly and concisely as possible and explain how the person falls short. Speak in the first person. Norma, 'I'm concerned that you called them "riffraff".'
- Step 3. *Give space to respond.* Let the supervisee react in their own time. People have different ways of reacting to the discomfort of being challenged and need time to respond. Listen carefully to what they say and show that you have listened by referring non-judgementally to what they have said. A challenge is more likely to escalate into an argument if the supervisee feels that she has not been listened to.

    Iris: It was only a 'turn of phrase', no offence meant.
    Norma: (gently) Perhaps no offence intended, but it may still be taken.

- Step 4. *Explain the relevance.* Sometimes it might be useful to explain the relevance and to say why you are bringing the issue up at this point in time.

    Norma: (gently) Maybe this is the key to the problem you talked about last time: you know, some patients complaining to the GPs about you. If they pick up that you think they are riff raff then perhaps they have a right to complain.

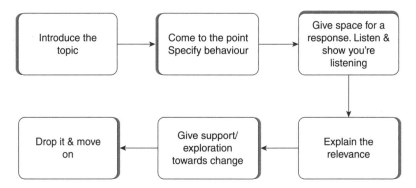

Figure 6.4 Challenging the supervisee-Level 1

- Step 5. *Support.* Follow up quickly with some support to help the supervisee explore the meaning of this situation and to develop awareness and change, without taking back your challenge or undermining it. Offer support appropriately.

> Norma senses there is some unacknowledged difficulty underlying the prejudice: 'I wonder if you ever feel unsafe when you're working in the satellite surgery? I do sometimes when I'm working in that area.'

- Step 6. *Drop it.* There may be times when it is appropriate to drop the subject for a while. Your aim is to enable the supervisee to develop awareness and to change, not to win an argument or get your way. Give the supervisee the chance to think about it and save face, perhaps by changing the subject.

> (Iris is very red but is acting defensively)
> *Iris:* Well, of course not, I'm an experienced practice nurse, why should I feel unsafe? And anyway, this isn't what I came here to talk about, this is a waste of time.
> Norma wonders if Iris's aggression may parallel the patients' aggression too, but feels this is too much for Iris to absorb at this time.
> *Norma:* (gently) OK, let's put that aside for now. The next thing on your agenda was . . .

Steps in challenging: Level 2

- Step 7. *Persist.* Follow through the challenge with persistence if the supervisee is side-tracking or the issue is unsafe practice that cannot be dropped, or you have dropped it and the supervisee does not spontaneously return to it herself. See Figure 6.5.

> Iris seems more collected and has been happier discussing something less awkward. When that topic seems to have been covered, Norma brings it back to the challenge.

> *Norma:* (gently) I'd like to go back to what we were discussing earlier. You know, there's nothing wrong in admitting you're feeling unsafe sometimes, however experienced you are. Perhaps many of the residents of the estate are afraid too, especially your vulnerable patients?

> They go on to discuss why some of Iris's patients act aggressively when asked to come to the surgery rather than have the district nurse visit. At the next session, Iris apologizes for 'being so bolshy' and seems to have discussed her concerns more openly with her colleagues at the surgery and they have worked out a better security system for staff.

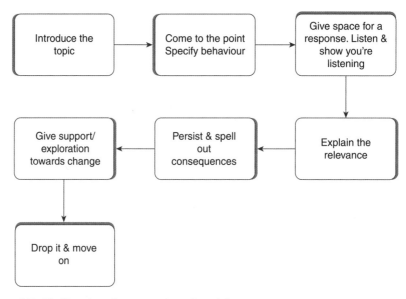

Figure 6.5 Challenging the supervisee, Level 2

Completing the examples of challenging

A number of scenarios were introduced earlier to illustrate topics for challenging and this section goes on to complete scenarios B to H. There are a lot of examples but course members have found them useful for reference. A note about the tone of these examples: we have often used these scripts as role-plays on courses: group members analyse them and enact them as play-readings to trigger discussion. We have found that when we do not write 'gently' in the scripts, the people role-playing the clinical supervisors usually read the words harshly, which changes the whole tenor of the dialogue. While there can be a tendency to overact in role-plays on any courses, this harshness has been especially consistent on most supervisor skills courses and discussion shows that there is a strong assumption that challenging is harsh. We have left the 'gently' instruction in all these examples, which may seem excessively repetitive, but is to emphasize the intended tone while you are reading.

Scenario B. In this example the clinical supervisor, corrects the supervisee's mistake.

> To recap: Brenda is a staff nurse on an accident and emergency unit, who recently returned to work after a career break. In her clinical supervision she is reflecting on another issue when, in passing, she mentions that she was about to show a student how to treat a patient with hypothermia with a space blanket, but couldn't find one. The scenario continues:
>
> *Toby:* (gently) You said you were looking for the space blankets to teach a student about hypothermia treatment?

Brenda: Yes.

Toby: (gently) We don't use space blankets any more, they've been proved to be OK for prevention but by the time people get to us with definite hypothermia, they're not effective enough.

Brenda: Well, that one passed me by. What are we supposed to do now?

Toby: It was a long time ago, but can you remember what we did before we had space blankets?

Brenda: Yes, we just had to rely on warming everything, blankets, oxygen, IVs and so on.

Toby: That's it, we're back to that, the studies have shown it's more effective.

Brenda does not show any curiosity about the evidence base for the change and does not mention anything about updating herself on this topic.

Toby: (gently) I think it's very important that you do some updating on this or patients could be at risk during this next cold spell and you could be teaching students the wrong approach. I'll let you have a couple of references if you like, to start you off.

Scenario C. This example does not appear to have a particularly positive outcome. The clinical supervisor does not have the authority to intervene between the colleagues (that is the manager's responsibility) but she fulfils her role in attempting to raise the supervisee's awareness of her responsibilities. It is possible that she has given the supervisee food for thought. In either event, the clinical supervisor has her own clinical supervision as a place for support.

To recap: Charlotte is telling her clinical supervisor Pauline about a conflict with her new manager. Charlotte does not see it as her responsibility to negotiate annual leave with her colleagues. The scenario continues:

Pauline: (gently) I can see that the change of approach is difficult for you, but I think that your manager has every right to expect three senior practitioners to cooperate enough to organize their annual leave cover between them. What's the problem between you?

Charlotte: But I've told you, we tick along very nicely if we keep our distance. We just don't see eye to eye and it's best this way.

Pauline: How do you manage to cooperate for other things, like covering clinics if someone's off sick or having to deal with a client crisis?

Charlotte: Well, the other two box and cox between them, they both have their own large families and are for ever having to take time off for this and that. I'm single, I never have any sick leave and I don't have crises with the families on my caseload, I can anticipate them, I manage my caseload properly. So I keep myself to myself.

Pauline: (gently) It sounds to me as if there are some difficulties in dealing with differences in ways of managing your caseloads and in your different lifestyles and that leaves you quite isolated.

Charlotte: You could say that.

Pauline: (gently) Look, the session's almost over for today, and we don't have time to explore it, but I'm really concerned for you: I think there may be a crisis looming for you, because your manager would have the right eventually to discipline you and your colleagues if you do not get adequate cover organized for your annual leave, and I don't want that to happen to you. Will you think about how you can at least raise the issue with your colleagues?
Charlotte: I suppose so.
Pauline: (gently) If you'd like an earlier session than the one we've planned for next time, to talk it through, just let me know. I really want to help you to prevent this blowing up.

They finish the session and Pauline resolves to take this to her own clinical supervision as she is dreading the next session!

Scenario D. This example illustrates the importance of being prepared to break confidentiality in the case of unsafe practice that is apparently not being dealt with. Every qualified nurse should understand their own accountability when they become aware of any situation of risk and should be aware of the process of what to do, but we have summarized this process in the context of clinical supervision in Figure 6.6. Dimond (1998a) highlights the point that you are obliged to put aside any other considerations, such as confidentiality or wanting the supervisee to like you, and ensure the safety of the patient or the public with an appropriate level of urgency.

To recap: David tells his clinical supervisor Hannah about having witnessed a colleague repeatedly slapping a patient with learning difficulties. David has reported this verbally to his line manager who appears to have done nothing about it. He feels that he has fulfilled his responsibilities. The scenario continues:

Hannah: (gently) Do you really think that your responsibilities end there?
David: Yes, it's up to them now.
Hannah: (gently but firmly) David, it's really important that you take this further. You really do have a professional ethical responsibility to keep at it, to persist until the abuse has been stopped for good. You are also accountable for what you witness. Do you understand that?
David: Well, what else can I do?
Hannah: (gently) Can *you* think of anything else you can do to take it further?
David: I suppose I really should write something down. But I don't want to get my team leader into trouble.
Hannah: (gently but firmly) You've done the right thing in talking to your team leader and, yes, now you need to put it into writing. You need to describe exactly what you've seen and when you saw it and ask that it is investigated. Then give it to your team leader and if you don't get a response, send a copy to her manager.
David: Oh okay, I'll do it tomorrow.

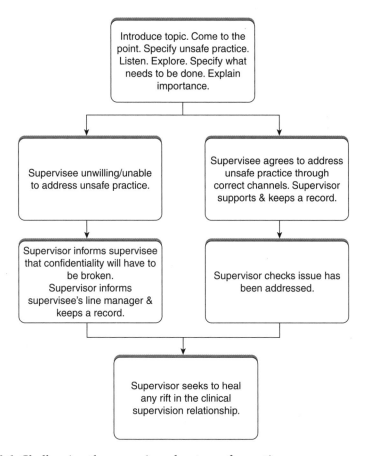

Figure 6.6 Challenging the supervisee about unsafe practice

Hannah: (gently but firmly) I know this is a really difficult thing to do and I'm behind you all the way. But it needs to be done now. I'll help you draft it if you like.

They go on to work out a letter and Hannah explains that she will have to use the 'exception to confidentiality' ground rule that they agreed at the outset of clinical supervision, in order to check that David's team leader has received the letter and that some action has been taken. They agree to bring the next clinical supervision session forward so they can debrief and re-establish their clinical supervision relationship. David leaves the session with the letter to hand to his team leader and Hannah telephones her an hour later to check she has received the letter. It turns out that the team leader has begun to address the issue with the abusive staff member, and there are other disciplinary issues involved but she is unable to tell David about them. She was unaware that the abuse had continued and is grateful to have the information in writing. This is the first time that Hannah has needed to do this and she is anxious about doing it correctly. Afterwards she anonymously telephones a professional adviser at the NMC and is reassured. If David had not agreed to write the letter, Hannah would have had to inform him that she would have to break confidentiality and contact his line manager and share the information he had given her.

Scenario E. In the next example, the clinical supervisor challenges procrastination over implementing action plans and seeks to explore the underlying reason. She brings what is happening between them in the present situation to the fore and links it to one of the supervisee's problems.

To recap: Evelyn is procrastinating about challenging a colleague who is not pulling her weight in the team. The scenario continues:

Zara: (gently) Your action plan was that you'd talk to Tiffany about this, but you've been putting it off for months. What's the problem?
Evelyn: Well, I couldn't face it. I've got enough on my plate at the moment without dealing with her as well.
Zara: (gently) Well, a lot of your time with me is spent on my supporting you with the stress of dealing with an unnecessarily high workload. I don't think you'll ever be able to manage your time properly until you've challenged Tiffany and you both have a more equal share of the work. What makes it especially difficult for you to challenge her?
Evelyn: I just can't face upsetting her, she tends to go really over the top.
Zara: It sounds as if it's verging on bullying. (Evelyn looks up sharply when she hears the word 'bullying') Would you call it bullying?
Evelyn: No it's not that bad, but she just makes a fuss and creates an atmosphere (Evelyn looks upset).
Zara: Have you ever been bullied at work?
Evelyn: No, I haven't, but ... (Still looks upset. Zara leaves a silence to give Evelyn a chance to speak but she looks down and stays quiet).
Zara: (acting on a hunch) Have you ever been accused of bullying?
Evelyn: Yes.
Zara: Do you want to tell me about it?

Evelyn recounts an event three years before, when she challenged a colleague who was not doing her share of the work. The colleague put in a formal complaint of bullying and there was an investigation that Evelyn found very traumatic. The outcome was that Evelyn was justified in challenging the colleague and she was not found to have bullied but that she had been overly aggressive in making her point.

Evelyn: Where I come from, we just speak our minds, but here it's taken as being aggressive. So since then I've just kept my mouth shut. (Crosses her arms and legs)

Zara: (gently) But that's not working is it, you've now got the problem of Tiffany. And last month you told me that your manager said he found you uncommunicative. (Evelyn stays silent)

Zara: (gently) We've got a complex issue here to think through. It's not only a matter of dealing with Tiffany. There's different cultural expectations. There's the difference between aggressive and assertive. There's the problem that your manager finds you uncommunicative. Which of those would you like to focus on? (Evelyn stays silent. Zara leaves the silence for some time in case Evelyn needs the space to think)

Zara: (gently) And now you've stopped communicating with me. Have I offended you?

Evelyn: No, it's not you, I'm just fed up with the whole thing.

Zara: (gently) Well, it is difficult but I'm here to support you and to help you think it through. (Another long silence)

Evelyn: You said something about being assertive. I've heard of assertiveness training. Do you know anything about it?

Zara suggests that Evelyn gets some information from her local authority adult education college and from a colleague responsible for professional development. Evelyn makes a firm commitment to follow this up. Also, in the meantime, they look in detail at what Evelyn could say to Tiffany. She rehearses how to gently but assertively approach Tiffany, considers how to deal with any over-reaction and plans exactly which day she will do this. She will also ring the clinical supervisor for support if she's tempted to put it off again. Zara does not usually offer extra contact, but on this occasion she thought it might help to set Evelyn on the right track.

Scenario F. This example shows the clinical supervisor bringing to the fore the supervisee's present behaviour towards him as clinical supervisor.

To recap: Fergus tends to describe a problem to his clinical supervisor Mohammed in a manner that implies: 'There it is, now see if you can sort it out'. The scenario continues:

Mohammed: (gently) You seem to me to be expecting me to come up with a solution to this problem.

Fergus: Well, that's what you're here for isn't it?

Mohammed: (gently) I'd like you to think back to the agreement we made in our first session in April. Remember, my role is to help you to think it through and come to your own decision, and yours is to take responsibility for that.

Fergus: But I've thought it through and I don't know what to do about it.

Mohammed changes to an informative mode and offers to talk Fergus through a problem-solving cycle, making a drawing of the cycle as he speaks. Fergus becomes quite interested and the session becomes productive. However, at the beginning of the next session, Fergus is late, seems grumpy and is still expecting Mohammed to solve his problems.

Mohammed: (gently) Fergus, I get the impression that there's still something wrong, this supervision isn't going as well it could.

Fergus: What do you mean. I'm here, aren't I?

Mohammed: (gently) Well, you're still bringing practical issues that you need to ask your colleagues or your manager about, rather than the reflective issues we discussed in our contract. And you seem to be increasingly grumpy with me.

Fergus: (opening up a bit) It's not actually *you.* It's just that getting the time and cover to make it to supervision is so difficult, it hardly seems worth the bother.

It turns out that Fergus feels overwhelmed with the pressure of his work and making the time to get to clinical supervision is a great strain on him. They go on to explore how Fergus can manage his time, asking for more help from colleagues and letting the manager know about some totally unacceptable aspects of his workload, rather than just struggling on non-assertively.

Scenario G. This illustrates the importance of the clinical supervisor having their own clinical supervision to support them in raising the difficult issue of diversity in the relationship.

To recap: Gamada has repeatedly brought topics to clinical supervision about conflicts with senior colleagues and his manager, who are white women. Although Catherine is of the same grade as Gamada, she is white and Gamada had little choice about having her as his clinical supervisor. Catherine is hesitant about discussing this with him. She is unsure whether there is any significance to the theme or whether it has to do with her own feelings about having a black male supervisee. The scenario continues:

Before she says anything to Gamada, in her own clinical supervision Catherine discusses her unease. There she finds herself recalling the experience of a close colleague of hers who had been accused of racism when correcting a junior nurse who was making errors. Catherine could see that the junior nurse was indeed making mistakes and it would have been racist not to correct him because he was black. It did not get as far as a formal complaint (as there was no justified case to make) but it was very unpleasant and Catherine's colleague was very stressed about it. Catherine wonders if this contributes to her feeling disabled in speaking about diversity issues with her supervisee. She decides to wait to see if his grievances reappear again in his sessions and plans how to respond. They do almost immediately, during the next session. After Gamada has ranted about being challenged for being half an hour late for work, she decides to test out her hunch.

Catherine: (gently) Gamada, I want to acknowledge your sense of injustice that you have consistently brought to clinical supervision sessions and I notice that it all seems to involve conflicts with white women who are senior to you. And I'm aware that I am another white woman, and may be seen to be senior to you. I wonder what you think about that.

Gamada gives vent to more feelings about the injustice of always being the subordinate to these people despite his many years of experience, his superior academic qualifications and even winning a national award for a project he ran. Catherine gives him a chance to air the grievances, which begins to clear the air: he becomes less spiky.

Catherine: (gently) Of course I'm not your actual senior, but nevertheless I am your clinical supervisor and you had only a take-it-or-leave it choice about working with me. I wonder how you feel about that.

They explore how Gamada felt about the lack of choice and the atmosphere continues to improve. Catherine is able to return to the point about the confrontation about lateness and suggests the manager was justified in raising it, which Gamada admits to be true. In later sessions, trust continues to develop and they are gradually able to discuss the diversity issues between them that Catherine had named, but which they both had sidestepped: their colour and gender differences. These are uncomfortable but valuable discussions and according to Gamada's accounts, his relationships at work also began to improve.

Scenario H. This example illustrates how a challenge can inadvertently uncover a personal problem which affects practice, and the need for compassionate emotional first-aid, thereafter returning to the purpose of clinical supervision.

To recap: Fran notices that her supervisee Holly (a nursery nurse) is complaining a lot about the parents she works with on a mental health mother and baby unit, whereas she used to speak about enjoying this aspect of her work. Fran has tried to explore this catalytically but Holly is going round in circles, seemingly stuck in a cycle of repetitive complaining and criticizing. The scenario continues:

Fran: (gently) I haven't heard you speak kindly about any of the parents today, just criticizing. You used to enjoy working with them. I wonder what's gone wrong?'
(Holly blusters, then bursts into tears and tells Fran about her recent miscarriage)
Holly: It all seems so unfair, some of these parents act as if as if they didn't really want their children, and people like me and Nathan really wanted to have a child and we're devastated about losing this one. I feel so stupid about getting upset like this, my mum says I'm over-reacting, lots of women have miscarriages.
Fran: (gently) You have a right to be upset . . . People often underestimate the impact of a miscarriage . . . And your work reminds you about it all the time.

Table 6.4 Pitfalls in challenging in clinical supervision

- AVOIDANCE – Putting off making the challenge until it is too late
- PUSSYFOOTING – Making half-hearted hints, over-using support and catalytic skills and never quite coming to the point
- SLEDGE-HAMMERING – Being too harsh, non-supportive and punitive
- SMILING DEMOLITION – Trying to soften a heavy challenge with a smile which contradicts the seriousness of what you are saying
- 'SMILING DILUTION' – Giving a gentle challenge with a smile and the challenge loses its importance; the supervisee cannot take you seriously
- JOKEY PUT-DOWN – Insensitive tease or sarcastic comment
- TALKING TOO MUCH – Saying too much for the supervisee to take in, repeating yourself and not giving supervisee space to react
- WIN-LOSE PUSHINESS – Inappropriate persistence in order to win and the supervisee loses face
- LACK OF FOLLOW-THROUGH – Inappropriate lack of persistence

Holly talks for about 20 minutes about her personal trauma and Fran shows her support by listening and providing emotional first aid. She checks that Holly has someone else to talk the problem over with (she has Nathan, two close friends and an aunt that she could turn to, though up to now she hasn't liked to trouble them). Apart from that, she does not probe into Holly's private life. Eventually she brings things back to working with parents in the unit.

Fran: (gently) I don't want to sound uncaring here, but I think my role in clinical supervision is eventually to help you think about how you can keep working effectively with the parents on the ward, in spite of feeling so raw about this. Are you ready to think about that now or shall I make you a cup of tea so you can have time out?
Holly: No, I'm fine, thanks ever so much for letting me go on about it, you've been very kind. Yes, let's get back to the subject.
Fran: (gently) What did you used to enjoy most about working with the parents?
Holly: Well, I suppose what I used to enjoy most was showing the parents how to settle the babies and to cuddle them calmly without jiggling them about a lot. It makes such a difference to the baby's sleep and to their relationship.

Holly has been able to collect herself and is able to discuss her work with the parents more positively. She plans to use her strengths more in working with them in the near future, and to accept more personal support from the people close to her. In this case, that's all she needed from Fran to get back on track.

Pitfalls in challenging

Most of the pitfalls in challenging arise from the clinical supervisor's own anxiety about doing it: the anxiety can be allowed to get in the way of steering a supportive mid-line between over- or under-doing it. This highlights the importance of having your own clinical supervision.

1. *Avoidance.* One of the most common pitfalls is avoidance of challenging and we have highlighted in Chapter 2 and elsewhere how widespread this is and that it is a serious concern within the nursing profession as a whole. It needs to be reiterated that supportive challenging between nurses should be the norm and this includes during clinical supervision. While you are likely on many occasions, using your support and catalytic skills, to enable the supervisee to come to a realistic self-assessment, there comes a point when you need to be prepared to challenge.
2. *Pussyfooting.* In other words, making half-hearted hints, over-using support and catalytic skills and never quite coming to the point. If you hear yourself waffling, pause and start again. This time start off the challenge with 'I'll come to the point … '. If the best time for the challenge has passed, you might still retrieve the situation by going back to the point, for example: 'I've been thinking about what you said earlier about … '.
3. *Sledge-hammering.* This is the opposite: being too harsh, non-supportive and punitive. Sometime this happens because the clinical supervisor has pussyfooted and built up such a level of tension that her belated challenge comes out too strongly. Alternatively, the situation might remind her of something difficult that she herself has experienced. This especially highlights the need for clinical supervisors to have their own supervision.
4. *Smiling demolition.* Inappropriate smiling can result from your nervousness: 'smiling demolition' is when you try to soften a heavy challenge with a tense smile the supervisee can interpret as your enjoying their discomfort.
5. *Smiling dilution.* This is when you give a challenge with a smile which contradicts the seriousness of what you are saying. The challenge loses its importance and the supervisee cannot take you seriously.
6. *Jokey put-down.* In an attempt to make the challenge with a light touch, use of humour may end up as a jokey put-down, insensitive tease or sarcastic comment.
7. *Talking too much.* Your anxiety may make you say too much for the supervisee to take in, repeating yourself and not giving the supervisee space to react. If you have a tendency towards this pitfall, it might be helpful to practise giving hypothetical challenges, or to pre-rehearse for a real situation, if you have time.
8. *Win-lose pushiness.* The clinical supervisor's determination to get the issue tackled may lead to 'win-lose pushiness', until she has won and the supervisee has lost face. A more forceful version of this can turn

into bullying. To avoid this pitfall, remember that the purpose of the challenge is to raise awareness and support the supervisee towards change. Developing increased awareness and changing usually take time, so try to give the supervisee space to reflect. If the issue is not urgent, be prepared to drop it temporarily until the supervisee is more ready to work with it.

9. *Lack of follow-through.* On the other hand, lack of persistence and follow-through may happen through timidity, over-sympathizing or allowing yourself to be side-tracked by a supervisee who responds to challenge by trying to divert you away from the point. One way to avoid this is to hold the issue in your mind when the discussion moves on, and to come back to it when appropriate.

10. *Blame.* This is about forcing the supervisee to take responsibility in a punitive way, with no underlying support to manage the shame of making a mistake and no support to rectify and learn from it.

Note that there are also some starter phrases which include challenges in the section on self and peer review in Chapter 7.

Summary

We have given challenging skills a lot of attention in this chapter because nurses often tell us they feel under-skilled in this area and ask for guidance. Equally important is the fact that managers and practitioners are justifiably concerned about risk management and accountability issues when clinical supervision has such well-defined boundaries that leave them feeling shut out and when the clinical supervision ethos seems to emphasize the facilitative and appears to ignore the authoritative elements. We hope that we have set the record straight here and in the code of practice we propose in Chapter 10.

As a clinical supervisor or member of a clinical supervision group, your use of your skills in giving information, advice and challenge arises from your authority as a professional nurse and colleague and is non-hierarchical. The authoritative approach, when linked appropriately with support and catalytic skills, allows for an appropriate symmetry in the clinical supervision relationship that is a fundamental part of the working alliance that we advocated in Chapter 3.

7 Skills of group clinical supervision

Group clinical supervision is advanced clinical supervision. When group members have the skill, time and commitment to attend, group supervision can be even more valuable than one-to-one supervision: intensely supportive, stimulatingly challenging, creatively reflective, full of ideas and information. You can learn an enormous amount from each other's in-depth reflection.

For it to be effective, all group members need to have developed the skills of being a supervisee, a clinical supervisor and a group participant, and the facilitator needs to have group facilitation skills. The 'frame' for a clinical supervision group needs to be even more rigorously set up than one-to-one clinical supervision because:

- the issue of self-disclosure is magnified: many nurses find it more difficult to self-disclose in a group setting as opposed to one-to-one;
- there is more potential for confidentiality leaks;
- the dynamics of the clinical supervisor–supervisee relationship are more complex since each group member is a clinical supervisor to the others in the group;
- the dynamics of the group as a whole is an added layer of complexity;
- the practical issues of commitment and attendance are greater than in one-to-one supervision.

This chapter looks at the skills required to be a participant in, and to be the facilitator of, a clinical supervision group, but it cannot stand alone: the skills involved in building the working alliance and being a supervisee and clinical supervisor, which we examined in Chapters 3, 4, 5 and 6, are as important in group clinical supervision as they are in one-to-one supervision. As a member of a clinical supervision group, you are building multiple clinical supervision relationships: with each of the other group members, with the facilitator and with the group as a whole. Given that any group develops its own identity, its whole becoming more than just the sum of its parts, you will have a sense of the group as an entity in itself and will also have a relationship with 'the group' which is over and above the relationships you have with individual members. Many of the psychological processes outlined in Chapter 2 also apply to this relationship and can help or hinder its effectiveness, with the added layer of group dynamics to complicate the relationship even further. If the aim of a group is to study these group dynamics, then most of the activity of the group is unstructured, to allow these issues to surface and be enacted. The main purpose of a clinical supervision group is not to study group dynamics; therefore we suggest some structures which aim to help you acknowledge some of the complexity of the group clinical supervision working alliance, and minimize the potential for deeper issues to sabotage the work of the group.

This chapter offers frameworks for understanding and building group skills and some structures for carrying out group clinical supervision that are intended to enable you to work with your clinical supervision group members towards building a secure enough psychological base for effective clinical supervision to take place (see Figure 7.1).

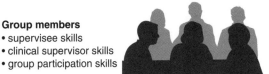

Group members
• supervisee skills
• clinical supervisor skills
• group participation skills

Facilitator
• clinical supervisor skills
• group participation skills
• group facilitation skills

Figure 7.1 Skills needed for effective clinical supervision in a group

Defining group clinical supervision

To begin we wish to clarify what group clinical supervision is and what it is not. First, misunderstandings can occur about the concept of a 'group'. We define a 'group' as: three or more people who come together and interrelate cooperatively with each other towards their common purpose. Therefore, a clinical supervision group is: three or more people who come together and interrelate cooperatively with each other towards their common purpose of giving and receiving clinical supervision (see Figure 7.2). We provide an expanded definition later in this chapter.

For instance, in Room 1, five people are sitting in a circle receiving information from the speaker about Trust guidelines for clinical supervision. They are not a *group*: they are an audience sitting in a circle. There is no interaction towards that common purpose: this is a briefing meeting. We are not suggesting there is anything wrong with briefing meetings – combined with written handouts, they are an effective method of passing on information within an organization, but they are not a clinical supervision group.

In Room 2, five people are sitting in a circle waiting for their turn to have clinical supervision-type attention from the leader. Again, they are not a *group*: they are in the same place for the same purpose (to get clinical supervision), but they are not interrelating specifically towards that goal. This is one-to-one supervision with an audience. The value in this method lies in being a one-off demonstration or masterclass, but it is not appropriate for ongoing clinical supervision: it is a time-consuming way to provide one-to-one clinical supervision.

In contrast, in Room 3, five people are meeting and communicating with each other by taking turns to be the supervisee and using the skills, knowledge,

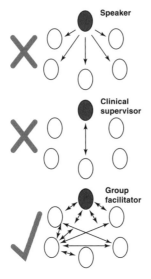

Briefing meeting
The speaker is presenting information to an audience who happen to be sitting in a circle.
This is not group clinical supervision.

One-to-one clinical supervision with an audience
The leader is the clinical supervisor and is providing clinical supervision for each person in turn, while the others listen and wait their turn.
May be useful as a demonstration during training.
This is not group clinical supervision.

Group clinical supervision
The group members take turns to share an issue and reflect on it, with supportive, catalytic, challenging and informative help from other group members. The facilitator facilitates the process of group interaction.

Figure 7.2 Interaction in group clinical supervision

experience and qualities of all those present who all cooperate together as clinical supervisors to provide clinical supervision for each person. When each person takes their turn they have at least 45 minutes. This is a clinical supervision group.

A second misunderstanding can relate to the nature of the collaborative work a group does together. We have found that some groups which meet for professional purposes have been mistakenly dubbed clinical supervision, when the work they do together, though valuable, is not actually clinical supervision. For instance, an intensive therapy team which meets to debrief after a traumatic incident on the unit may be doing something essential for the mental health of staff members and for the cohesion of the team, but they are not a clinical supervision group because the sessions are not regular and individuals do not have an hour or so of air time each. A group of health visitors who work in isolated rural GP surgeries meet to make human contact, give each other general support, share information about organizational issues and discuss current topics of concern in the profession: they may be having very valid, necessary and constructive meetings, but they are not a clinical supervision group because they are not taking turns to have facilitated in-depth reflection on practice. A group of mental health nurses who are working with a group analyst as facilitator may be learning a lot about group dynamics, especially about unconscious processes in groups, but they are not a clinical supervision group because, again, they are not taking turns to have facilitated in-depth reflection on practice. A group of staff nurses and students who meet when they are able, during quiet spells in the afternoon, to share their reading of the nursing journals, may be functioning very well as a journal group, but they are not a clinical supervision group.

To become clinical supervision groups, these groups would have to have a more regular pattern of planned meetings, fixed months ahead. The membership of each group would need to be fixed in order that there is enough continuity to allow the group members' relationships with each other to develop into a secure enough psychological base. The actual work done together would have to change so that each person gets at least 45 minutes for in-depth reflection on their own practice and on the part they as individuals play in the complexities and quality of that practice, facilitated in that reflection by the supportive, catalytic, challenging and informative interventions of the other group members.

So, our definition of a clinical supervision group is: three or more people form a fixed membership group and have planned, regular meetings in which each person does in-depth reflection on complex issues relevant to their own practice and on the part they as individuals play in the quality of that practice, facilitated in that reflection by the other group members who cooperate as joint clinical supervisors.

Skills of group participation

In addition to advanced skills in being a supervisee and clinical supervisor, members of a clinical supervision group also need to have advanced skills in being a group participant. It cannot be assumed that every nurse has the ability to be an effective member of a group which is as rigorous as clinical supervision and which involves so much self-disclosure. In order to highlight these group skills, we have adapted two frameworks which describe aspects of group dynamics. Firstly, a framework adapted from Johnson and Johnson (2008) which focuses on impulse management (see Figure 7.3). It suggests that you are using the skills of managing your individualistic, competitive and cooperative impulses, and

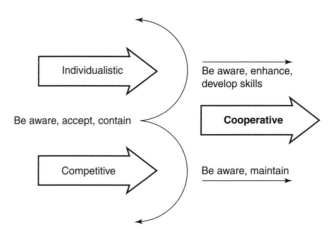

Figure 7.3 Managing your own impulses as a group participant

using predominantly collaborative skills in your communication with others in the group.

Managing your goals and impulses as a clinical supervision group member

It is important to be aware of your own individual goals in attending the group and of the impulses which lead you towards those goals. Each type of goal plus its impulse is termed a 'goal structure'. Johnson and Johnson (2008) describe three categories of goal structure: cooperative, individualistic and competitive. They suggest that each person brings all three to any group to which they belong, whether that person is aware of them or not.

- *Cooperative goal structure.* Your individual goal is similar to everyone else's in the group, and your goal is not achieved if others do not achieve theirs (e.g. to receive and give effective clinical supervision). Your impulse will therefore be towards ensuring that you have your air time and some useful facilitation from others, and that this is reciprocated with everyone in the group. This explains why it is humanly impossible to be cooperative if you are attending a group meeting unwillingly, do not understand the purpose of the meeting or disagree that the purpose is a valuable use of your time.
- *Individualistic goal structure.* This is when your individual goal is not related to anyone else's and you achieving yours does not depend on others achieving theirs (e.g. to satisfy your curiosity about what is happening in another unit and find out if the rumours you have heard are true). Your impulse would be towards diverting the interaction away from clinical supervision into having a gossip session instead.
- *Competitive goal structure.* Your individual goal is only achieved if others do not achieve the same (e.g. to be seen as the one who is best at something, such as knowing the most models of clinical supervision, thinking of solutions to problems or asking the most clever questions). Your impulse would be not so much to help the person having air time for their problem, but to find an opening in which to insert your competitive comment.

The skills of an effective group participant are those of awareness, acceptance and selective impulse containment and enhancement (see Figure 7.3). Being aware of your own goals and impulses goes hand in hand with self-acceptance: every human being has these impulses and goals and you are not a bad person if you become aware of your negative ones. You can use your awareness to enhance and give full rein to your cooperative goals and impulses for your own and the group's benefit, while containing your individualistic and competitive ones. A group participant who is unable to contain their individualistic and competitive urges will damage the group and render it ineffective. A group analytic therapy group is an appropriate and useful setting to give free rein to these impulses, but a clinical supervision group is not.

Next we will look at how you can enhance and maintain your cooperative impulses as a group participant.

Skills of cooperation

To set the context of the group participation skills that we suggest are important for cooperation in a group, we need to consider the dynamics of an effective clinical supervision group. There are many phase theories which describe the energy phases of groups, and Jacques (2000) provides a good overview of a wide range of them (but beware of playing competitive 'let's see who knows the most group dynamics theories' games!). Our clinical supervision version simplifies the main phases referred to by most of the theorists. We find there are three main enabling phases which support the collaborative clinical supervision work of an effective clinical supervision group: first, settling, then energizing, then, after the collaborative clinical supervision work, completing (see Figure 7.4).

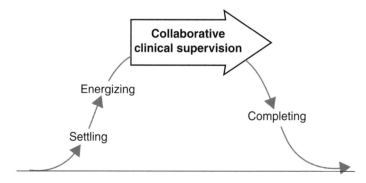

Figure 7.4 The enabling phases of an effective clinical supervision group

If these enabling phases are effectively attended to by the group, then the quality of the collaboration and the work of the group towards its purpose is greatly enhanced. Collaboration goes wrong when the enabling phases are not attended to.

There are also many role theories which describe the various roles that group members can take in a group. Belbin's (2010) is probably the most widely quoted, though it is most useful when applied to work teams of 8 to 10 people. Randall and Southgate (1980) incorporate role theory into their phase theory. They suggest that individual group members are each likely to have a tendency to contribute more at one or other of the phases of group energy. We adapt their framework here. As a clinical supervision group participant, it can be useful to clarify your own tendency and to take this into account when working in your group: that is, do you have more skills in 'settling', 'energizing' or 'completing'?

Settlers

People who are predominantly skilled at settling tend to be good at the skills of establishing and maintaining relationships. They are the people who make sure that people get welcomed and introduced and help people feel included in what's

Table 7.1   Examples of additional ground rules for group clinical supervision

---

1. *Confidentiality:* the ground rule outlined in Chapter 4 is augmented by the clause that anything personal which anyone shares is kept confidential to the context in which it was disclosed, i.e. any work in pairs or subgroups is kept to that context and not disclosed in the whole group, unless permission is given to pass it on. There are two exceptions: disclosure of unsafe or illegal practice
2. *Autonomy and choice:* each person can decide for themselves how much to disclose or keep private and can stop any process that is causing undue pressure on them
3. *Speaking for self:* trying to speak in the first person, i.e. 'I think/feel/find in my experience...' rather than 'you', 'one' or 'we' when speaking about own opinions, feelings and experiences
4. *No put-downs:* no judgements about other colleagues' personalities, feelings, shared experiences, vulnerabilities
5. *Commitment:* making the group clinical supervision sessions a priority and bending over backwards to make the necessary arrangements to attend punctually each time, sending a message if unable to do so. Also, being willing to take what is, for you, some risk in speaking up in the group, and being prepared to feel somewhat awkward at times in order to try something different and so to learn
6. *Reciprocity:* each person taking part agrees to take their turn to be both giver and recipient of clinical supervision

---

going on: they chat easily and the group relaxes. Settling skills include checking that everyone understands the purpose of the group, and establishing and maintaining ground rules (such as those in Table 7.1). They also include clarifying what resources are needed and available for doing the work together, offering relevant new information needed for the collaborative work and ensuring everyone understands it. Suggesting a plan or 'order of play' as a framework for the group's activity and providing 'tools' to help people grasp what is going on are both settling skills. People skilled at settling are able to influence other group members through sharing useful information and through their openness. They are easy to get to know in a group, being comfortable with the skills of self-disclosure and of listening to others non-judgementally.

However, if the 'settlers' in a group are in a majority, or are especially influential and the settling phase goes on too long, then the group atmosphere becomes too comfortable. It can degenerate into non-productive, cosy chat and eventually the group energy falls flat. People feel smothered, there is avoidance of nitty-gritty discussion and a fear of rocking the boat through disagreement or surfacing conflict. There is little motivation to get the work done so the group action is half-hearted, if done at all. This atmosphere is unhelpful in clinical supervision, as you need to stay alert to each other's areas of practice that need developing and especially be willing to challenge unsafe practice.

If you are skilled at settling, your initiatives are very much needed in the establishment of the group, when people do not know each other well and are especially nervous. Your taking a lead near the beginning of each group session will be useful, to help everyone put aside the busy-ness of activities before the session and settle into being a group again. During the other phases of the group, your contributions can continue to remind the group of its purpose and ground rules, and your ability for self-disclosure and listening can oil the wheels of real communication. Look out for any tendency to 'mother hen' the group: if you are encouraging the group to linger over or slide back into a cosy settling phase, then sit back and let the 'energizers' take more of a lead, however uncomfortable this might make you feel.

Energizers

Skilled energizers are likely to feel impatient with the settling phase and want to get on with things. They do not like sitting around gently chatting and want to charge the group with energy. Energizing skills include being able to excite a meeting with enthusiasm and being full of ideas and creative possibilities. They also include being able to stimulate some creative tension through playing 'devil's advocate', stirring up some indignation in the less energetic until they take a more active part. Making logical and intuitive connections and formulating and articulating arguments are energizing skills, along with the quality of being not easy to put down. Skilled energizers are able to influence other group members through reasoned argument, persuasion and impassioned speeches. They can usually assert their own needs, for example, for air time, and can be good advocates for others in the group who are less assertive.

However, if people predominantly skilled at energizing dominate the proceedings, the more reflective people give up when they can't get a word in edgeways or when their constructive contributions are undermined or shouted down by compulsive 'devil's advocates'. There can be too much non-focused discussion, with ideas going in too many different directions and some group members becoming overwhelmed by it all. The quality of listening falls and some people get locked in endless argument while those who attempt to break the cycle get attacked for their efforts. A cold atmosphere develops and there's a reluctance to attend next time. Again, the task of the group does not get done with full cooperation and is therefore not done properly, if at all.

If you are skilled at energizing, your input is very much needed in the energizing phase of the group, but try not to jump in too near the beginning or get too carried away during the energizing phase. Attempt to focus your and the group's energy onto the task of effective clinical supervision or, if you find it hard to get focused, allow others to do this. Your contribution in any of the other phases can be helpful to keep the energy going or move along a group that becomes stuck. The combination of skilled settlers and energizers taking leadership roles in the group can make for a very positive and energetic start, and the collaboration in doing clinical supervision together can develop very well from this basis. However, when the main body of the work has been done, the completers can help tie it all together.

Completers

These are usually calm and reflective, and are possibly the quietest people in the first few phases of the group. They are the people who can see the totality of the work that has gone on and their group participation skills include clarifying themes, making summaries, clarifying decisions that have been made, drawing conclusions and making final links. Their 'helicopter' vision may lead them to see more clearly the process of the group and this can be useful feedback. They help to cool out a meeting and to clarify what has and has not been achieved. They may be able to suggest plans that need to be made for next time and a way of ending the meeting on a positive note.

In contrast with the other two enabling phases, we find that it is common in groups of nurses for the completing phase to be under- rather than over-emphasized. This leads to puzzlement for some group members about what was achieved, or feelings of being taken for granted. The energy is focused into rushing off to the next thing without finishing the group, and there is difficulty arranging further meetings while half the group are rushing out of the door. There is little regard for group successes and the group can become undervalued, with decreasing motivation to attend each time. In contrast, in academic nursing settings, there are often more completers in a group and the pitfall can be 'analysis paralysis' whereby analysis of the group's work and process is drawn out beyond its usefulness.

We find when working with practitioners that completers often undervalue and hold back their contribution. If you are predominantly skilled at completing, it is important that you push yourself forward at the appropriate time as your perspective can stimulate and clarify an essential part of the learning that is done in the clinical supervision group. During other phases, you can contribute positively by sharing your 'helicopter' vision of the proceedings, validating the way the group is working together or highlighting when it is going off track.

This framework for looking at roles in a group is not fixed: we do not anticipate that you will always use your collaborative skills in the same way every time your clinical supervision group meets. As you consider the three enabling phases and the roles that people play in a group, you are likely to find that you are able to contribute to more than one phase. You might find that your style of participation differs according to the people you are with or according to how you are feeling on a certain day. We suggest this framework as a way of raising your awareness of the skills you already have, the possible pitfalls in terms of your effect on the group's energy and flagging up some group participation skills that you may wish consciously to develop in order that your clinical supervision group can have an effective balance between the three enabling phases of group energy.

Skills of group facilitation

The person whose role is to facilitate a clinical supervision group needs to have more than the clinical supervision skills we outlined in Chapters 4, 5 and 6: group facilitator skills are also necessary in order to ensure that the group is effective. Our definition of a group facilitator is:

Someone who works with a group to enable the members to communicate and cooperate with each other towards achieving their common purpose. Hence the facilitator of a clinical supervision group facilitates the group process in order that the group members can each take a turn and the other group members cooperate as clinical supervisors.

Bentley's (1994: 31) definition emphasizes the autonomy of the group: '[group] Facilitation is the provision of opportunities, resources, encouragement and support for the group to succeed in achieving its objectives and to do this through enabling the group to take control and responsibility in the way they proceed'. The concept of a 'group facilitator' underpins the framework we are presenting here.

Some clinical supervision groups have a regular facilitator whose role is to facilitate the group each time and does not take their turn to receive clinical supervision: they have theirs elsewhere. The options for who should be this person are similar to those we have outlined in Chapter 9, with the added requirement that they should have skills in group facilitation. We emphasize that this person should not have any line management relationship with anyone in the group: our rationale for this is given in Part I. In other groups, members take turns to be the group facilitator. There are advantages and disadvantages in having an outside group facilitator or being peer-facilitated and these are also outlined in Chapter 9.

As a framework for examining the skills of a group facilitator, we offer an adaptation of Heron's (2001) modes of group facilitation (see Figure 7.5). It focuses on the question: who manages the tasks and the process of the group? In a clinical supervision group, attention needs to be paid not only to the clinical supervision that is given and received but also to how the process of communication and cooperation between group members is handled. Heron's model suggests three main options that you have as facilitator at any point when deciding what needs to be done:

1. To be directive and take charge of some of the tasks or process, *for and on behalf of the group.*
2. To be coordinating and manage some of the tasks or process *with the group.*
3. To be space-giving and let the group manage the tasks or process for *themselves.*

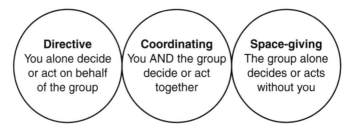

Figure 7.5 Three modes of group facilitation

The three modes are not static: you can move flexibly from mode to mode as appropriate, from moment to moment. Examples of this flow are given later in the chapter. Overall, a rule of thumb in clinical supervision groups is to move from short periods of being directive, in order to set the scene, to being predominantly coordinating, then predominantly space-giving when the group members become settled and able to communicate and cooperate effectively with little active intervention from you as group facilitator. You may need to become directive for a moment to remind the group of ground rules or to point out that they are going off the point. Occasional coordinating prompts may be needed. You may need to become more directive to keep people to time and bring the session to close, though the group can become responsible for these things in time.

There is no intention to suggest that any one of the three modes is 'better' than another: all have their time and place. Some nurses practising group facilitator skills can sometimes feel uncomfortable with coordinating or space-giving since they believe that they are not 'doing' enough in these modes. Others can feel uncomfortable with the directive mode since they believe that group facilitators should be totally non-directive, that a group should wallow or revel in the chaos until it finds its own level. Our view is that these positions are too extreme for clinical supervision, though appropriate in some other types of group. The urge towards too much direction is a common but mistaken tendency in a hierarchical culture such as nursing, and destroys the effectiveness of a clinical supervision group: motivation to participate and turn up to sessions diminishes. This tendency is a two-way process if the group facilitator is in a position of managerial authority over the group members: however non-directive the facilitator tries to be at the outset, the group members will tend to respond better to the more directive interventions and subliminally push the facilitator into being directive.

On the other hand, there can be an urge towards extreme non-direction in facilitators of some clinical supervision groups. This sometimes seems to arise from a backlash against hierarchical control in which the pendulum swings too far the other way. It can also arise from misapplication of some group analytic methods which are intended for group therapy, not learning groups such as clinical supervision. Again, too much non-direction can make a clinical supervision group ineffective and people lose their motivation to participate and attend.

Looking at these modes, we urge you to develop skills which allow for a flow between being directive and being non-directive from moment to moment when facilitating a clinical supervision group (see Figure 7.6). Two scenarios illustrate this movement between modes: Group Scenario A, with Lisa as facilitator and Group Scenario B, a clinical supervision group facilitated by Bryony.

Directive group facilitation

The group facilitator directs, does things and makes decisions for and on behalf of the group. They take responsibility for and make decisions about some of the tasks or the process. However, these decisions and actions are done with the intention that they will ultimately enable the group to cooperate more in working together

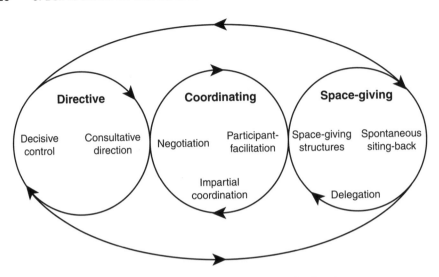

Figure 7.6 Flowing between the three modes of group facilitation

and therefore need less direction. So, for instance, while you may be directive in giving some necessary information, you keep it brief and you're careful not to project so much charismatic energy that the group members become captivated into becoming an attentive audience.

This mode can be subdivided into two: *decisive control* is the most directive, and *consultative direction* slightly less so. Decisive control is where you make the decision or carry out some action without any consultation with the group beforehand, perhaps spelling out take-it-or-leave-it options, maintaining your bottom line, insisting on something which you know to be important. This is all done in a way which gives people the genuine choice to accept it or not.

A. Lisa decides the venue of the first clinical supervision group meeting. It would be a waste of time for her to send memos to the group participants to coordinate their views on a venue: someone needs to get on with it or the group will never get started.

B. In a more established group, Bryony is facilitating a group clinical supervision session in which Karen is being disruptive: she is bad-tempered and is being negative about everything, including being destructively critical of one member of the group who is feeling vulnerable. Bryony has tried a supportive approach, giving Karen the chance to talk about what's making her so grumpy, but to no avail. So Bryony decides to confront her: 'Karen, it seems to me that your grumpiness and negativity are getting in the way of what this group is here to do. I'd like you to work more cooperatively, or at least stop hindering others in doing so, or accept some support for what's bugging you.' Karen sulks for a while, but at least the others are able to get on with the work. She later apologizes and during the following meeting is able to accept some support for the very considerable stress she is under in her job.

Consultative direction is when you collect and listen to information and views from group members and make your decision afterwards.

A. Lisa invites potential group members to let her know which dates they would be available for the first few in the series of clinical supervision sessions. She decides the best dates which suit the most people, including herself.
B. In the last few minutes of Bryony's group session they plan the next meeting (this group likes to have an 'order of play' worked out beforehand). She asks group members what their preferences are for the order in which they work. She bears in mind what they have said and then decides the sequence.

The pitfalls involved in being directive are to do with being directive too much or too little or in an inappropriate manner. Too much of this mode can result in a passive and dependent group (though sometimes they may be content with this, since it may be what they are used to) or a resentful/sabotaging group. Group members lose their self-direction and potential for cooperating together. Taking on an 'expert' role in group clinical supervision, perhaps by making a lot of clinical supervisor interventions, can leave the group expecting that you are there to do the job rather than to enable the group to do it for themselves: it can become a 'taking turns to have one-to-one clinical supervision, in front of an audience' format instead of true group clinical supervision.

Too much skilled direction of the group process can turn the group into amazed observers, marvelling at your skill and going along with you, but feeling that they could never do what they are doing unless you are directing them.

Your manner may slip into an authoritarian, aggressive, abusive, bossy, critical or patronizing style. Most of us have had plenty of such role models in nursing. On the other hand, you may develop a charismatic, captivating style and people are happy to follow you, or at least are unwilling to challenge your directiveness because they like you. This can be equally disabling of real communication within a group.

At the other end of the scale, your manner may be apologetic about being directive. This flabbiness can leave the group feeling sorry for you and going along with you to make you feel better, or irritated by your ineffectualness and likely to sabotage. It is necessary to be directive at times, and some facilitators feel they are failing when they are doing so, perhaps because of a legacy from the days when facilitator training veered too much towards the non-directive. Too little direction can create unnecessary confusion and lack of safety, and deprive the group of some of your knowledge and expertise or support and protection.

Coordinating group facilitation

Here the facilitator shares power, does things and decides with the group. You guide and enable collaborative action and decision-making. There are three main types of coordinating, in decreasing order of directiveness: negotiation, impartial coordination and participant facilitation. You can negotiate with the group, share your own views which may be influential but not final, and enable group members to negotiate with you and with each other.

> A. Lisa suggests an 'action learning set' structure for the clinical supervision sessions and receives comments. Two group members want to push the design away from clinical supervision towards an unstructured support group. Lisa spells out her bottom line, which is the need to have some pre-agreed structure, such as set amounts of air time for each person agreed beforehand, but she is willing to negotiate on other aspects, such as making the support element of the feedback explicit. Together she and the group adapt the structure to take in her concerns and those of the two group members.
>
> B. Bryony's group has degenerated from giving air time to one group member, Sam, into a general discussion in which no one is listening to one another, especially not to Sam. Bryony says, 'I get the impression that you're discussing red herrings and having difficulties listening to each other. Why do you think that's happening?' The group discusses this and eventually agrees that the subjects they are discussing are interesting but are diversions from Sam's problem and that their listening has gone down the plug-hole. Bryony goes on: 'I wonder if it's because the problem that Sam brought has shocked you and reminded you of your own limitations but that's too painful to admit? That's my interpretation of the situation: what's yours?' Bryony and the group discuss this and, in effect, negotiate a common understanding of the group process.

Impartial coordination is when you actively facilitate the group's interaction towards their objective, but you do not have any direct input yourself into the topic/task they are working on. This is often the official role of a chairperson at a meeting (though in practice the chairperson often loses impartiality and tries to influence the outcome). It is especially useful when facilitating in this mode to pay attention to the three enabling phases of group energy that were outlined earlier in the chapter and draw in or interrupt group members who have strong tendencies to a particular type of energy, according to the phase of the meeting.

> A. Some members of Lisa's group wish to finish the clinical supervision meeting early, so the whole group starts arguing about this. Lisa has nothing to say about the actual decision since they are progressing well through the plan for the session. She intervenes only occasionally to ensure that the quieter people have the chance to have their say. Then she points out to

them that they seem to have come to a decision yet the discussion is going round in circles unnecessarily.
B. Bryony's group has become stuck in gloom about Sam's problem. She asks Jean (who is usually full of ideas) an open question to refocus attention on the problem-solving cycle and actively encourages the other members to add their thoughts. She does not offer any answers to the questions.

Participant facilitation is when you take an active part in the process, sharing your own contribution as if you were a participant, not actively facilitating the group process but modelling good participation. However, you remain aware of what is happening in case you need to shift mode to get the group back on track.

A. Lisa's group is working in two groups of three at either end of the room. Lisa joins in as a participant in one of the sub-groups. However, she has her antennae out, having some awareness for how well the other triad is coping and she is ready to change mode if necessary.
B. At the beginning of the first meeting after the Christmas break, Bryony suggests people take a turn at describing their hopes and dreads about the clinical supervision sessions in the coming year. She takes a turn as a participant in this exercise by sharing hers.

Again, the pitfalls in coordinating are about using this mode too much, too little or in an inappropriate manner. Too much can waste time and effort when some direction is appropriate. You may be avoiding being directive (especially when challenge is needed) because you want to be liked. Conversely, not moving on to space-giving can result in your subtly maintaining some inappropriate control, while appearing to be caring. Your always being part of the process in such a likeable way can inhibit group members doing it on their own when they are capable. Too much skilled coordination can again leave the group amazed at your skill and dependent on you to coordinate their activities rather than move towards autonomy.

You might slip into a manipulative approach, 'facipulation', giving the appearance of enabling the group, but actually getting them to decide/think/act exactly as you want, without laying your cards on the table. A common example is when the facilitator is writing things up on a flip chart, ostensibly to collect the group's ideas but actually only writing up the points she had in mind. This causes cynicism and reduces commitment to participate.

Too little coordination can mean that the group is being directed too much or feels abandoned to get on with it, or swings between these two extremes, without the intermediate stage of establishing how to work together cooperatively with your support.

Space-giving group facilitation

Here the facilitator gives the group the freedom to find their own way, do the work of the group themselves, sort out their own difficulties, make their own mistakes and learn from them. Space is given for group-directed decision-making and action. This is not intended to be a laissez-faire option: you choose the time when they are ready and do not abandon the group to get on with it, but instead let them know where and when you will be available to them if they need you or want to draw you in. You have three main options in aiming to be space-giving: setting up space-giving structures, delegating some for the facilitation and spontaneous sitting back.

Space-giving structures give the group members the chance to work in pairs, small groups or in the whole group without your presence, but you need to be clear about where you will be so that you can be available in the room or nearby should they wish to consult you.

> A. Lisa is using a hands-off approach to the clinical supervision in her group. She has set up pairs, where the group members have a period of one and a half hours. After checking that they understand the task, she leaves them in privacy to take turns to have 45 minutes air time with the other taking the clinical supervisor role. She clarifies where she will be and that she will be available if they want some help.
> B. Bryony's energetic clinical supervision group are having some more problems: two group members, Pat and Eva, seem to have some unfinished conflicts to resolve and are taking up the group's time with irrelevant bickering. Bryony suggests that they have half an hour to sort it out in another room while the group gets on with its work, and report back to the group afterwards. Again, she is not involved in their interaction but she states where and when she will be available to help if necessary.

Delegation is a second option for space-giving. This is when you delegate some aspect of the facilitator's role to a specific person or persons in the group.

> A. Lisa identifies a time-keeper in each pair for the co-supervision structure and asks them to ensure that the pair have equal air time each and that they reconvene at the agreed time for the last part of the group session.
> B. Bryony's group has been discussing the issue of very differing interruption rates between the men and women. It is agreed that one group member will monitor the subsequent rates of contributions and interruptions for a set period, and report periodically, especially if there is a recurrence of the problem they had originally.

A third option for space-giving is when you spontaneously sit back when the group are doing fine without your intervention, or are quite capable of working through any issues that arise out of your lack of intervention. You maintain your concentration on the group process but you give your support through silent attention.

A. Lisa has been coordinating the sharing of what they have learned from their clinical supervision session that day. She says nothing for over five minutes, because the group are doing well at cooperating with each other in their sharing and discussion.
B. Bryony has been discussing with the group some of the problems they have been having in keeping to the point and in doing effective clinical supervision together. She stays in the circle but is silent while they consider what they have learned in previous discussions they have had with her about their group process and how they can prevent these blocks in their next session. They get tense but Bryony gives supportive space for them to work through it themselves. They come up with an excellent plan for the next session, that they own and to which they seem to be very committed.

The pitfalls of space-giving in group facilitation can again be described as either too much or too little of this approach or using an inappropriate manner. Too much space-giving may degenerate into a laissez-faire approach, abandoning the group without adequate preparation, facilities or support. This is likely to result in the group wallowing in confusion, misconception, ignorance, defensiveness, avoidance of the task, chaos, abuse, negative hierarchies or leadership battles. Too little space-giving stifles the group's potential. They become dependent on the facilitator to guide or rescue them from the inevitable difficulties of working collectively, and the potential creativity of a cooperative clinical supervision group is not sufficiently explored. Their sense of ownership and commitment to the task can diminish. The manner of your space-giving could be punitive. Your underlying message could be, for instance, 'So you think you know it all, then get on with it without me and see what a mess you make'; or 'If you can't be bothered then I can't either'.

Putting it all together

You will move between the three modes of group facilitation from moment to moment as you work with the clinical supervision group. Most of the time you will not be aware of your intentions or the skills you are using to facilitate. However, this three-mode framework can help you to focus your thoughts when planning and when things are not going too well.

A. During the first meeting of the clinical supervision group, Lisa identifies the areas which she considers need to be covered, including sharing hopes and fears, previous experiences of clinical supervision, aims of the meetings, ground rules and practicalities such as timing. She takes about five minutes to outline these and list them on a flip chart as a starting point for the agenda. (*Decisive control:* she's deciding they need to draw up an agenda.)

She then throws it open for discussion and asks the group some open questions to encourage them to react to her proposed agenda. She gets no response and the long silence is uncomfortable. She rephrases the question and still there is no response. (Attempting *negotiation:* she was aiming to get a joint agenda.)

She realizes that the group members are not yet ready to speak out in the whole group and suggests they talk in pairs about 'What I want from this clinical supervision group' and 'What we need to sort out as a group so I can get what I want', discussing these points together in privacy. (*Space-giving structure.*)

Bringing them back together, she collects points from each pair, noticing which points had an impact, from the non-verbal reactions of the other group members. She invites specific people who reacted non-verbally to say something: 'You looked interested in what Frank had to say, Barbara. What's your view?' Then she signals with her hand for Barbara to speak directly to Frank, rather than to herself. (*Impartial coordination.*)

The discussion gets underway and Lisa sits quietly enjoying the way the group are sharing their ideas, experiences and feelings. They go off the point a little but it seems important to let them get to know each other. (*Spontaneous space-giving.*)

After a while, Lisa summarizes their discussion, adds two points to the list of topics to be covered and starts a list of ground rules, writing in two that arose spontaneously during the discussion. (*Negotiation.*)

She focuses on establishing ground rules: 'Ground rules seem the most important topic for you at this point, so let's look at them in more detail.' (*Consultative direction.*) 'What other ground rules would you like to have?' She encourages people to contribute and writes up what they say. She adds one ground rule that she would like to have, then asks people to clarify a little more what they meant by each point, checks if everyone understands and then asks whether everyone agrees to the list of ground rules as their contract for working together as a clinical supervision group. (*Negotiation.*)

Lisa then suggests they focus on sharing experiences of clinical supervision (*consultative direction*) and invites each person in turn to let the others know what their previous experiences of clinical supervision have been. She takes her turn (*participant facilitation*). And so on.

B. Bryony stays silent while Karen, a senior sister on a cardiac surgery ward, recounts a traumatic experience. (Spontaneous sitting back.) Karen describes how the family of a seriously ill patient tried to abduct the patient against his will to take him back to their home country to die, becoming verbally abusive and threatening towards Karen and the registrar when they intervened. Hospital security staff and eventually the police were involved. Having heard the account, the group are stunned and silent. A few tentative attempts at support are made but these come out in the form of factual questions and do not seem to be experienced as supportive by Karen; in fact, she reacts rather defensively as if the questions imply that she has not dealt with all aspects of the situation.

Bryony manages to step asks the group, 'Having heard Karen's account of this very difficult situation, what strengths did you notice she used in dealing with it?' She then encourages group members to direct their explicitly supportive comments directly to Karen: rather than saying 'She did well with ...', to say '*You* did well with ... ' (*Impartial facilitation.*) This results in more explicit support and Bryony says nothing as they are doing well. (*Spontaneous sitting back*) Later, the group members seem to be using questions focused on problem-solving inappropriately, since all action had been taken and plans for the future are fully in place. Bryony realizes that it is more appropriate to focus on helping Karen to reflect on her learning from the experience: she suggests this and asks the group to bear in mind a 'learning from experience' cycle that they had used previously. (*Consultative direction.*) She then uses the framework as a way of focusing a question to Karen to help her reflect, and to help the group members understand what she is getting at. (*Participant facilitation.*)

Others in the group then take over helping Karen through the most appropriate stages of reflecting on the experience and on what she and her staff could learn from the perspective of a few weeks' hindsight. This goes well so Bryony sits back and says nothing. (*Spontaneous sitting back.*) And so on.

Some structures which might be used or adapted in clinical supervision groups

Action learning sets

An action learning set is made up of four to six people and a group facilitator who meet at least monthly for at least three months to explore the complex workplace problems or learning issues of each group member in turn, each meeting taking up one whole day. The set membership can be homogeneous or varied: all at a similar level in the same organization; all at a similar level in different organizations; a vertical slice through some levels of the same organization; a combination of people from client and provider groups; unidisciplinary partners in the provision of a service; multidisciplinary partners in the provision of a service; any group that feels it can work together in this way.

Background to action learning sets

Revans (1982) worked as a management consultant with the newly nationalized Coal Board, just after the Second World War. Engineers and miners were frustrated with expert-led change management and Revans set up action learning sets with mining engineers to increase the practical relevance of change processes, with considerable success. Although Revans found difficulty in gaining acceptance of the action learning approach in organizations and in higher education until the late 1960s, action learning sets are now widely accepted as a valuable approach to management and organizational development.

Meanwhile, humanistic psychology emerged as a 'third force' in psychology in the 1950s and 1960s (behaviourism and psychoanalysis being the first two). Humanistic psychology emphasizes the individual, subjective interpretation of experience and sees people as free decision-makers who can learn and change according to their own wishes. It has a particular emphasis on affective learning – i.e. learning about becoming aware of and constructively handling emotions rather than repressing them beneath intellect. 'Self-managed action learning sets' developed out of the humanistic psychology movement. It borrowed the structures of action learning sets pioneered by Revans to give a framework for a humanistic approach to learning, to be applied in educational as well as occupational settings.

Action learning sets are *not* useful when:

- participants require specific information from an expert;
- people attending are not motivated to learn, not willing to deeply reflect nor to disclose their vulnerabilities, or they believe that they have no more to learn;
- there are insufficient skills in facilitating each other's reflection;
- participants are authority dependent: they do not value learning from peers and are passively dependent on having a 'chalk and talk' teacher.

Typical format for a group clinical supervision session

This relates to the enabling phases we identified earlier in this chapter.

- *Phase 1* (settling and energizing): each person speaks in turn, taking a few minutes to share current top-of-the-head preoccupations, news, progress with any action plans made at the last meeting. Support and challenge are given to individuals about how they followed through their action plans. This phase might take about half an hour.
- *Phase 2* (collaborative work): each person in turn has the same length of time to have the attention and help of the other members. The person in the 'hot seat' defines how they can most use the time fruitfully and the rest comply as long as it is within their capabilities, ethics, any common agreement about content or process, etc. Each person has at least 45 minutes for in-depth reflection, and there is a lunch break.
- *Phase 3* (completing): about half an hour is spent on debriefing, reflecting on the process of the meeting, acknowledging achievements and learning, tying up ends, planning next meetings and ending.

The group facilitator is an outsider to the set and is experienced in group facilitation, though not usually with specific technical or clinical expertise in the area of work done by set members. She is a facilitator of the process and has no direct input into the problems which set members present to the group. She may give guidance on factors affecting the process of communicating and collaborating in the set. For instance, she might provide relevant theoretical underpinning of the process, structures for working together, guidance on how to be appropriately helpful to each 'hot seat' person and ways of understanding and dealing with process blocks and difficulties.

Two structures for use in Phase 2 of the action learning set

The first is the *present/observe* structure, which is useful with beginners, or in the early stages of a new clinical supervision group.

- The person in the 'hot seat' outlines her situation, e.g. 'These are my ideas for my project plan so far.'
- She then puts an open question to the group, e.g. 'What would you expect to see in my plan and how would you expect me to proceed?' She then sits back and stays quiet, taking notes, while the group discuss the question.
- Finally, she answers the question, 'What has been food for thought?', reflects on it and comes up with an action plan.
- She carries it out and reports back to the set at the following session.

The second is the *in-depth reflection structure*, which is the format to work towards. In-depth reflection is the essence of an action learning set.

- The person in the 'hot seat' outlines her situation.
- She reflects logically, intuitively and emotionally on what she has said, with the members of the set facilitating deeper reflection by supporting explicitly, being catalytic, challenging and being (minimally) informative.
- She formulates an action plan.
- She carries it out and reports back to the set at the following session.

The content of the work done by the action learning set

The opportunity that an action learning set provides is best utilized when the content of what is brought to the group by individual members includes most of these features:

- it is directly part of the individual's working life ('I am part of this issue and it is part of me');
- it is too big for tidy solutions;
- it involves complex issues with no single 'best' solution;
- it involves multiple factors and human relationships;
- it is a real-life issue which needs to be dealt with now.

The type of topics that an individual can bring can be agreed at the outset as totally up to each person on each occasion the set meets, or part of a joint work project or personal learning theme. For instance, members of an action learning set which is concerned with a change management programme in an organization will bring examples of complex problems related to that change programme. A self-managed action learning set which is made up of people on a professional training course might agree to bring examples of problems in applying the course theory to professional practice.

Guidelines for using the action learning set format for group clinical supervision

Group facilitator

Your task is to guide the group through the settling, energizing, collaborative clinical supervision and completing phases, keeping to the time limits agreed. Establish the sequence in which group members will take their air time. From time to time you might want to have an observer to identify the skills being used and the pitfalls. Allocate at least 45 minutes for the person to take a turn as supervisee and for the other group members to collaborate as clinical supervisors. If you have an observer, you will need to allocate additional time for feedback and discussion, perhaps 10 minutes. Ensure that the supervisee is given space and explicit support to outline the issue before people start questioning and that they are not swamped with too much questioning, advice, information, challenge, etc. Interrupt when this is beginning to happen. Ensure that the group work stays focused on the issue the supervisee brings, and that the exercise does not turn into a general discussion on the topic. If this begins to happen, interrupt and remind the group that each person will have a chance to have a say about their own personal involvement in the topic during the winding-down phase. Notice the interactions in the group, sit back if all is going well, or take part as a clinical supervisor if appropriate. If the group and the air time person seem stuck, raise this as a problem and suggest a way of dealing with it, or encourage the group to think of a way forward themselves.

Supervisee (or 'presenter')

Your task includes planning in advance to bring a complex topic which relates to your work in real life and upon which you'd like to reflect with the help of the action learning set members. Guidelines for choosing topics are given in Chapter 4. Explain your topic as clearly as you can, perhaps mapping it out on a flip chart to make it easy for group members to follow. Allow the group members to help you reflect in depth on the issue. If you find that you are getting overwhelmed by the number of questions or amount of advice, then say so and ask them to give you more space.

Other action learning set members as clinical supervisors

Give the supervisee space to outline the issue in their own words before you begin questioning. You can take notes if this helps you. Listen and show you are listening non-verbally and make explicit statements of support before you ask any questions or challenge. Use support, catalytic and challenging skills to enable the supervisee to explore the issue in depth. Refrain from giving any advice or information until later on in the session and only if it is wanted (check if you are not sure). Ensure that you do not swamp the supervisee by competing with other action learning set members to support, question, give advice, information, challenge, etc. At the end of the session give any notes you made to the supervisee or destroy them.

Observer

Your task is to sit back from the group and observe the supervisee skills that the person in the hot seat is using, the clinical supervisor and group participant skills the action learning set members are using and the group facilitator's skills. Identify any pitfalls and give feedback at the end.

Self and peer review

Self and peer review is a reciprocal process, carried out in pairs or groups, by which you:

- agree upon one aspect of professional life which you have in common;
- generate the criteria for effectiveness in carrying out this aspect of professional life;
- take turns to share your own self-assessment and receive supportive and constructively critical feedback from your colleague(s);
- make an action plan for development in this aspect of professional life.

Self and peer review was first described by Heron (1972) and has since been used in a variety of settings. Boud and Kilty (1983) provide guidelines for its use among teachers and researchers working in higher education. Heron (1981) describes its use with NHS regional education and training officers (educators of doctors) doing clinical audits. It is a model recommended by Pedler *et al.* (1991) for companies taking on the 'learning company' principles. The Institute for the Development of Human Potential pioneered its use as the assessment and accreditation method in its training of group facilitators, and various counselling training institutes have since adopted it. In nurse education, we have used it as a valuable adjunct to tutor assessments of students and staff appraisal schemes. Apart from in group clinical supervision and action learning sets, we have also successfully used it as a needs assessment and motivating tool for experienced staff embarking (initially unwillingly) on a staff development programme. We have also used it as a team-building tool, for bringing concerns about each other's work out into the open in a constructive and supportive way (see Figure 7.7).

Self-assessment is the fundamental element of the self and peer review process, indeed it is a most important component of any professional person's development: without commitment to your own learning and development, any

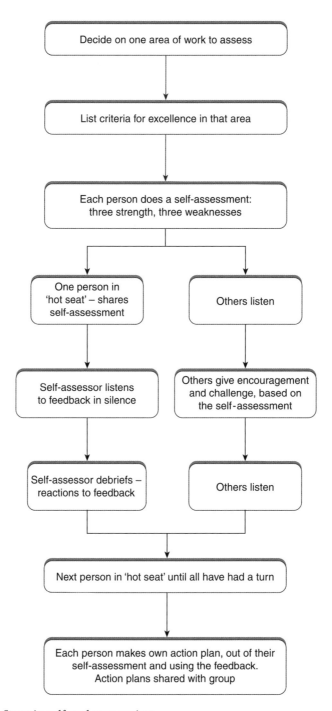

Figure 7.7 Steps in self and peer review

educational or management process imposed from outside cannot work. Clinical supervision which does not have this at its core is likely to have but transitory effects.

Gregory (1989: 2) states the aims of self-assessment:

> The aim of self assessment is to enable the person to integrate the ideal self (i.e. the fantasy of what I could be/would like to be, which tends to be unrealistic) and the denied self (our potential skills and gifted self which may have been suppressed in childhood and even in nurse training!) into the real self which is how we are and how we function within our socially constructed reality.

A structure for self and peer review in a clinical supervision group

1. *Decide which area of work to assess.* As a group, decide on one aspect of your work which all group members have in common.
2. *List criteria for excellence in that area.* In twos or threes, with a sheet of flip chart paper and felt pen, taking 7 to 10 minutes, make a list of phrases which would begin to offer answers to the following question: 'What abilities/skills/qualities/approaches/knowledge/attitudes/actions/results achieved make for a high standard of practice as far as (chosen area of your work) is concerned?' Be specific: rather than using one word, try to express each point in more than two words to clarify what you had in mind. For instance, rather than putting 'communication', put 'keeping colleagues informed about patients' changing needs'. Do not list descriptions of personality types; keep to specific abilities, etc. You do not have to agree with each other on each point: write all contributions onto the list, using one side of the paper only. At the end of the time, put all the lists together and display them so they are visible to everyone.
3. *Self-assessment.* Working alone, each person makes an individual self-assessment of their abilities. Out of all the criteria the group have produced, make a list of about 20 of the ones which you think are important. Reword them to fit your own words. Now pick out one of your strongest points from the list. If your confidence is having a bad day and you cannot think of a 'strength', then pick out something in which you think you are least hopeless! Then pick one of your weakest points from the list. If your humility is having a bad day and you cannot think of any 'weaknesses', then pick out one in which you are least brilliant. Then identify a second strength and a second weakness, then a third of each. Ensure that your list has an equal number of strengths and weaknesses. It is important to strike this balance: many nurses are often too ready to be over-critical about themselves and list more weaknesses than strengths. Others are afraid to admit to weaknesses. Working in a group where each person is revealing a few can help get over this reticence. Ensure that you do not choose or interpret any criteria as being about your personality: this is an assessment of

your *expertise* in the chosen area only. Write a sentence or two illustrating in concrete terms exactly how strong or weak you are for each particular criterion. Being vague is a common pitfall in this type of self-assessment. Vagueness can be a defence against challenging yourself to look at your abilities and weaknesses and making any concrete plans to change and develop.

4. *First person in the hot seat.* The next stage is to set up the peer feedback in the group. Plan the order of taking turns to be in the hot seat. Agree set amounts of time for each step. We suggest times here but more experienced groups may want to have longer. Taking your turn as the hot seat person, give the group your self-assessment (3 minutes). Then listen silently to the feedback for the agreed length of time (allow 1 minute per person giving feedback, so five minutes if the clinical supervision group is five people plus facilitator). Write down the feedback, or have someone else do this. Silently evaluate each item as one of three categories: (i) Valid – yes, you agree; (ii) Not valid – no, you disagree; or (iii) Partially valid – perhaps there's something to think about. Being silent can be very hard to do, since there is a tendency in most of us to explain or defend or to divert the process into a red herring discussion. If you find that the feedback is becoming overwhelming, with too much to take in, or is feeling unbalanced, with either too much cosiness or too much criticism, you can stop the process at any time. There is no purpose in continuing with something that is unhelpful. When the feedback phase is over, you can speak by way of a debriefing (2 minutes). You might want to say how you felt before, during or after the feedback, to describe your reactions to specific points or to the overall experience, or verbalise top-of-the-head insights that came to you as a result of the process.

5. *Next person in the hot seat.* And so on until everyone has had a turn. When you are one of the people giving feedback, listen carefully to the self-assessor and take brief notes of their self-assessment. Do not interrupt if there are any points you don't quite understand.

6. *Action planning.* When everyone has had a turn in the hot seat, each person takes time on their own to formulate a plan of action to develop not only each weakness, but also each strength (10 minutes). We find that people often tend to omit the latter in unstructured self-assessment. Be specific about what exactly you will do, when and how. Set realistic targets to prevent yourself slipping into patterns of negative thinking. Then get together again as a group and share action plans (5 minutes). Make a note of others' plans so you can review next time how they got on.

Giving feedback

During the feedback phase, link every piece of feedback in some way to the self-assessment. Give encouraging feedback and some challenging nudges to enable

Table 7.2 Self and peer review: starter phrases for giving feedback

Your personal reactions
– to your colleague's self-assessment, for
   instance:
'I liked most/least . . .',
'I agree/disagree with . . .',
'I notice you were more weighted towards
   the positive/negative',
'I am delighted/concerned that you
   said . . .',
'I'd like to encourage you to develop . . .'

Supportive challenging questions
– to give self-assessor something to think
   over, for instance:
"I wonder why . . .'
'Do you really think . . . ?',
'When did you last actually . . . ?',
'What makes you think . . . ?',
'Are you aware . . . ?'
(The recipient of the feedback just receives
   these questions silently and records them
   to think over later)

Constructive challenging feedback
Comment on action/approach, not
   personality, for instance:
'I noticed that . . .',
'I think/don't think that . . .',
'I get the impression that . . .',
'It seems to me . . .',
'I'm concerned about . . .',
'I felt . . . when you . . .', 'I wonder if you
   really . . .',
'I noticed a contradiction between what you
   said about . . . and . . .'

Exaggerated hunches
Exaggerate own imagination, mental pictures
   or perceptions, even if no specific evidence,
   for instance:
'I imagine that in such-and-such a situation you
   might . . .',
'If let my imagination run riot, I can picture . . .',
'My worst fear is that you would . . .',
'My highest hope is that you would . . .',
   'If I was your patient, I imagine that . . .'

Suggestions
– for instance, soft advice:
'Perhaps you could try . . .',
'One option/alternative/possibility could
   be . . .',
'You might try . . .',
'It might be useful to . . .',

or hard advice:
'It's very important that you . . . otherwise . . .',
'I strongly urge you to . . .'

Positive feedback
Comment on action/approach, not personality,
   for instance:
'I like the way you . . .',
'I valued/appreciated . . .',
'I felt pleased when you . . .',
'1 support . . .',
'You have a right to . . .',
'I noticed one of your particular strengths is . . .'

the self-assessor to think about doing something differently or changing their approach. Some forms of words by way of starters are suggested in Table 7.2. You will notice that most of the suggested forms of words are spoken in the first person: 'I think/feel', etc. This is important in this process. Speaking for yourself in this way acknowledges the subjectivity of your feedback, avoiding the pitfall of pseudo-objectivity which can make feedback patronizing or destructive.

Comments about your colleagues' personalities are not part of this process: you are giving feedback about their abilities, skills or approach. Often, when doing this for the first time, groups tend to be anxious and, contrary to everyone's expectations, become too reassuring and cosy, contradicting the self-assessor's identification of weaknesses. Think of your challenges as gentle nudges to help the person in the hot seat look at things another way and push their existing skills and competencies to even greater heights. Allow the self-assessor to identify their weaknesses and encourage them to develop their abilities in these aspects, even if you think they are already skilled enough. Overall, try to keep a balance between the challenge and support that the group gives, and end on a positive note.

After each hot seat exercise, note briefly the feedback that you gave and consider the extent to which each comment also applies to yourself.

Very occasionally, some groups can become gung-ho in giving too many challenges and not enough encouragement and support. We have found these are usually people who have recently learned how to be challenging and want to overuse their new-found skill. Where the group members work together elsewhere than in the clinical supervision group, sometimes the feedback session can degenerate into giving vent to criticism and frustrations that belong to other occasions and settings, and should be dealt with outside the clinical supervision group.

Reciprocal clinical supervision in pairs

Some clinical supervision groups resolve the difficulty of ensuring each person has enough air time by spending some time working in pairs. After settling as a whole group, you divide the time you have available in two, and during the first clinical supervision session one person in the pair is the supervisee and the other the clinical supervisor. Then at the end of the time, those who were clinical supervisors become supervisees and have their air time. At changeover time, you can either swap roles in the pairs or rotate with other pairs – we find the latter works better, because nurses have a tendency to let the first supervisee run over time and take up the second person's air time. It saves time to draw out the pairings on a board or sheet. For instance, in a group of six people:

Session 1: A is supervisee, B is clinical supervisor; C is supervisee, D is clinical supervisor; E is supervisee, F is clinical supervisor.
Session 2: B is supervisee, E is clinical supervisor; D is supervisee, A is clinical supervisor; F is supervisee, C is clinical supervisor.

This can be adapted to make training triads, whereby there is an observer with each pair. The observer's task is to sit back from the pair, out of the supervisee's line of vision and to note which supervisee and clinical supervisor skills are being used and identify pitfalls. The observer then gives feedback at the end. It is important that the observer does not become involved in discussing the topic, however interested they are. If the observer is part of the clinical supervision group, they should take a turn as supervisee and clinical supervisor.

The group facilitator can join in and take the clinical supervisor role when there is an odd number, or can visit the pairs or threes as an observer if that is agreed by the pair.

For the observers to get their turn as supervisees, there need to be three sessions, with changeovers in between. For this structure to allow some in-depth reflection, each person needs to have at least 45 minutes as supervisee.

After working in pairs or threes the whole group reconvenes to share action plans and finish the meeting together.

Some examples of clinical supervision group structures in action

Clinical supervision groups have adopted and adapted a variety of adaptations and combinations of these structures. The following examples highlight the need for close structuring and timing to ensure that clinical supervision does indeed take place and the group does not avoid the rigour of clinical supervision by sliding into general chat, open-ended support or abstract discussion. Examples of two groups are given here.

Group X, a peer group of six staff nurses from a number of different wards meet for two hours every six weeks. They each take a turn to facilitate the group, and the facilitator joins in with the activities. Each group member also receives one-to-one clinical supervision of one hour every six weeks, with a clinical supervisor who is not a group member. They have planned to experiment with various formats for group clinical supervision for the period of one year, and will decide then whether to continue with group clinical supervision and, if so, in what format, or to have only one-to-one supervision, but more often. They have had three meetings so far. For the last two meetings, their format has been:

Settling: news, progress reports on previous action plans, practicalities (10 minutes).

Pairs: two 45-minute sessions. Session 1: A is supervisee, B is clinical supervisor; C is supervisee, D is clinical supervisor; E is supervisee, F is clinical supervisor. Session 2: B is supervisee, E is clinical supervisor; D is supervisee, A is clinical supervisor; F is supervisee, C is clinical supervisor.

Completing: winding down, sharing action plans, planning next meeting (15 minutes).

A total of 5 minutes is allowed for changeover time between the various activities.

They have decided to try the self and peer review format for the next two meetings, so this format will be:

Settling: news, progress reports, practicalities (10 minutes).

Self and peer review: listing criteria (10 minutes); self-assessment (10 minutes); each person in the hot seat (3 minutes sharing self-assessment, 5 minutes feedback, 2 minutes debriefing) which is 6×10 minutes = 60 minutes.

Completing: winding down, sharing action plans, reviewing how they felt about this structure, planning next meeting (15 minutes).

A total of 10 minutes is allowed for changeover time between the various activities.

The next two meetings after that will have an adapted action learning set structure:

> Settling: news, progress reports, practicalities (10 minutes).
> Action learning set structure: one person (A) in the hot seat for 45 minutes, reflecting in-depth with the help of other group members.
> Next person (B) in the hot seat for 45 minutes, reflecting in depth with the help of other group members.
> Completing: winding down, sharing action plans, planning next meeting (15 minutes).
> A total of 5 minutes is allowed for changeover time between the various activities.
> At the end of the year, Group X reviews their experiments and decide on their structure for the next year

Group Y, a group of mental health nurses, five people plus outside facilitator, meets for two and a half hours every month. Every third meeting is half an hour longer to allow for a review of the atmosphere of the group, the way they work together and the effectiveness of the clinical supervision that is taking place. Their format goes as follows:

> Settling: news, progress reports, practicalities (10 minutes).
> Action learning set structure: one person (A) in the hot seat for 45 minutes, reflecting in depth with the help of other group members.
> Pairs and triads: two 40-minute sessions. Session 1: B is clinical supervisor, C is supervisee, with the group facilitator as observer; D is clinical supervisor, E is supervisee, with A as observer.
> Session 2: B and C reverse roles and have A as observer; D and E reverse roles, with the group facilitator as observer (total 50 minutes).
> Completing: winding down, sharing action plans, planning next meeting (10 minutes).
> Five minutes is allowed for changeover time between the various activities.

Group Z, a group of eight nurse teachers in a university meet monthly for three and a half hours. Their format is:

> Settling: news, progress reports, practicalities (10 minutes).
> Action learning set structure: the group divides into two groups of four, to take turns to be in the hot seat for 45 minutes, reflecting in depth with the help of other group members.
> A total of 10 minutes is allowed for changeover times, hot drink, loo break etc.
> Completing: back together as a whole group, winding down, sharing action plans, planning next meeting (10 minutes).

Pitfalls in group clinical supervision

Group clinical supervision is a complex process and there is potential for many aspects to go wrong. It takes a long time to do properly and it takes a number of people away from the workplace at the same time. If the process is not experienced as valuable, nurses will not prioritize the time to attend, therefore each session needs to make very good use of the time. The structures we have suggested may help do this. However, it may be useful to consider some potential pitfalls in order to be able to notice or prevent them.

1. The 'settling' phase turns into a general group discussion which takes up the whole session. No one gets a turn to present and reflect on her own topic.
2. Ai-li begins to present her account of the difficulties of managing a member of her team. Before she has finished her story, group members interrupt and ask lots of factual questions. Ai-li begins to feel she is under interrogation and retreats.
3. Brandon tells his story and the group members begin to give him advice. Then they start to argue between themselves about the various options. Brandon can't get a word in edgeways.
4. Chas shares a difficult situation about working with a client. Group members start to talk about their experiences, competing to tell the worst horror story. Tammy wins. The group becomes fascinated with Tammy's tale and forgets it was supposed to be Chas's turn.
5. Dorinda tells of her difficulties with managing conflict within her team. When she has finished, there is a long silence – no one wants to be the first to speak. Dorinda feels unsupported and that no one is interested, and says so. Eventually the group starts to tell her what she has done wrong, focusing only on the negatives. Dorinda is left feeling that the group was too negative and a waste of time (she can get better support elsewhere) and doesn't turn up the next time.
6. Eddie misunderstands the term 'presenting his topic to the group'. He gives a high-powered presentation about a project he's working on, using PowerPoint and other aids. The session turns into a lecture from Eddie. The group are so impressed by the presentation and handouts that they do not notice that there is a fundamental error in the way he is going about doing his project. Eddie confidently continues with his project oblivious to his mistake.
7. Feroza tells her story in about 5 minutes and asks for advice. She writes down the advice and finishes the session. The whole process took about 10 minutes and Feroza did no reflection or action planning of her own.
8. The group do not leave enough time for a completing phase, so no one can identify what they have learned from each other or how to improve

the process of the clinical supervision group. Dates for the next meeting are not clear and only half the group turn up next time.

9. Two members of the clinical supervision group get into a downward spiral about the workloads in their particular profession, and how 'things ain't what they used to be'. They both depress themselves so much that they cannot listen or allow others to have their say. They especially cannot allow any expression of optimism without cutting it down with cynicism. The group is not working and no one voices that fact. Few people turn up next time.

Summary

You will see that for group clinical supervision to stand on its own, without being combined with one-to-one, a considerable amount of time must be allocated to the meetings to ensure each person has enough 'air time' in which to reflect in depth on their practice.

We emphasize that group clinical supervision is not an easy, quick or cheap option: quite the contrary. We do not usually recommend clinical supervision in groups for nurses without also having one-to-one: meeting the need for continuity and sufficient air time is seldom possible. Creating a group of consistent membership, with the same people able to attend each time, is out of the question in most branches of nursing: it is just not possible to synchronize the availability of five or six people. It is seldom that cover for staff can be arranged to enable them to attend a clinical supervision group meeting of adequate length to allow each individual sufficient air time in which to reflect in depth. We examine in more detail the advantages and disadvantages of group clinical supervision as opposed to one-to-one in Chapter 9.

If, however, group clinical supervision is sometimes possible and preferred we hope this chapter has been useful in clarifying a picture of group clinical supervision, and has provided enough pointers for a new group to start or for an established group to review whether or not its structure is effective.

Part III

The big picture

8 Clinical supervision and clinical effectiveness: what works, what do we think works, what do we need to do to demonstrate it?

In this final part of the book, we wish to bring some of the themes together to focus on the practicalities, challenges and implications, for the organization as a whole, of setting up clinical supervision systems. The perceived benefits of this have been referred to throughout the book. It is time to explore if and how this has been demonstrated and what is needed to develop it further. It makes sense to have a systematic, rigorous implementation of a supervision system that places clinical supervision firmly in the picture alongside, but separate from, line management and safeguarding supervision. When this is done well it can enable staff to be demanding, thoughtful, more aware practitioners, who know what the shortfalls in the delivery of client-centred care are in their areas of specialty, as well as the strengths that need to be built upon.

This chapter explores how clinical supervision sits within the 'economy of care', so that purchasers can be clear about its benefits. In other words, what works, what do we think works and what do we need to do to demonstrate it? Chapter 9 assesses the ways in which managers and organizations can practically implement clinical supervision systems, and in Chapter 10 we consider what the future may hold and suggest a code of ethics and practice for clinical supervision, that empower nurses to have a stronger profile and be centre stage of health care delivery.

Nurses need more personal and professional confidence to take a more active role in innovative and clinically relevant health care initiatives that set good practice for improved standards. The rhetoric of all the policies and commissions that are advocating this will remain empty unless health care organizations and managers facilitate it with commitment via ordinary, everyday development mechanisms such as clinical supervision.

We are concerned that conditions for effective implementation will fade under the competing pressures not just on individuals but within areas of the workforce and organizations. We want to reiterate the themes of the introductory chapters: the need to ensure a balance in implementing the principles of clinical supervision and, in so doing, seek to diminish the adverse effects of resistant forces. Effective clinical supervision systems need to see a merging of practical endeavours from both those individuals on the ground who will be most directly involved and those within the managerial and organizational structure who can help enshrine them in the fabric of the culture.

> If clinical supervision is to get the sponsorship it deserves, it has to demonstrate to all stakeholders that things become much worse if practitioners lose their supervision time to other pressures and priorities. In order to do this, the Trust must ensure that the system it designs is focused on the contribution that it can make to health care in its widest sense, and to the metrics of cost, quality, service and speed.
>
> (Wolsey and Leach 1997: 24)

This extract from Wolsey and Leach was written the year the first edition of this book was published. We were not as impatient as those authors to see this happen at this time conscious of Butterworth's sensibly cautious reminder that 'it appears fashionable to make no progress on any new development unless they can somehow be tied to patient-led outcomes and evidence based practice, as though these laudable aims can be achieved overnight' (Butterworth *et al.* 1997: 186). Over 10 years on since the first edition, we hoped there might have been more rigorous studies, perhaps even a comparative or longitudinal framework, to make correlations between implementation of effective systems of clinical supervision and client outcomes. In Butterworth *et al.*'s (2008) literature search analysis, they describe work that may benefit professional practice and they also identify two 'new' messages. The first underscores the responsibility of health care organizations to sustain and develop clinical supervision and the second points to the potential benefit that clinical supervision may have to patient outcomes. Although this is rightfully demanded throughout many areas of nursing, the Commission on the Future of Nursing (2010) makes it clear, that although many examples of good evidence based practice do exist, illustrations from nursing are not as extensive as they might be.

So, what does exist in the literature on clinical supervision? There are numerous descriptive studies of small or Trust-wide introductory and established clinical supervision programmes, not only from the UK, but also from areas of Europe, such as Scandinavia and Holland, as well as Canada and Australia. These studies explore and identify key components of clinical supervision, and make best practice recommendations as well as highlighting factors to support effective clinical supervision. For simplicity we are going to be selective and give illustrations of some of these findings by dividing them into three main areas, along with small 'taster' examples to illustrate these themes. A further discussion will follow.

Studies focusing on the relationship in supervision

These are linked to the importance of reflective practice and its impact on professional well-being and job satisfaction, including self-reporting of improved competence and confidence, interpersonal relationships, reduction of anxiety, stress, burnout and teamwork. Many were very positive, and suggest that this improved satisfaction and focus could have a positive influence on staff retention, sickness rates and overall workforce resource implications.

Tasters

Butterworth (1997) describes a large-scale (23 sites) national evaluation of nurses using the Manchester Clinical Supervision Scale. They reported overwhelmingly positive results from supervisees: supervision had been beneficial and improved clinical competence and confidence. It emphasized a much needed opportunity for reflection and advancement of skills and support.

White *et al.* (1998) conducted an exploratory study, funded by the Department of Health and the Scottish Home and Health Department, over an 18-month period in 23 selected sites in England and Scotland. They also explored the experience of a small sub-sample of 34 nurses engaged in clinical supervision as supervisors and supervisees. Interviews were undertaken to help better understand some of the issues involved in terms of the domains of structure, process and outcome. Respondents reported an enthusiasm for the opportunity to talk meaningfully to a trusted colleague about their personal circumstances at work. Nurses who wished to reflect upon their own practice with clients, especially when dealing with their clinical conditions, which were upsetting, or otherwise challenging, and sometimes harrowing, particularly welcomed such opportunities. The study identified improved staff morale, strengthened relationships with work colleagues and reduced feelings of isolation as organizational outcomes. Supervision was deemed a recruitment incentive and 'a brake on staff leaving'.

Malin (2000) identified that clinical supervision improved team relationships and helped nurses to reflect on the care they provided. It enabled them to cope with change, to improve service delivery, to prioritize workload and be more focused in their clinical care.

Kelly *et al.* (2001) reported that 83 per cent of all staff in their study of community mental health nurses believed that clinical supervision relieves the isolation implicit in the work environment.

Williams *et al.* (2005) performed an evaluation of a group clinical supervisor programme and identified that the group had successfully developed a supportive environment, but an independent observer reported that there were minimal attempts by group members to challenge each other. Peers agreed to find ways of doing this.

Begat and Severinsson (2006) synthesized three studies to deal with the research question, 'How does clinical supervision enhance nurses' experience of well-being in relation to their psychosocial work environment?' The results suggested very positive influences on well-being and in turn on nurses' commitment to practice. The value of work becomes clearer when nurses reflect on themselves as professionals and as authentic human beings in supervision, and have this witnessed and responded to by their supervisor.

Cutcliffe and Hyrkas (2006) investigated multidisciplinary attitudes to clinical supervision. They surveyed 72 professionals from a mixture of nursing specialties and related professions and asked them to rank 17 statements in order of their perceived importance. There was unanimous agreement from all professions except the health visitors (due to their accountability for child safeguarding) that the most important element to clinical supervision was that confidentiality should be assured and agreed on. However, there was no further explanation of the confidentiality terms and when it would be appropriate for a clinical supervisor to discuss a clinician's work with a manager. There was also universal agreement that the clinical supervisory relationship must be separate from the management system.

Studies focusing on setting up systems to support supervision

These include standards, policy development, documentation such as contracts with clear roles and responsibilities, selection of supervisors, and education and training. Access, support and resources are key essentials for clinical supervision and are critical to quality health care practice. Many of the barriers identified in the literature can be overcome by having a practical structure in place to ensure effective clinical supervision.

Tasters

Jones and Partington (2007) document details of an action study in the development of a community nursing clinical supervision programme. Nearly half reported that it had assisted in a practice change.

Edwards *et al.* (2005) used the Manchester Clinical Supervision Scale with community health nurses in Wales. Those who had chosen their supervisor, whose sessions took place away from the workplace, and especially where sessions were over an hour and at least once a month, most positively evaluated supervision.

Barriball *et al.* (2004) report on an audit of clinical supervision in one Primary Care Trust. Data was collected by telephone interviews with 44 respondents from a range of professions occupying different clinical and managerial grades in the organization. Clinical supervision varied both in terms of its availability and management between different professional groups and teams, reflecting, in part, differing levels of motivation towards supporting clinical supervision by individual practitioners and managers as well as a perceived lack of Trust leadership. Respondents also reported several potential and actual benefits of clinical supervision, including the improvement and standardization of practice and the facilitation of learning and professional development. It was widely agreed that the introduction of mechanisms for monitoring both the process and outcomes of supervision, greater protection of time allocated for supervision and more training opportunities to increase the skill and number of available supervisors were needed.

Rafferty *et al.* (2003), in a rigorous qualitative study (using a modified Delphi technique, experiential and collaborative, collecting narratives from practitioners), developed provisional standards for supervision for clinical nurses and health visitors. These standards include: appropriate time, environment, contract, relationship, atmosphere; reflective interventions; retaining and recording; organizational support; feedback via supervisee; competency; maintenance of good clinical standards; enabling emotional competency, transition and change; collaboration; affirmation; prevention of harm; promotion of reflective practice; education about supervision; and focus of clinical supervision as a professional activity that is not disciplinary or counselling. It is noteworthy that the list of standards does not include any evaluation process.

Kavanagh *et al.* (2002) reported that trained supervisors were more likely to relinquish power by encouraging active involvement of their supervisees in supervision, than supervisors who had not participated in training. This is likely to support more confidence and autonomous thinking.

Kelly *et al.* (2001), in a pilot study of community mental health nurses in Northern Ireland, concluded that important training and education deficits exist at the interface between management and clinical supervision due to problems with resourcing. They reported that 81 per cent of the workforce was involved in clinical supervision but 63 per cent had not received preparation for the process. Of the 37 per cent who had, only 19 per cent had preparation in supervisee skills. Managers, supervisors and supervisees agreed that preparation for the role is essential and should be planned, and that without appropriate education clinical supervision may not be effective. Kelly *et al.* emphasize the importance of keeping managerial supervision separate from clinical supervision and the importance of confidentiality. They caution that any merging between the two roles would dilute an effective support system.

Teasdale *et al.* (2001) investigated the contribution clinical supervision made in the management of critical incidents, burnout and workplace support using three instruments: i) Critical Incident Questionnaire, ii) Maslach Burnout Inventory, iii) Nursing in Context Questionnaire. This study found no significant differences on levels of burnout between supervised and unsupervised nurses. However, the Nursing in Context Questionnaire results indicated that supervised nurses reported feeling more supported and demonstrated higher coping abilities than unsupervised nurses. This was more evident in the junior nurses.

Malin (2000) performed a small qualitative study to examine how clinical supervision was operating, its strengths, its weaknesses and where improvements might be made. The study followed the introduction of clinical supervision nine months earlier for nurses and carers employed in three community homes and one community multiprofessional team. The method consisted of direct observation of individual and group supervision and staff completing critical incident questionnaires, followed by semi-structured, audio-taped interviews with seven registered nurses and four community team members, including a social worker, psychologist and physiotherapist. Outcomes were expressed in two ways: in terms of the benefits of clinical supervision or of its ambivalence. The range of matters brought for discussion, or resolution, in supervision reflected some of the difficulties or dilemmas staff faced working in this area, for example promoting empowerment and assisting clients to make choices, and dealing with clients' challenging and inappropriate behaviours. As for the role of supervisor there was some evidence of nurses expressing apprehension or unpreparedness and a perceived general concern over the relatively low status of clinical supervision, thought to be due to absence of visible management approval or failure to articulate properly the objective of supervision.

Studies focusing on measurement of patient outcomes and clinical effectiveness

There is little research measuring direct client outcomes, although there is a lot of inferential reporting of the likely positive impact of other outcomes on this. There is a growing recognition of the importance of research to measure outcomes of both supervision preparation and the focus of the interaction, and its implications for improvements in practice and related clinical governance.

Tasters

Cutcliffe and Hyrkas (2006) agree that it is important to link the two processes of clinical supervision and management in local policies – for example, involving management in evaluation processes and service benefits.

Bambling (2003) investigated the impact clinical supervision had on psychotherapy practice and the outcomes of treatment for clients with depression. She hypothesized that a stronger working alliance would result, along with better patient outcomes. A total of 127 therapists were randomly assigned to three groups, one process-based, one skills-based and the third unsupervised. Measures included patient drop out, symptom scores, satisfaction and psychosocial stress, and Beck depression scores. This study concluded that clients who were treated by a supervised therapist, irrespective of the type of supervision, showed greater reduction in their symptoms, were more satisfied with their treatment and were more likely to continue with treatment than those clients treated by an unsupervised therapist. In fact the study indicated that a single session of supervision had a major impact on the working alliance between the client and the clinician. Although this is an example from Australia and from psychotherapy, albeit in a community mental health setting, we offer it as a method that could be adapted by some nurses.

Discussion

There are a variety of evaluation tools used within the studies, the most common being self-completion questionnaires providing quantitative and qualitative data (Teasdale *et al.* 2001); semi-structured interviews (Barribal *et al.* 2004); focus group interviews (Williams *et al.* 2005); Delphi technique (Butterworth *et al.* 1996; Rafferty *et al.* 2003); and existing evaluation instruments such as the Maslach Burnout Inventory and the Manchester Supervision Scale (Edwards *et al.* 2006). Action-based studies were rarer (Jones and Partington 2007), while randomized controlled trials, apart from Brambling (2004) are very scarce on the ground. There are also methodological difficulties associated with what outcomes to measure and how to measure them (Coleman and Lynch 2006), and suggestions of methodological flaws in much of the research, sometimes with no agreed operational definitions of key constructs (Wolsey and Leach 1997).

The bulk of the studies concentrate on the quality and outcome of the clinical supervision relationship and its focus. It is likely that improvements in the ability to reflect on and improve situations, improving satisfaction in both individuals and teams, will have an impact on patient outcomes, just as they are related to organizational gains in workforce stability. Each is interrelated and can impact on the other. It makes sense – or at least contributes to useful research questions – that there is a likelihood that improvements in nurses' well-being, connectedness to their work, stimulation and satisfaction can have a related positive impact on their relationships with patients and the meaning they can make together.

One thing we know from 40 years of extensive, replicated attachment research is that people who build more secure and consistent relationships *with* others are more able to replicate this *for* others. And we know that being able to depend on something secure as a back-stop and place to go in difficulty, breeds an independence and creativity of spirit and of mind, not a mindless dependence or cosiness.

We suggest that the occasional jaundiced or snide attacks in some of the literature which diminish the importance of more relational outcomes compared to 'proper' research may well indicate yet more defensiveness about the importance of these outcomes. Kavanagh *et al.* (2002), although not dismissive in tone, state that the literature on supervision is very light on good evidence since it has few randomized controlled trials and much of the evidence relies on rated feedback from supervisors and supervisees. We believe that we need to continue to explore the debate about what constitutes 'good' research. We know that at a national level 'good' can also mean 'what we want to prioritize and afford'. Hawkins and Shohet (2006) state that action research is the most suited methodology for clinical supervision evaluation since it seeks to improve practice as well as share similar ethical principles. A more narrow and reductionist methodology may limit the exploration of the more creative, qualitative and relational aspects of supervision that may lead to clinical change. The Commission on the Future of Nursing and Midwifery in England (2010) has expressed concern about the loss of more compassionate, reflective and thoughtful care if a more mechanistic climate were to prevail.

Ham (2003) strongly states the importance of building capacity for change from the bottom up rather than from the top down, harnessing the energies of clinicians in the quest for innovation and improvements, where professionals feel they are leading the process. He believes that strategies that motivate are more likely to be successful than those that focus on tighter control of service delivery. However, he states that it is essential to develop a better balance between autonomy and accountability. He also advocates collaborative approaches, linking clinicians who are close to clients and the point of care with managers and organizational support. An action research model which focuses on learning through doing, and derived from reflection through real experience, is suggested as a model.

None of this means to say that the vital requirements to monitor, measure and evaluate patient outcomes are not an absolute priority. They are, and more studies are needed, but the principles need to be congruent with the principles of clinical supervision.

Summary

This chapter has outlined some useful studies that indicate the potential benefits of clinical supervision such as improved job satisfaction and a positive influence on staff retention and sickness rates.

Other studies have highlighted some elements which enable effective use of clinical supervision, such a ensuring it is kept separate from line management supervision, held in a place away from the workplace, that the supervisee has an hour for individual reflection and is held at least once a month. Monitoring both the process and outcomes of supervision, greater protection of time allocated for supervision and training opportunities to increase the skill and number of available supervision were also highlighted.

This outline and critique of the existing literature and its gaps has set the scene for the next chapter in which we suggest some practical ways of setting up and maintaining clinical supervision systems.

9 The practicalities of setting up clinical supervision systems

Before we consider the options open to you in terms of organizational systems or modes of clinical supervision, we want to place the relationship between supervisee and clinical supervisor at the centre of any strategy for developing clinical supervision. Within the studies that included setting up clinical supervision, which was almost all, the pros and cons of the managers understanding and enabling this emerged constantly.

Conditions necessary for an effective clinical supervision relationship

It is important to consider the conditions that need to apply for the working alliance to develop. Unacknowledged concerns about self-disclosure can negatively influence the implementation of clinical supervision, creating the conditions for superficiality and resulting in a lack of support and rigour. We suggest that seven conditions need to apply to give the opportunity for an effective relationship to develop (see Figure 9.1).

1. *Sufficient frequency of protected sessions to provide enough face-to-face time together.* There needs to be enough contact time structured into the delivery system for face-to-face contact between the supervisee and clinical supervisor so that a relationship can be built and skills of clinical supervision can develop. Delivery systems that offer one hour three or four times a year are merely paying lip-service to the concept of clinical supervision: there is no chance to get to know each other within the special context of clinical supervision and to build enough trust for effective in-depth reflection. For instance, Johnson (1995), despite supporting the range of opportunities and merits of clinical supervision, goes on to advocate, from a management perspective, a minimum frequency of a mere two sessions a year. This may achieve a target but it misses the point. Admittedly his suggestion is only a minimum, but minimum recommendations can become the depressing norm.

    Having planned the time in, it needs to be protected by all concerned: management backup is needed to allow the supervisee to get away from the demands of the work setting, and the supervisee and clinical supervisor need to give priority to punctuality, especially if travelling time has to be taken into account. Attendance is a crucial issue here: the relationship

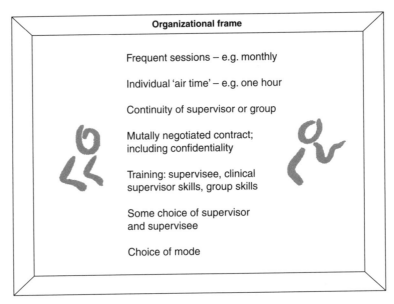

Figure 9.1 Conditions for an effective clinical supervision relationship

cannot happen if the people involved are not there. There can often be a vicious circle as far as this issue is concerned. At an individual level, someone who is not committed to clinical supervision is less likely to make the arrangements necessary to be able to turn up: their time management will be poor and they will not assert their need for cover from their colleagues or manager and will therefore always have the excuse of being too busy to attend on time or at all. At an organizational level, managers who are not committed to clinical supervision will not make explicit the expectation of attendance nor provide the backup resources to ensure that clinical work is covered in order to release staff. Ragged attendance means an unsatisfactory experience of clinical supervision, with further loss of commitment and so on, until the reality of clinical supervision disappears into thin air.

2. *Enough protected air time for in-depth reflection at each meeting.* Another dimension of the time issue is air time, the time each individual supervisee has to reflect on their practice and the part they play in the quality of that practice, facilitated by the clinical supervisor or group. The supervisee needs blocks of reflection time of at least 45 continuous minutes in order to engage in facilitated in-depth reflection on their practice and on the part they play as a person in the quality of that practice. This is seldom available when the group mode of clinical supervision is chosen on its own: one-to-one offers more likelihood of meeting this criterion. We recommend that one hour per month should be the target: this allows for a session to cover a review of progress and agenda-setting, 45 minutes

in-depth reflection, and finally some action planning to be reviewed at the next session. In the consultation discussions prior to the publication of the UKCC (1996) position statement on clinical supervision, there was much agreement on this issue, although the paper did not include this figure. The one-hour-per-month rule of thumb is increasingly coming into play. Unfortunately, we still occasionally encounter employers who pay lip service to the provision of clinical supervision. One organization offers one hour of one-to-one clinical supervision for three sessions a year, which pans out at 15 minutes per month on average, which is woefully inadequate. Likewise, we have come across a 'group clinical supervision' system where 11 people meet for one hour per month: this averages out at a maximum of four and a half minutes per person of 'air time' per month!

3. *Continuity of clinical supervisor or group membership.* Knowledge of the attachment needs of adults, touched on in Chapter 2, illustrates the need for continuity, reliability and establishing and maintaining boundaries. The supervisee needs to have the same person or people at each clinical supervision session, otherwise relationship-building goes back to square one each time there is a change. This continuity is usually easy to maintain in one-to-one clinical supervision but many clinical supervision groups end up having variable composition because of difficulty in fixing dates suitable for all, with the problem being exacerbated the larger the group is. This is illustrated in a study by Butterworth *et al.* (1997), where a clinical supervision group of five members was usually attended by only three of them each time. Continuity of venue should be attempted too, reducing the stress of getting there due to knowledge about travel time, route, etc. The reliability of having the same person or persons, who are committed to the process of clinical supervision, and can be punctual and settled enough to pay attention, is a vital part of building the relationship.

4. *A clear, mutually negotiated working contract.* The contract and boundaries of the relationship need to be mutually understood and accepted, clearly established, worked within and regularly reviewed, as we outlined in Chapter 3. This contract especially needs to include confidentiality, with very clear understanding of the conditions in which it could, in theory, be broken. It is important that the people involved have some chance to use their own wording for the contract, in order to ensure they fully understand each other and feel ownership of it.

5. *Training in supervisee, clinical supervisor and group skills.* Training in the skills of clinical supervision is usually essential. Indeed, in the study by Butterworth *et al.* (1997), this was found to be the principal 'hot issue' identified by those involved, who emphasized the need for appropriate educational preparation for clinical supervisors. However, in our experience, training for supervisees is equally important and very often overlooked. Not all nurses have had significant training in reflective skills, and most nurses need some training in the skills we identified in Chapters 3 and 4. It could

be argued that if all supervisees had enough understanding of the aims of clinical supervision, and were skilled enough at reflection and assertiveness, they could take charge of the clinical supervision sessions and train their clinical supervisors on the job, though this would take time and they may get a raw deal for the first few years.

In terms of the training needs of clinical supervisors, virtually all research studies examining the nurse/patient or teacher/learner communication skills of nurses have highlighted that non-directive skills are lacking across the board. Any clinical supervision system that assumes a body of staff with enough skills in the facilitation of another's reflection is likely to founder, even in fields where such skills are often assumed to be stock-in-trade, such as mental health nursing, health visiting and nurse education. Our experience in training workshops bears this out. An increasing number of nurses have also trained as counsellors or psychotherapists, but we find that this group often need training in incorporating more challenging and informative skills, and need to focus on the aims of improving practice, and on maintaining clearer boundaries regarding probing into the personal issues of supervisees. Another vital dimension to address, if group clinical supervision is being considered, is the area of group skills. We attempted to highlight in Chapter 7 that the group option is not the easiest one, as is often mistakenly assumed: skills of group participation as well as advanced supervisee and clinical supervisor skills are required by all involved, as well as good group facilitator skills for that individual.

6. *Choice of mode of clinical supervision.* If group clinical supervision is a practical possibility (given the time it takes to do it properly), individual members of staff need to be able to choose whether to have group or one-to-one clinical supervision. Self-disclosure in a group is more difficult for most nurses than one-to-one and it can be detrimental to slot people into a form of clinical supervision which does not fit, when another could be more fruitful.

7. *Choice of clinical supervisor.* Having a real choice of who to see as clinical supervisor is essential to building a working alliance, although we have recommended which types of people to exclude from the list of choices (see Chapter 3 and the code of practice in Chapter 10). Clinical supervision is inevitably a process in which self-disclosure needs to happen and a supervisee may not feel empowered by or trusting enough of the clinical supervisor who has been allocated. Nurses often avoid the choice issue in case a clinical supervisor's feelings are hurt if they are not chosen, but the quality of clinical supervision and ultimately the quality of care must not be compromised because of this fear. If one person is consistently not being chosen, this may highlight issues which need to be addressed about them as a clinical supervisor, whether these are to do with their individual abilities or qualities or the position they hold in the organization. Where people are employed expressly to be clinical supervisors, there is a special problem about choice. Some staff will not want to have this person

as supervisor because they may be seen as too intimately connected to the immediate management structure, but may be willing to see another similar clinical supervisor in another hospital or locality, or arrange their own supervision with a peer colleague. Likewise, the clinical supervisor should have the choice about whether or not to work with a particular person. Membership of a clinical supervision group must be afforded the same attention. Allocation of members is unlikely to lead to success: members need to have some choice. When we emphasize choice, we realize that total free choice is impractical and, in some cases, undesirable. A choice of two or three clinical supervisors is preferable, or perhaps the freedom to express first and second choices from a list of possible supervisors. As we stated in Chapter 3, we see this as an equal opportunities issue.

Developing clinical supervision as a distinct entity

Clinical supervision needs to be established, developed and protected as an entity in itself, as does line management supervision. Figure 9.2 places clinical supervision in relation to other types of supervision and monitoring and Tables 9.1 and 9.2 expand on this. We need to use effectively and develop the other communication systems in their own right. For instance, there is much concern to strengthen the authority of the ward manager or equivalent, and that of community nursing team leaders. Combining clinical supervision with their roles can dilute their authority in their line management role: the nature of the clinical supervision is a relationship of peers, whatever their respective levels in the hierarchy. The line management relationship is not: the senior person has distinct responsibilities in relation to the management of the subordinate and a manager who strives to be 'one of the girls/boys' is abdicating their authority and responsibilities. This has long been the view in nursing in the British armed forces, where clarity about lines of authority is an explicit priority, and since clinical supervision was first introduced it has always been separate. This has applied even in mental health nursing in the forces, whereas in civilian life the tradition has been to use the social work model of combining the two forms of supervision.

In using authority and supporting and developing staff, a manager uses the whole range of leadership styles, from very authoritative to very facilitative. It is the overall emphasis which differs from the clinical supervisor's role. Table 9.3 illustrates this, and can be compared to Table 6.1 which highlights the emphasis in the clinical supervisor's role.

As a manager, you personally may feel ready to distinguish between line management and clinical supervision and you may feel that you could hold distinct meetings with your staff to fulfil the separate functions. However, your staff are unlikely to be so ready, given the realities of the line manager's authority. In Parkinson's (1992) study of the effectiveness of this type of combined supervision, nurse managers reported no difficulties in separating their managerial role from their advice and support role, but did admit that they thought that some staff had

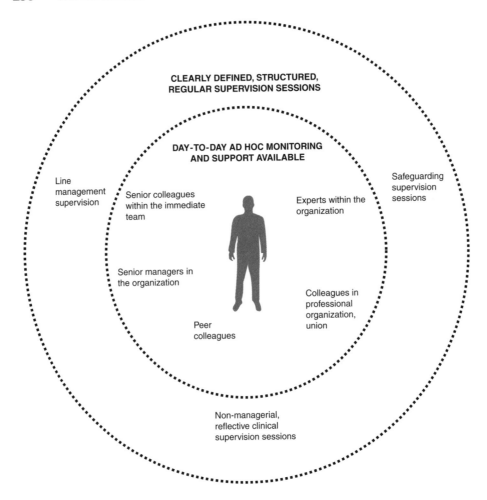

Figure 9.2 The place of clinical supervision within the whole picture of supervision and monitoring of nurses

difficulty responding to the latter. Their staff agreed, tending to see the potential disciplinary and control function as predominant.

Letting go of their personal involvement with the clinical supervision of their own staff will be difficult for many managers, who feel that they are committed to clinical supervision and combine these roles within the system they have already set up. In the early days of developing clinical supervision, many proactive, supportive and caring managers set up systems which they hoped might reflect support and professional development principles and yet, by combining or confusing clinical supervision with forms of management supervision, they have unwittingly skewed these systems towards a mainly normative function.

Table 9.1   Emphasizing the distinctive place of clinical supervision

Clinical supervision	Management monitoring	Support and development
Clinical supervision is distinct from these other communication systems. It should augment them. Clinical supervision should not be amalgamated with any of these systems. Nor should it replace or undermine any of these important means of communication between staff.	• Complaints procedure • Day-to-day monitoring of standards • Performance management • Disciplinary procedure • Management by objectives • Managers briefing staff • Performance appraisal (Individual Performance Review) • Staff giving accounts of service delivery information to managers • Team meetings • Work hand-over meeting	• Ad hoc peer support • Ad hoc support from manager • Case conferences • Clinical teaching • Consultation exercise for developing strategy, policy • Debriefing sessions after traumatic events • Educational assessment • In-service training and development • Mentorship • Occupational health backup • Personal counselling • Preceptorship • Specialist clinical advice, e.g. infection control; child protection; HIV; hospital/community liaison • Staff support group

The logistics as well as the ethics of combining the two would place an enormous strain on already depleted numbers of clinical managers. In Parkinson's (1992) study many managers did admit that they really did not have enough time to combine the roles due to an excess of competing demands from their other management responsibilities. Managers who have attended our courses have also reported that the amount of anxiety it causes them to hear of the uncertainties and vulnerabilities of large numbers of their staff is too much to expect of someone whose responsibility lies in managing the overall service. They find it a relief to articulate the impossibility of combining the role of an effective clinical supervisor with their diverse spread of functions, and begin to see their role as facilitators, enablers and sponsors of clinical supervision systems. These roles taken on by managers provide a crucial link between implementation in practice, and the structural acceptance and development of clinical supervision in the larger organization.

In many organizations that set up separate systems, managers have described to us how various positive effects of separate clinical supervision have been directly manifested in line management supervision. For instance:

- managers often find that their team members are more focused and come to the point during their line management and staff meetings;

Table 9.2 Distinguishing between clinical supervision and line-management supervision

	Clinical supervision session	Management supervision meeting	IPR meeting	Disciplinary interview
Agenda setting	Agenda mostly defined by the supervisee. Clinical supervisor may highlight items arising from the content of sessions or about the way the working relationship is going	Agenda defined by manager and practitioner together	Agenda defined by IPR document, devised by manager, possibly with some input from practitioners	Agenda defined by manager
Confidentiality	Almost total, with exceptions of legal or professional ethics. Possibly a record of attendance dates and times. Record of content negotiated between practitioner and clinical supervisor, for their eyes only	Not necessarily confidential, but discretion used in passing on information about practitioner, e.g. to selected team members in order to ensure effective team functioning. May be recorded in manager's own notes and/or in personnel file	Not confidential, but discretion used in passing on information about practitioner. Copy of IPR document may be kept in manager's file and/or in personnel file	Not confidential, but discretion used in passing on information about practitioner. Recorded in manager's file and personnel file
Information giving and advice	Some information, advice, guidance offered to supplement the supervisee's own expertise, to help the supervisee see options available and make own informed decision	Information, advice and guidance given to direct the practitioner towards team and organizational objectives. Information given about policy directives	Information, advice and guidance given to direct the practitioner towards team and organizational objectives and training opportunities within the organization	Information given about the disciplinary procedure and to direct towards improving the performance which is being challenged. Information about consequences of not improving

Challenging	Based on evidence gained during the clinical supervision session s only. Challenging technical mistakes, inadequate clinical standards, contribution to problems with team work, more personal issues such as unhelpful or self-defeating behaviour or attitude, blind spots, broken contracts	Based on evidence gained/ observed in any work situation. Challenging technical mistakes, inadequate clinical standards, contribution to problems with teamwork, lack of achieving pre-agreed objectives	Based on evidence gained/observed in any work situation. Challenging technical mistakes, inadequate clinical standards, contribution to problems with team work, lack of achieving pre-agreed objectives	Based on evidence gained/ observed in any work situation. Challenging severe and/or repeated technical mistakes, inadequate clinical standards, contribution to problems with team work, lack of achieving pre-agreed objectives
Support	No practical help given outside sessions, except reporting unsafe practice. Support for the supervisee as a person and encouragement given to help supervisee recognize and use own expertise and personal abilities towards developing their professional expertise	Practical help may be given outside the meetings. Support and encouragement given to help supervisee recognize and use own expertise and personal abilities towards meeting specific team and organizational objectives	Practical help may be given outside the meetings. Support and encouragement given to help supervisee recognize and use own expertise and personal abilities towards meeting specific team and organizational objectives	Practical help may be given outside the meetings. Support offered: often not a situation in which the practitioner can easily accept support from the person involved
Catalytic help	Enabling reflection on issues ultimately affecting practice, learning from experience, problem-solving, pinpointing ways of dealing with difficult emotions, decision making and planning and reviewing application to practice	Manager elicits information from practitioner about work done and standards achieved. Enables problem-solving on team and management issues	Manager elicits information from practitioner about standards achieved in the areas of practice outlined on the IPR document. Enabling overall performance review, problem-solving, goal setting	Manager elicits information from practitioner about the issues under discussion. Enables goal setting

Table 9.3 A leadership matrix, indicating examples of the range of leadership characteristics within the authoritative/facilitative dimension, highlighting the emphasis on the line manager's authority

CONTINUUM	AUTHORITATIVE ──────────────────────────── FACILITATIVE			
LEADERSHIP CHARACTERISTIC	DIRECTIVE	NEGOTIATING	CATALYTIC	SPACE-GIVING
LEADERSHIP TASK	DECISION-MAKING			
Whose responsibility is it to make the decision?	Yours / Mostly yours	Yours & staff	Mostly staff	Staff
Who decides?	You decide / You decide, then consult, then change decision or not / You consult, then decide	You decide then negotiate compromise / You give a few options from which staff can decide / You explore options together & jointly decide	You indicate the overall boundary & enable staff to decide within that. / You give information or possible options to enable staff to decide	You impartially & catalytically enable staff to decide for themselves / You do nothing, wait for staff to decide, but stay alert to what decisions are made or not.
LEADERSHIP TASK	INITIATING ACTION BY STAFF			
What do you do?	You give an unequivocal order / You direct / You persuade	You request then negotiate compromise / You give limited options, staff choose which ones to act upon	You indicate the overall parameters & enable staff to get things done within them. / You provide the necessary information & give staff space to act upon it in their own way.	You enable staff to reflect in-depth, use intuition, knowledge, feelings, & motivation & give space to carry out the action in their own way. / You do nothing, wait for staff to do what needs doing, but stay alert to what's happening or not happening.

- Staff have felt more equipped to use appraisal or individual performance review (IPR) constructively, in contrast to many other Trusts, where staff attend IPR sessions unwillingly or avoid them if possible;
- staff bring more thoughtfulness to operational issues: 'they bring me solutions now, not moans';
- one group of paediatric nurses developed time-saving measures to create the time for their clinical supervision sessions: they reduced by almost half the time it took to give handovers between shifts by instigating a more focused and reliable system.
- Managers also report noticing less unfocused chit-chat between staff during the course of a day's work.

Roles of people involved in setting up and maintaining a clinical supervision system

We outline here the possible roles of the various people within the organization who are involved in setting up and evaluating a clinical supervision system (see Table 9.4.) Further guidance about this strategy is provided later.

Business or senior manager

The senior manager's role as sponsor of the clinical supervision system involves providing the organizational backdrop while others take centre stage. This management role involves being an advocate for genuine clinical supervision within the political climate of the organization, to establish and maintain the integrity of the system, resisting pressure from powerful elements within the organization who misunderstand or wish to misapply clinical supervision. Inevitably, this requires you to make a case for, win and manage a budget to cover the costs of training and backup resources to allow unit, ward or team managers to release staff from their work areas to attend clinical supervision sessions. You will need a framework for calculating additional staffing resource needs, though this needs to be offset by considering how much time is saved by there being less unfocused chat in the workplace.

You could be involved in initiating the first steps in setting up a clinical supervision system – if the initiative has not already come from staff themselves – and perhaps the initial coordination of the system. Ultimately, you will have the responsibility for ensuring that monitoring and evaluation of the clinical supervision system are carried out.

Yours is the task of educating the purchasers about the added value of a genuine clinical supervision system within your organization's portfolio for purchasers. Cuts in management systems are being demanded by purchasers as management is seen as expensive: it is timely to insert your case for clinical supervision at times of

Table 9.4 Roles of people involved in setting up and maintaining a clinical supervision system

Senior manager	Unit, ward or team manager	Coordinator
• Be the sponsor of the clinical supervision system, not directly involved but providing management backup • Initiate the setting up of a clinical supervision system, if the initiative has not already come from staff themselves • Make a case for, win and manage a budget to cover costs • Be an advocate of clinical supervision within the political climate of the organization and maintain the integrity of the system, resisting pressure from powerful elements within the organization who misunderstand or wish to misapply clinical supervision • Provide backup resources to allow unit, ward or team managers to release staff from their work areas to attend clinical supervision, training sessions • Describe the clinical supervision system for inclusion in the organization's portfolio for commissioners • Monitor and evaluate the system	• Initiate the setting up of a clinical supervision system if the initiative has not already come from the staff themselves or from elsewhere in the organization • Train as a clinical supervisor and provide clinical supervision to members of other units, wards or teams (not your own) and possibly to peer colleagues at your grade • Enable staff to be released from their work to attend clinical supervision, or training sessions • Continue to use and develop your day-to-day managerial supervision with your staff. Avoid the temptation to try to pass on your management problems to the clinical supervisor of any of your staff • Avoid the temptation to intrude on the confidentiality of your staff's clinical supervision by asking their clinical supervisor about the content of discussion • Take on the role of coordinator if appropriate • Ensure that you receive and use your own clinical supervision to cover the whole range of your work, with someone who is not your line manager • Ensure that you have supervision of the clinical supervision that you provide, with someone who would not compromise the confidentiality of your supervisee	• Initiate the setting up of a clinical supervision system if the initiative has not already come from the staff themselves or from elsewhere in the organization • Investigate the level of interest and expertise in clinical supervision among staff • Convene and facilitate a working group comprising people who are interested in clinical supervision, at various grades and as multidisciplinary as possible • If there are other similar working groups within the organization liaise between them and share information • Provide or seek backup managerial sponsorship, so the working group can implement the strategy for setting up clinical supervision

Table 9.5 Extract from recommendations by Butterworth *et al.* (1997: 4)

- Trust Boards should ensure that business plans contain a strategy for the development of clinical supervision... This should address issues of allocated time and resources.
- Purchasing authorities should seek evidence of clinical supervision... in providing services as confirmation of good quality practice.
- Employers should recognise and capitalise on the benefits of clinical supervision... as it will form part of a human resource strategy that facilitates recruitment, retention and continuing professional development.
- Staff must be given time for clinical supervision and a suitable location in which to carry it out.
- Attention must be given to the preparation and education of clinical supervisors... Employers will need to attend to these needs through their own training resources or approach educational purchasing consortia for additional support.
- The training and development of supervisors... must prepare them to deal with the wide range of content which will be presented to them, and ongoing support should be provided to enable their continuing work.

---

management cuts, as purchasers are more likely to accept its cost and its increased necessity. Professionally there is an even greater need for clinical supervision at such a time, though it can be difficult to get across this quality issue if the people you are dealing with on the purchasing side do not have nursing backgrounds, as is usually the case. This is the setting to emphasize the normative function: how clinical supervision is the only formal system so far which provides a window through which one nurse can get an in-depth view of the professional knowledge, thinking processes and values behind the other nurse's practice and be in a position to offer acceptable support and influential guidance (and, if necessary, bring serious concerns to light). Thus the safety, risk management and clinical effectiveness element can be highlighted. The detail and subtlety of how this is achieved is unlikely to be of interest given all the other priorities that have to be addressed at this level. To back up your case, you could cite the research summarized in Chapter 8, along with the specific recommendations to purchasers and employers included in the Department of Health's (1993a) *A Vision for the Future* and especially the report of the evaluation study by Butterworth *et al.* (1997), of which the summary recommendations are shown in Table 9.5.

You will need to appoint a manager to lead not only the setting up of a new or revised clinical supervision system, but to maintain it.

Unit, ward or team manager

We are aware that in many Trusts, particularly in the community, the nursing management structure has become so 'flattened', with layers being eradicated, that the same senior practitioners who need to be considered and trained for the role of clinical supervisor also have the additional responsibility for organizing the entire setting up of local clinical supervision systems. Although they do not have management responsibilities as reflected in grading and pay, they have become a very cheap option for Trusts and have the enormous stress of having organizational development responsibilities grafted onto their practice caseloads and team leader roles. If you are in this position we acknowledge the difficulties you face and offer some pointers to highlight which aspects of the setting up and development of a clinical supervision system may be especially pertinent to you.

If the initiative has not already come from junior staff or from elsewhere in the organization, you may need to set the ball rolling. You may be required to take on the role of coordinator if appropriate. You also need to train in the skills of the clinical supervisor and provide clinical supervision to members of other units, wards or teams (not your own) and possibly to peer colleagues at your grade.

You need to make arrangements to enable your staff to be released from their work to attend clinical supervision, training sessions, and to make a case to your business manager for resources to be allocated to provide increased staff cover.

As the team, ward or unit manager, you need to continue to use and develop your day-to-day line management supervision with your staff. Avoid the temptation to try to pass on your management problems to the clinical supervisor of any of your staff. You need to monitor whether or not your staff are actually attending and find out the reasons if they do not get to the clinical supervision sessions, but avoid the temptation to intrude on the confidentiality of your staff's clinical supervision by asking their clinical supervisor about the content.

It is important that you ensure that you receive and use your own clinical supervision to cover the whole range of your work, with someone who is not your line manager. You may wish to combine this with supervision of the clinical supervision that you provide, but you need to be alert to the need to keep confidential the content of the work you do with your supervisees, so it is preferable that your own clinical supervisor does not know your supervisees.

Coordinator/clinical supervision lead

Who the coordinator of a clinical supervision system is varies: it might be a senior manager, team manager or senior practitioner. If you are taking on the coordination of a system, you need to set your sights realistically by designing a process which you feel you can handle, which seeks to meet the clinical supervision needs of an appropriate number of staff, whether a small team of four, or all nurses within a whole Trust.

You may need to be the person who initiates the setting up of a clinical supervision system if the initiative has not already come from elsewhere in the organization. The type of system you set up needs to be appropriate to the numbers and needs of the staff involved. Guidelines about developing a strategy are summarized in Figure 9.3 and outlined next.

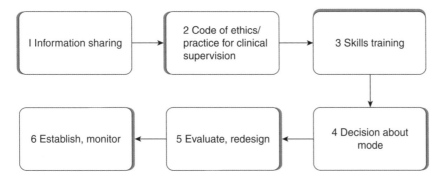

Figure 9.3 Strategy for implementing a new or revised clinical supervision system

Strategy for implementing clinical supervision

We provide guidelines here for starting a clinical supervision system from scratch, which may be useful if you are setting up a completely new service, or a new organization to deliver an existing service. In many settings, clinical supervision will have been implemented in some way, but these guidelines can still be useful for reviewing progress or taking a new look at your system.

In the first edition of this book we wrote about pilot projects, but the time for this has passed. There is enough evidence that clinical supervision is effective and enough written about various delivery systems to just get on with it.

General principles are offered by Kohner (1994), as shown in Table 9.6 and are still relevant. Swain (1995) suggests that managers address four main issues, an approach which mirrors good management practice in determining and planning for the health needs of clients: (i) the search for health needs of staff; (ii) stimulating an awareness of health needs; (iii) the influence of policies affecting staff health; and (iv) the facilitation of health-enhancing activities. We have attempted to incorporate the main principles identified by Kohner and Swain into a practical six-stage framework for setting up and maintaining a clinical supervision system.

Information-sharing

Investigate the level of interest and expertise in clinical supervision among staff. Those who have had experience of clinical supervision in previous posts or who are trained as counsellors, and those who have studied clinical supervision during basic nurse or postgraduate training courses, are valuable people to have on board. The medically allied professions, such as physiotherapy, occupational therapy, speech and language therapy and so on seem also to be interested in developing non-managerial clinical supervision and we have found that it is very fruitful to share information, training and, in some cases, a clinical supervision system, between the professions.

Table 9.6 Guidelines for the introduction of clinical supervision: a summary

1. Before introducing clinical supervision, its purpose should be discussed and clearly defined. This definition should be informed by a theoretical understanding of the role and function of supervision and, equally, by a practical understanding of the circumstances and needs of the unit and its staff
2. All staff should be involved in the process of planning and introducing a system of clinical supervision
3. Careful consideration should be given to the qualifications, skills and experience required of supervisors, and to their ability to meet the individual needs of supervisees
4. All supervisors should be given opportunities to receive training and learn the skills that are needed to provide supervision that is both constructive and supportive. Those who receive supervision should have similar opportunities to learn about their role as supervisees
5. All supervisors should also receive supervision, in order to monitor and develop the quality of supervision they provide
6. Supervision should be available to all practitioners, regardless of seniority
7. The content of supervision should be carefully defined, with boundaries agreed about what is and what is not to be dealt with in supervision time. The processes to be supervised should also be made clear
8. The relationship between supervisor and supervisee should be formally constituted. Ground rules should be negotiated and agreed
9. It is essential that clinical supervision is monitored and evaluated. Supervisees and supervisors should play an equal part in these procedures
10. Individual units need the support of their employing authority to implement and maintain a system of clinical supervision

Source: Extracted from Kohner (1994).

Encourage staff to share books and journal articles on clinical supervision that they find useful for understanding and potentially for implementing clinical supervision, avoiding those which baffle or seem written for the sake of the author's academic CV rather than the practitioner. Focus your discussions on gaining enough understanding to begin to embark on a clinical supervision system, rather than aiming to understand everything about clinical supervision at once. There comes a point at which you cannot really understand any more unless you accept the uncertainty and just do it.

A code of ethics and a code of practice

In Chapter 10 we propose a code of ethics and practice for clinical supervision. We suggest that key members of staff who have experience of clinical supervision use the code as a pointer for discussion in formulating their organization's own codes from which to develop clinical supervision systems. At the centre of any code should be consideration of accountability, how staff are to be treated in using the non-managerial clinical supervision, and addressing the sensitivity required for appropriate self-disclosure in clinical supervision.

Skills training

Practical training in the skills of being a supervisee and a clinical supervisor are necessary and we have discussed the reasons for this in Chapters 2 to 7. If your remit is to cover numbers of staff larger than, say, 12, this can be done by buying in an outside education and training consultant, as it will be more cost-effective than sending so many people to outside courses. It also has the advantage that the courses can be tailor-made for your staff and you have the chance to monitor the content and the standard of training. If you get the cooperation of the training or human resources department, a rolling programme of skills training courses could be set up to meet the training needs of new staff in your Trust and also to generate income by selling places to nearby Trusts. Multidisciplinary training offers more flexibility and can be very useful, provided that the other professions are committed to using a non-managerial model of clinical supervision: we find this in some allied health professions but not in social work, for instance. Although nurses are usually reticent to begin with, they value the experience of learning clinical supervision skills with other professionals once they have tried it. Multidisciplinary skills training can help to focus on the skills of interaction rather the nursing content.

Some important criteria to look for in commissioning training are:

- Is the trainer currently receiving their own equivalent of non-managerial clinical supervision and also giving it?
- Will the group size be under 22?
- Will the teaching style be facilitative?
- Are there structured skills-practice exercises based on real-life issues for the individual course members?

The time for conference-style information-sharing on clinical supervision has passed since enough has been written about it, so it is more cost-effective for staff to share information between themselves. You may wish to consider training some of your experienced clinical supervisors as trainers, in order to maintain a rolling programme of staff induction and updating.

Self-training triads

Using self-training triads can be a cost-effective, though slow, method of skills training. Three people meet at least monthly for three and a half hours. They take turns to be supervisee, clinical supervisor and observer. After each (real, not role-played) clinical supervision session of one hour, the observer gives feedback to both the supervisee and the clinical supervisor on the skills they used and the pitfalls they fell into. The recipients of the feedback take notes and consider it between sessions. If this is the chosen method, it is useful during the information-sharing stage of this strategy to compile a lengthy checklist of skills and pitfalls in relation to the supervisee and supervisor (the evaluation tools shown in Chapter 9 suggest some criteria, and lists of pitfalls in Chapter 6 indicate some pitfalls). Observers in the triads then have a common framework from which to give feedback. Two essential ground rules are: that the observer stays absolutely silent throughout the session, sitting back out of eye contact; and that the observer does not comment upon the content of the session, except to illustrate an example of a skill or pitfall, and definitely does not give any last-minute advice, however tempting.

Mode and structure

If you wish to offer more than one-to-one clinical supervision, your system needs to give individual supervisees a choice about the mode – i.e. whether one-to-one, group or a combination. The options are as outlined in Table 9.7.

Ensure that all clinical supervisors are included as supervisees in your structure. It is vital that they receive as well as give clinical supervision in order to build their understanding of the nature of the process and especially to enable them to deal with the added stress of being a clinical supervisor. Butterworth *et al.* (1997)

Table 9.7 Modes of clinical supervision

Pairs
- One-to-one with supervisor more experienced in the same field as the supervisee, not line manager, but in the same locality
- One-to-one with supervisor more experienced in the same field as the supervisee, not line manager, and in a different locality
- One-to-one with supervisor from another discipline (e.g. clinical psychology) but supervisee has access to someone in own speciality for ad hoc sessions as necessary
- One-to-one with peer colleague, reciprocal in pairs
- One-to-one with peer colleague, in circular arrangement: A supervises. B who supervises C who supervises D who supervises A

Triads
- One-to-one, with a third person observing the supervisor, with a coaching role to enable supervisee and supervisor to develop skills

Groups
- Group with peer colleagues within the same discipline, led by supervisor who is more experienced in the same field of the supervisees and has group facilitation skills too
- Group with peer colleagues within the same discipline, led by supervisor who has specialist expertise within supervisee's own field (e.g. child protection, HIV) and has group facilitation skills too
- Group with peer colleagues of mixed disciplines, led by supervisor who has group facilitation skills
- Group with peer colleagues of same discipline, led in turn by group members
- Group with peer colleagues of mixed disciplines, led in turn by group members

Combination
- The circular arrangement of one-to-one, monthly for 5 months, then all meeting as a clinical supervision group for the 6th month, facilitated by someone from outside the group. Repeating that 6-month cycle.
- Meeting monthly as a whole group, settling together, then working in pairs dividing the time between them, then as a whole group to share action plans.

Table 9.8 Pros and cons of one-to-one clinical supervision as compared to group

Advantages	Disadvantages
• More practical, easier to arrange mutually convenient times • Supervisee more likely to get an appropriate amount of 'air time' in which to be able to reflect in depth • Preferable for beginners, as less complex than group clinical supervision • Self-disclosure can be less frightening for more introvert individuals than in group situation • More continuity, the same clinical supervisor each time • May be preferred by individuals who have had bad previous experiences in learning groups • Gives more of a sense of being listened to as an individual, cared for by the organization • The working alliance, the clinical supervision relationship, can develop more deeply more quickly	• Can be too intense a setting for supervisees who are not used to and afraid of self-disclosure • The choice issue is more critical: there must be some choice for the supervisee as to who to have as clinical supervisor. This is difficult if someone has been appointed to do clinical supervision. Even where there is choice, some nurses may choose someone in order not to hurt their feelings about not being chosen, rather than out of genuine preference, which gets the clinical supervision relationship off to a wobbly start. The supervisee may choose someone as an easy option, who they know will not challenge them. It being a one-to-one situation, there is no one else to do the challenging • No one else there to referee if there is an argument or to dilute the effect of a personality clash • Supervisee gets the perspective of only one other person

showed that supervisors who themselves did not receive clinical supervision were significantly more stressed than those who did.

As an individual supervisee choosing a mode, you need carefully to consider the pros and cons of each and to decide according to your priorities and needs (see Table 9.8).

Advantages of one-to-one clinical supervision over group supervision is that it is more practical and easier to arrange mutually convenient times. This means that there is more continuity than is usual in group clinical supervision, since you are with the same clinical supervisor each time. The other main factor to take into account is that you are more likely to get an appropriate amount of air time in which to reflect in depth. One-to-One clinical supervision is less complex than group and is therefore usually a better choice of mode for people who are new to non-managerial, reflective clinical supervision.

One-to-one clinical supervision may suit certain personality types: for more introvert individuals self-disclosure can be less frightening than in a group situation, or it may be preferred by individuals who have had bad previous experiences in groups. This mode can give more of a sense of being listened to as an individual, of being cared for by the organization. The working alliance – the clinical supervision relationship – can develop more deeply and more quickly when there is only one person to get to know.

Disadvantages of one-to-one clinical supervision

The choice issue is very critical: there must be some choice for the supervisee as to who to have as clinical supervisor. This is difficult if someone has been appointed to do clinical supervision. Even where there is choice, some nurses may choose someone in order not to hurt their feelings about not being chosen, rather than out of genuine preference, which gets the clinical supervision relationship off to a wobbly start. The supervisee may choose someone as an easy option, someone they know will not challenge them. It being a one-to-one situation, there is no one else to do the challenging if that one person colludes.

If there is a disagreement or even an argument, there is no one else there to referee or to dilute the effect of a personality clash. The supervisee may feel trapped, working with someone to whom they cannot relate and they may not be assertive enough to make alternative arrangements. A final disadvantage is that the supervisee gets the perspective of only one other person on the issues brought to the session.

Disadvantages of clinical supervision in a group

Moving on to group clinical supervision (Table 9.9), we strongly caution you to consider carefully the criteria which need to be thought through before embarking on the group model. We find that this model is often chosen because it might appear, incorrectly, to be more time- and cost-effective than one-to-one supervision: one clinical supervisor can 'do' five supervisees at once. Group clinical supervision is diluted and ineffectual when this is the only criterion for choosing this model. Other criteria need to be considered: here we will highlight some disadvantages in choosing group clinical supervision, as they are often underestimated.

If the mistaken criterion of 'one clinical supervisor can do five supervisees at once' is applied, then each supervisee will get less than one fifth of the air time that she would have received if she had been having one-to-one supervision. For example, if a clinical supervision group of five people and one group facilitator meet for one hour every month, then each group member gets 10 minutes of air time per session: this scanty amount of time pays only lip-service to the aim of 'in-depth reflection' that is intended in clinical supervision (this timing allows for five minutes to settle in together as a group and five minutes to wind down and make plans for the next meeting). Many of the complicated issues that supervisees would want to bring to clinical supervision would take 10 minutes or more just to explain to a group, there being no time for reflection at all. Some groups have a system of taking turns to be the supervisee: each week, one person has the whole 50 minutes to present an issue to the group and receive clinical supervision from them. This, however, means that each member of a group of five only receives clinical supervision once every five months, which is also woefully inadequate if not combined with one-to-one sessions as well.

If clinical supervision in a group is to provide sufficient air time, then many would consider that it is time-consuming rather than time-effective in comparison to one-to-one. Another factor to take into account is the time needed to build

Table 9.9 Pros and cons of group clinical supervision as compared to one-to-one

Advantages	Disadvantages
• Setting for pooling of professional knowledge and expertise, by getting an insight into how individual group members manage their relationship as individuals with their practice • Self-disclosure can be less frightening for more extrovert individuals than in a one-to-one situation • May be preferred by individuals who have had good previous experiences in learning groups • Builds a sense of belonging to the team or organization • Reduces isolation and enhances feeling of being supported by the organization: especially useful for practitioners who work on their own • Learning, changing and application to practice can be enhanced by the support and challenge of a group; the supervisee gets a variety of perspectives • Group dynamics can be exciting and stimulating if all group members are very committed and skilled	• Time-consuming for each person to have adequate 'air time' and additional time needed for group dynamics • In reality, individuals often get scanty amounts of 'air time' • High level of skills needed: participants need supervisee skills *and* clinical supervisor *and* group participation skills; facilitator needs clinical supervisor skills *and* group facilitation skills • Self-disclosure can be more frightening for more introvert individuals or those who have had bad previous experiences in learning groups • Easier for non-committed individuals to 'hide' and say very little • More difficult to arrange times for sessions which are convenient for all • Difficult to get continuity, since different people attending each time therefore less trust, less of a sense of a working alliance in which to reflect in depth • More likely to slide into becoming a session for chat, general discussion, support or professional information updating rather than focusing on each individual's in-depth reflection • Group dynamics can go wrong, and sabotage everyone's clinical supervision

and maintain positive group dynamics and to deal with the likely group dynamic problems that will arise from time to time. So, our group of five would need to meet for a session of five hours each month to allow enough time for five people to have 45 minutes each, and to have settling time at the beginning, breaks and winding down time at the end. While we have found one group of senior managers able to make this time commitment, we have not yet come across any groups of practitioners who have been able to sustain it.

Receiving clinical supervision in a group setting will not suit every nurse's personality. Self-disclosure in a group can be more frightening for more introvert individuals than in a one-to-one situation. Dealing with the inevitable conflicts that arise in ongoing groups can be too scary for such nurses. Some nurses have had bad experiences in groups and this has negatively coloured their expectations of the value of groups as a learning environment, even those with the most extrovert personalities. Others not committed to clinical supervision might choose a group mode in order more easily to hide and just go through the motions of participation.

A crucial disadvantage of clinical supervision in a group rather than one-to-one is that it requires more skills. Participants require not only supervisee skills, but also clinical supervisor and group participation skills. The facilitator needs group facilitation skills as well as clinical supervisor skills. Finding or training people to possess these skills can be especially problematic when setting up clinical supervision from scratch, with few or no staff having had any previous experience of it.

Another practical disadvantage is that it can be more difficult to arrange times for sessions which are convenient for all. Usually this results in a lack of consistency in attendance, which not only exacerbates the practical problem of lack of air time, but also interferes with the consistency that is required for enough trust to be built up to enable in-depth rather than superficial reflection, and can make the dynamics of the group difficult. Varied group composition usually results in less cohesion and motivation to attend and the group can peter out.

Lastly, the group dynamics can go wrong and thereby reduce the effectiveness of the clinical supervision that each person receives. For instance, one member can sabotage the others' clinical supervision if, say, they are antagonistic towards clinical supervision or towards another person in the group. One group member who has difficulty in disclosing their own problems can hold back the development of safety in the group, so others will be reluctant to share anything significant and therefore the level of reflection that goes on in the group is superficial. Or, too much time can be taken by one person being given all the space because they are particularly stressed.

Advantages of clinical supervision in a group

However, there are some definite advantages to choosing group rather than one-to-one clinical supervision. These relate to the potential for greater sharing of expertise, belonging, support and energy. The group can provide a setting for pooling of professional knowledge and expertise. This can work well if group members can contribute different perspectives from different professional experiences, such as mixing newly qualified practitioners with very experienced ones. The experienced practitioners can be brought up to date with recent approaches and the new practitioners can learn from the real-life experiences of the others. You might want to have a mix of experiences from different branches of nursing.

You may wish to have clinical supervision as a team for the team-building effect. Brown and Bourne (1996) describe this effect in social work teams. However, we caution against this because of self-disclosure issues and because part of the normative function is lost, as individual team members are not getting the value of benevolent scrutiny from an outside clinical supervisor. Team-building is more effectively addressed by 'awaydays', which focus explicitly on the team dynamics and working through those systematically.

The clinical supervision group could be made up of people from different teams within a hospital or locality, and this can build a sense of belonging within a wider sector of the organization. Group clinical supervision can be especially useful for practitioners who work alone a lot, reducing isolation and enhancing a feeling of being supported by the organization.

Nurses whose personality suits working in groups may prefer clinical supervision in a group setting. Self-disclosure in a group can be less frightening for more extrovert individuals who might be more scared by being closeted alone in a room with one other person. Previous positive experiences of group work might lead even the quietest nurses to prefer group clinical supervision.

Tangible changes in practice can be more likely to occur in an effective clinical supervision group than in one-to-one supervision. The challenge of a group can help the individual to accept difficult realities and get through defensiveness that might otherwise have led to the supervisee to dismiss a solo clinical supervisor's challenge. The support of the group can help the individual to have the courage to carry out difficult changes.

The dynamics of a clinical supervision group can be exciting and stimulating if all group members are very committed and have the necessary skills. The stimulation of being challenged by a supportive group can stretch and strengthen each member's reflection on their practice and can enhance their motivation for clinical supervision and for developing their practice.

Choosing a facilitator for a clinical supervision group

If you choose a group mode of clinical supervision, then there is the decision to be made about whether or not to have an outside facilitator or to take turns to facilitate the group. Some options for an outside facilitator are:

- a person from another discipline (e.g. clinical psychology) or another specialty within nursing;
- a person appointed to a post in which the job role includes being a clinical supervisor (e.g. professional development workers, practice development nurses);
- a person with specialist expertise within the supervisees' own field (e.g. child protection, HIV), however, the content of the clinical supervision session can include any other topics supervisees wishes to bring;
- a senior person who is not line manager to any of the group members (e.g. manager of another group or unit);
- a colleague at peer level who belongs to another clinical supervision group.

In other clinical supervision groups, members take turns to be the group facilitator. There are advantages and disadvantages in having an outside group facilitator or being peer-facilitated, and these are summarized in Table 9.10.

There are three further decisions to be made about the organizational structure of the delivery system of clinical supervision: whether or not it is to be compulsory to attend, how to recruit clinical supervisors and what records should be kept.

Compulsory or voluntary?

One of the main problems arising from making attendance compulsory is that it may raise resistance, exaggerating the fears of clinical supervision being a

Table 9.10   Advantages and disadvantages of having an outside or peer group facilitator

Outside group facilitator	
Advantages	*Disadvantages*
• May be more skilled at group facilitation • Has more authority, easier to challenge negative group processes • People not experienced at clinical supervision may find it useful to learn from the group facilitator's modelling • Especially useful with group members not used to collaborative work and self-disclosure in groups • Especially useful when there are interpersonal tensions already existing between members of the group	• Payment usually needed • Has to get own clinical supervision elsewhere • Group may be dependent on group facilitator, invest her with too much authority • Group members do not learn how to facilitate groups

Group members take turns to facilitate the group	
Advantages	*Disadvantages*
• No payment needed • Group members learn how to facilitate groups • Some group members may find it easier to collaborate and self-disclose in the group • Especially useful when group members are experienced at clinical supervision and/or collaborating and self-disclosing in groups • Group members may have more commitment to making the group work well, owning the process	• Has less authority, can be more difficult to challenge negative group processes • May not have enough skill in group facilitation to deal with the difficulties arising in the group • May be a tendency to avoid taking a directive role

management tool. Secondly, few organizations have yet developed such a smoothly running system that appropriate training and genuine choice of supervisor exists, and it would be unreasonable to force someone into a clinical supervision relationship with an inappropriate clinical supervisor. On the other hand, the problems of having a voluntary system include the fact that probably the staff most needing professional development will not volunteer. When some then face disciplinary proceedings about instances of poor practice, they are likely to be required to attend clinical supervision in the future. As Dimond (1998a) points out, 'Nothing would render clinical supervision more infamous and unacceptable [than] for it to be seen as part of the disciplinary process'.

On balance, we recommend that it becomes compulsory to attend clinical supervision, but within that, maximum choice is built into the system including choice of mode (one-to-one, or a group, or combination) and crucially, choice of clinical supervisor. We find that most staff attend happily if it is compulsory as this gives them permission to make it a priority and they feel less guilty about leaving the workplace for an hour a month.

You may wish to introduce compulsory attendance gradually, with all new contracts of employment including such attendance, provided there is real opportunity for some choice of supervisor and for training. Any staff applying for promotion would be required to show evidence of attendance and a brief statement from the clinical supervisor or group to the effect that commitment to the process had been displayed (without revealing anything about the content). In some staff have to attend clinical supervision in their own time, during lunch breaks or outside working hours, because there is no management sponsorship to provide the necessary cover. In these cases, the organizations give up their right to make attendance compulsory. However, registration bodies in other professions require attendance at clinical supervision for maintenance of professional registration; we look to the NMC for leadership in this respect in the future.

Recruiting clinical supervisors

The stumbling block in many organizations is not having enough clinical supervisors, as staff who feel under pressure do not want to prioritize this additional demand on their time. There can be four approaches to recruiting clinical supervisors. Firstly to publicize the benefits by engaging existing clinical supervisors in a publicity campaign. Some benefits that course members have described are shown in Figure 9.4. Secondly to reward clinical supervisors in some way, whether with a token financial bonus, by public acknowledgement of their value or by including a comment of appreciation in any job references. Thirdly, becoming a clinical supervisor could be made a requirement in new employment contracts or when

Wider insight into other people's work
Learn a lot from the supervisee about practice
Learn a lot about different ways of reflecting
Sense of solidarity with professional colleagues
Stimulates me to reflect on own practice differently
Very satisfying to support & help someone develop
Reassuring to know other's have feelings too
Opportunity to practise skills differently
I feel less isolated too
Builds my own self-esteem
Contributes to moving the profession ahead
Builds transferable skills
Helps my career: experience, CV, reference from supervisee about my skills
Contributes to retention of good staff

Figure 9.4 Some benefits of becoming a clinical supervisor, as reported by course members

applying for promotion. A fourth option is to set up a clinical supervision arrangement with a nearby organization. Having a clinical supervisor who is not employed in your own organization is usually an attractive option for many staff. One group of black nurses told us that this was their preferred option, and specialist nurses who need a clinical supervisor in their own field benefit from going outside their own locality. There are three management concerns about this option: payment, accountability and organizational confidentiality. To address the payment issue: if you make a reciprocal arrangement, no money need change hands. For example, Ward Manager Jan Doe from Bloggsbridge NHS receives her clinical supervision from district nurse team leader Sue Smith from Bloggsbridge Care Trust. Sue Smith receives her clinical supervision either in a reciprocal arrangement with Jan Doe, or from Jason Jones from Bloggsbridge NHS.

The issues of accountability and organizational confidentiality can be addressed by an organizational contract with the external clinical supervisor. An example is shown in Table 9.11. The individual clinical supervisor and supervisee would need to agree their own separate contract about how to work together within that arrangement (as described in Chapter 3).

Record-keeping

As far as records of clinical supervision are concerned, the same legal principles apply as with any other records. The client has a right of access to any records which bear their name. The employer has a right to any records that are written about sessions that take place during work time, and can use them in disciplinary proceedings. The employer has a right of access to records of attendance. Any employer that invests resources into a clinical supervision system also has a right to a record which indicates the benefits or otherwise of clinical supervision. As Dimond (1998b) points out, in theory, courts can subpoena witnesses to bring any relevant records to court, including personal diaries, though this is unlikely and such personal records hold little weight.

Therefore, we recommend that under normal circumstances, only one record is essential:

- attendance date and time of each session and who was present.

A second and third are desirable if they can contribute to an audit of clinical supervision:

- written by the supervisee: brief list of benefits to the supervisee's practice and development, after each six sessions, without revealing any of the details of the discussions held in the sessions, so that the supervisee's confidentiality is upheld;
- written by the clinical supervisor: brief list of benefits to the supervisor's practice and development after each six sessions, without revealing any of the details of the discussions held in the sessions, so that the supervisee's confidentiality is upheld.

Table 9.11 An example of an organizational contract with an external clinical supervisor outside the organization

---

Contract for clinical supervision for .... (name of supervisee)

This is to confirm an agreement between ......(name of clinical supervisor) and .....(name of supervisee's line manager) for ....(name of clinical supervisor) to provide the following programme of reflective clinical supervision for ......(name of supervisee).

Format

The supervisee will attend monthly 1-hour, one-to-one sessions for a period of 12 months (10 sessions held during that time), renewable. This will be 'clinical supervision' in the sense of facilitated in-depth reflection on practice. The supervisee would be expected to continue to receive line management supervision from his/her line manager and to seek specific clinical advice and guidance from the relevant sources as necessary.

This clinical supervision will be on a reciprocal basis in that .....(name of supervisee's employing organization) will provide an equal number of clinical supervision sessions for a member of staff from .....(name of clinical supervisor's employing organization). Hence there is no financial fee.

Cancellation and postponement of sessions

If the date and time of a session has been agreed between supervisee and clinical supervisor but is not attended by the supervisee for any reason, then the clinical supervisor will, in an emergency, attempt to reschedule to a mutually convenient time but if this is not possible, the clinical supervisor will have fulfilled his/her obligation towards the supervisee in terms of providing that session. The next monthly session will be mutually agreed at the time of cancellation.

Accountability and confidentiality

The clinical supervisor will provide, on request, a record of the supervisee's attendance to their line manager. If any unsafe practice, failure of risk management or any other breach of the NMC (2008) Code of Standards of Conduct and Performance becomes evident during clinical supervision sessions that seems not to be being addressed through the required channels, and if the supervisee is not willing or able to set about going through the required channels with appropriate haste, the clinical supervisor will provide an urgent report to the supervisee's line manager with the knowledge of the supervisee. Otherwise, the content of the sessions remain confidential and no record will be kept of the content of the sessions. This applies to all personal, professional and organizational information disclosed.

Contact details

.........(name and contact details of clinical supervisor)
.........(name and contact details of supervisee)

Signed by ....(name of supervisee's line
       manager)

on behalf of ....(name of supervisee's
       employing organization)

Signed by ....(name of clinical supervisor)
as confirmation of the above agreement

as confirmation of the above agreement

Signature ....

Signature ....

Date ....

Position ....

Date ....

The following records of clinical supervision may kept if it is the supervisee's choice, without mentioning any client's name or any specific details of the content unless unsafe practice has been disclosed:

- an aide-memoire: we suggest that you write only general topic headings such as 'case review; stress management; time management; team work', etc. and some specific action plans; what is written needs to keep the details of the discussion confidential;
- personal reflective diary: written on supervisee's own stationery and kept confidential to herself and in her own home;
- references: brief statement by those involved by way of a reference for promotion of the supervisee or the clinical supervisor, about level of commitment to and skills of clinical supervision, but not about any content discussed.

However, of course it is vital that an extraordinary record is kept under circumstances of risk. A record must be kept of any unsafe practice that has been disclosed and this information must be passed on if the supervisee is unable or unwilling to deal with the matter through the required procedures.

Evaluation

Attempts to evaluate clinical supervision systems are notoriously difficult, as outlined in the previous section. As Butterworth (1996: 96) suggests, the ideal research answers will, of course, be those in which clinical supervision is shown to have an impact on client outcomes, but Butterworth has not yet been able to devise such an evaluation tool. He goes on to state that: 'at this early stage, a more measured and wide-ranging approach is likely to produce more satisfactory and reliable results. The "feel-good" factor for staff may well be central to high standard performance, and recent encouragement to care for and develop the workforce has some merit'.

This qualitative dimension may be difficult to capture but is likely to be more important than the alternative quantitative measures. The entire project could be set up as an action research project following guidelines suggested by Hart and Bond (1993) and Hawkins and Shohet (2006). Specific groups of staff could set up a cooperative enquiry, using models suggested by Reason (1988). Focus groups facilitated by an impartial outsider could be used to evaluate staff responses to their clinical supervision.

Butterworth (1996) presents a range of tools and research methods linked to potential benefits to be accrued in each of Proctor's (1986) three key functional areas – for instance, existing mechanisms of sickness rates, absence, recruitment and retention, and complaints could be used to audit staff satisfaction in the normative dimension as well as including client responses concerning satisfaction, complaints and health gain. Stress and burnout scales could be used to evaluate the support (restorative) sphere. The most widely used are the General Health Questionnaire (Goldberg and Williams 1988) which is a brief, 12 item self-administered questionnaire that takes a few minutes to complete and the Maslach Burnout Inventory

(Maslach and Jackson, 1981) which consists of 22 items and takes approximately 10–15 minutes to complete. Learning profiles and clinical skills development could be used to assess professional development in the formative component. Structured or unstructured one-to-one interviews from an outside researcher could be used to evaluate all three functional areas. The 'rich pictures' (Checkland 1970) approach could be used to feed back the information collected. The Manchester Clinical Supervision Scale contains 36 items and is applied after staff have attended at least six clinical supervision sessions (Winstanley 2000).

We also maintain that anecdotal evidence has it's value amongst other measures. The 'feel good' factor, for instance, in Swain's (1995: 56) overview of the monitoring and impact of supervision states that: 'The difference is somehow tangible; there is a sense of more openness and a positive approach', and in Model 3: 'the practitioner is more confident and assertive, begins to decide objectives, begins to see goals and progress. It is easy to think that nothing has happened, as often the milestones reached are only small. However sickness rates have been seen to drop while in supervision, and to rise for one recently qualified practitioner when supervision had to stop'. In Parkinson's (1992: 52) study the 'managers . . . noted the beneficial effects on safe practice which had been achieved particularly in terms of working more openly with families, record keeping and better report writing. One manager also thought a large number of staff felt safer in their work'. Clearly anecdotal evidence such as this is inadequate by itself but we hear a similar range of positive responses in early reviews of systems. As we observed earlier, there may still be a long way to go before links to staff satisfaction, increased competence and confidence may be translated into demonstrable benefits for clients, but meanwhile anecdotal evidence has its place.

Patient stories are gaining credibility as useful indicators of quality of practice (see Gullick and Shimadry 2008). One relevant example is the experience of one of the authors of this book, who did her own small evaluation while a patient on a surgical ward:

> I knew that clinical supervision was available to the staff on this ward, and that attendance was voluntary (I supervised the person coordinating it!). I made a list of the staff who nursed me over the period of my stay and rated how much trust I had in their professionalism: not an objective measure, but the most important criterion to me as a patient. The staff fell into two distinct categories: those I trusted and those I didn't. Those I trusted had good communication, aseptic technique and time management skills and were responsive when I needed help. Those I didn't trust were poor in all these skills and unresponsive to my requests for help because they were 'too busy', yet spent much time in loud aimless chatter and sexually harassing the junior male nurse at the nurses' station. I predicted that the individuals I trusted attended clinical supervision and the others didn't (I privately called the latter the MINCS – most-in-need-of-clinical-supervision).
>
> Towards the end of my stay I asked each in turn if they attended clinical supervision and I was 100 per cent correct in my prediction. The reasons given for not attending were: 'didn't know it was available' (there was a poster on the staff noticeboard within my sight as she spoke); 'too busy to be able to make the time'

(if the time spent chatting at the nurses' station during my short stay had been added up, this would have totalled more than an hour each); and 'don't need it' (no further comment!). To extrapolate: it left the chicken-or-the-egg question: does a voluntary scheme mean that the best nurses take up clinical supervision and others don't? Or does it mean that the nurses who take up clinical supervision subsequently perform better?

There may be potential for an evaluation project involving nurses who become patients, using similar indicators or eliciting their own priorities as patients.

Some evaluation tools

This book emphasizes the working alliance between the supervisee and the clinical supervisor, and on the specific skills of both roles; therefore our contribution to the body of evaluation tools has this focus. Tables 9.12 to 9.15 show some questionnaires for assessing your own skills, asking for feedback and for discussion, and Figure 9.5 summarizes the process of using these tools. The background to these questionnaires comes from the concerns managers have about evaluating clinical supervision. One manager asked us for something with tick boxes to show the Trust board in order to make a case for more funds for clinical supervision. It did

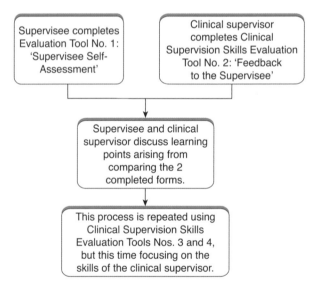

Afterwards, you can use your learning to:
1. Decide how you will develop your clinical supervision
2. Demonstrate your learning in your PREP portfolio and/or in your appraisal meetings with your line manager.

Figure 9.5 How to use the clinical supervision evaluation tools

Table 9.12   Clinical Supervision Skills Evaluation Tool No. 1: Supervisee self-assessment

For the supervisee to complete after at least 3 sessions with the same clinical supervisor.

This questionnaire is offered as a way of assessing how you are progressing as a supervisee. Ask your clinical supervisor to complete Evaluation Tool No. 2, based on the same criteria. Compare your sheets and discuss any emerging points of interest. It is not intended that anyone else would have access to this completed document: and the discussion is part of the confidential clinical supervision relationship.

Please tick one box for each point

As a supervisee in clinical supervision, I.....	No	Yes
Chose my own clinical supervisor rather than expected to be allocated one		

As a supervisee in clinical supervision, I.....	Never	Some-times	Mostly	Always
1. Prioritize the time needed for clinical supervision				
2. Assert myself in making the time to get to clinical supervision				
3. Maintain the boundary between clinical supervision & counselling				
4. Stick to appointments & am on time				
5. Protect the space: ensure there are no interruptions from telephones or people walking in				
6. Have clarified to the clinical supervisor what I expect of him/her & agreed ground rules				
7. Stick to the ground rules				
8. Decide which topics to bring to my clinical supervision and think about them before I attend				
9. Clarify what I want in particular from my clinical supervisor at the beginning of each session				
10. Take responsibility for any actions I take in practice as a result of the sessions				
11. Give feedback to the clinical supervisor about what they do that is most and least helpful				
12. Use the time to reflect in-depth on issues affecting my practice and avoid non-productive conversation				
13. Can tell my story in an articulate way				
14. Accept support from the clinical supervisor				
15. Express & explore my own opinions about the topic I bring to clinical supervision				
16. Express & explore my emotional feelings related to the topic I have brought				
17. Discuss personal concerns affecting my concentration at work				
18. Speak in a free-flowing, intuitive, uncensored, unstructured way and stop and reflect on what has emerged				

(continued)

19. Regain focus when I go off the point				
20. Analyse my topic logically				
21. Explore my professional strengths, knowledge & competencies				
22. Clarify my objectives relating to the topic I have brought				
23. Take responsibility for thinking of my own solutions to problems				
24. Explore my professional weaknesses, mistakes & limitations				
25. Explore my personal strengths & qualities & how these influence my work				
26. Explore my personal limitations & vulnerabilities & how these influence my work				
27. Identify themes which emerge over many sessions				
28. Explore implications & consequences of my actions				
29. Am open to challenge if I do not stick to the ground rules				
30. Seek & accept feedback from the clinical supervisor on my performance as a supervisee				
31. Am open to being challenged to explore topics or aspects of my work that I avoid talking about				
32. Am open to being challenged if my clinical supervisor thinks I have made a mistake or error of judgement				
33. Open to listening to the clinical supervisor's opinions on what I am saying				
34. Open to being challenged to stretch myself by tackling something difficult or learning something new				
35. Willing to listen to and evaluate the occasional suggestion or guideline from my clinical supervisor				
36. Challenge my clinical supervisor if s/he is giving too much advice, suggestions, information or guidelines				
37. Work out my own action plans arising from my reflection during clinical supervision sessions				
38. Clarify key questions to reflect upon after a session				
39. Use humour appropriately during clinical supervision				
40. Am open about my own feelings about how we are working together				
41. At the next session, inform my clinical supervisor about how my action plans were carried out				
42. Finish the session on time				
43. (*Space to add any other criteria for being an effective supervisee*)				

My clinical supervisor might be able to help me to expand and deepen my supervisee skills by......

Table 9.13 Clinical Supervision Skills Evaluation Tool No. 2: Feedback to the supervisee

---

For the clinical supervisor to complete after at least 3 sessions with the same supervisee.
This questionnaire is offered as a way of assessing how your supervisee is progressing in their use of clinical supervision. Your supervisee will have a self-assessment tool based on the same criteria. Discussing & comparing your sheets may be useful for developing your supervisee's ability to use clinical supervision time effectively and to consider how you might help him/her to do so. It is not intended that anyone else would have access to this completed document: the discussion is part of the confidential clinical supervision relationship.

My supervisee......,	No	Yes
Chose me as her/his clinical supervisor rather than expected to be allocated one		

My supervisee......,	Never	Some-times	Mostly	Always
1. Prioritizes the time needed for clinical supervision				
2. Asserts her/himself in making the time to get to clinical supervision				
3. Maintains the boundary between clinical supervision & counselling				
4. Sticks to appointments & is on time				
5. Protects the space: ensures there are no interruptions from telephones or people walking in				
6. Has clarified to the me what s/he expect of me in clinical supervision & has agreed ground rules or contract				
7. Sticks to the ground rules				
8. Decides which topics to bring to clinical supervision and appears to think about them before they attend				
9. Clarifies what s/he wants in particular from me as clinical supervisor at the beginning of each session				
10. Takes responsibility for any actions s/he takes in practice as a result of the sessions				
11. Gives me feedback about what I do that is most and least helpful				
12. Uses the time to reflect in-depth on issues affecting her/his practice and avoids non-productive conversation.				
13. Can tell their story in an articulate way				
14. Can accept support from me				
15. Expresses & explores her/his own opinions about the topic brought to clinical supervision				
16. Expresses & explores her/his emotional feelings related to the topic				
17. Reflects on personal concerns affecting concentration at work				
18. Reflects in an intuitive, uncensored and unstructured way				

(continued)

Table 9.13   Clinical Supervision Skills Evaluation Tool No. 2: Feedback to the supervisee (*Continued*)

19. Regains focus when s/he goes off the point				
20. Analyses the topic logically				
21. Explores his/her own professional strengths, knowledge & competencies				
22. Clarifies his/her objectives relating to the topic				
23. Takes responsibility for thinking of their own solutions to problems				
24. Explores his/her own professional weaknesses, mistakes & limitations				
25. Explores his/her own personal strengths & qualities & how these influence professional effectiveness				
26. Explores his/her own personal limitations & vulnerabilities & how these influence professional effectiveness				
27. Identifies themes which emerge over multiple sessions				
28. Explores implications & consequences of their own actions and attitudes				
29. Is open to challenge if s/he is not sticking to the ground rules				
30. Seeks & accepts feedback from me about how well I think they are using the clinical supervision sessions				
31. Is open to being challenged to explore topics or aspects of their work that they avoid talking about				
32. Is open to being challenged if I think they have made a mistake or error of judgement				
33. Open to listening to my opinions on what they are saying				
34. Open to being challenged to stretch him/herself by tackling something difficult or learning something new				
35. Willing to listen to and evaluate the occasional suggestion or guideline from myself				
36. Challenges me if I am giving too much advice, suggestions, information or guidelines				
37. Works out his/her own action plans arising from reflection during clinical supervision sessions				
38. Clarifies questions to reflect upon after a session				
39. Uses humour appropriately during clinical supervision				
40. Is open about her/his own feelings about how we are working together				
41. At the next session, informs me about how the action plans were carried out				
42. Finishes the session on time				
43. (*Space to add any other criteria for being an effective supervisee*)				

As clinical supervisor, I might be able to help my supervisee to expand and deepen his/her supervisee skills by....

Table 9.14 Clinical Supervision Skills Evaluation Tool No. 3: Clinical supervisor self-assessment

For the clinical supervisor to complete after at least 3 sessions with the same supervisee.
This questionnaire is offered as a way of assessing how you are doing as a clinical supervisor. Your supervisee will have a feedback tool based on the same criteria. Discussing & comparing your sheets may be useful for your development as a clinical supervisor.

Part 1

As a clinical supervisor, I.....	Never	Some-times	Mostly	Always
A. Keep clinical supervision separate from management supervision				
B. Maintain the boundary between clinical supervision & counselling				
C. Am reliable: stick to appointments & am on time				
D. Help the supervisee to finish the session on time				
E. Protect the space: ensure no interruptions from telephones or people walking in				
F. Settle myself: am able to focus on the supervisee when we start the session				
G. Help the supervisee to feel at ease with the clinical supervision process				
H. Help to make clinical supervision a constructive learning experience for the supervisee				
I. Have clarified to the supervisee what I expect of him/her in clinical supervision & have agreed ground rules or contract				
J. Maintain confidentiality (except in instances of unsafe practice that the supervisee cannot or will not address appropriately)				
K. If I have to break confidentiality, I first of all inform the supervisee				
L. Stick to the other ground rules we agreed				
M. Encourage the supervisee to decide which topics Is/he wants to bring to clinical supervision				

Part 2   *Please note that the scale has changed*

As clinical supervisor, I....	Not at all	A little	Just right	A bit too much	Much too much	Don't know
1. Give the supervisee space to tell their story in their own way & listen attentively						
2. Support the supervisee non-verbally						
3. Support the supervisee verbally, explicitly						
4. Encourage the supervisee to express & explore their opinions						
5. Encourage the supervisee to express & explore their feelings						
6. Enable the supervisee to discuss personal concerns affecting his/her concentration at work						

(continued)

Table 9.14 Clinical Supervision Skills Evaluation Tool No. 3: Clinical supervisor self-assessment (*Continued*)

7. Enable the supervisee to reflect intuitively and clarify emerging issues, insights, learning points and their own intuitive solutions						
8. Help the supervisee to focus when s/he goes off the point						
9. Enable the supervisee to analyse their topic logically, by prompting & questioning						
10. Enable the supervisee to explore their professional strengths, knowledge & competencies						
11. Help the supervisee to clarify objectives						
12. Prompt the supervisee to think of their own solutions to problems						
13. Enable the supervisee to explore their professional weaknesses, mistakes & limitations						
14. Enable the supervisee to explore their personal strengths & qualities & how these influence their work						
15. Enable the supervisee to explore their personal limitations & vulnerabilities & how these influence their work						
16. Help the supervisee to identify themes which emerge over many sessions						
17. Enable the supervisee to explore implications & consequences of their actions						
18. Challenge the supervisee if s/he does not stick to the ground rules						
19. Seek & accept feedback from the supervisee on my performance as a clinical supervisor						
20. Challenge the supervisee to explore topics or aspects of their work that they avoid talking about						
21. Let the supervisee know if I think is/he has made a mistake or error of judgement						
22. Give my own opinion on the situation the supervisee is describing						
23. Challenge the supervisee to stretch her/himself by tackling something difficult or learning something new						
24. Make suggestions or give guidelines						
25. Provide information						
26. Enable the supervisee to work out action plans						
27. Enable the supervisee to clarify questions to reflect upon after a session.						
28. Challenge the supervisee to carry out their action plans						
29. Take the supervisee & their issues seriously						
30. Use humour appropriately						
31. Am open about my own feelings about how we are working together						
32. Maintain objectivity about the supervisee's work situation.						
33. Maintain optimism						
34. (*Space to add any other criteria for being an effective clinical supervisor*)						

Any other comments

Table 9.15   Clinical Supervision Skills Evaluation Tool No. 4: Feedback from supervisee to clinical supervisor

For the supervisee to complete after at least 3 sessions with the same clinical supervisor.

This sheet is offered as a way of giving feedback to your clinical supervisor. S/he will have completed self-assessment sheet based on the same criteria. Discussing & comparing your sheets may be useful for the development of your working alliance and for the skills of your clinical supervisor.

Part 1

My clinical supervisor...	Never	Some-times	Mostly	Always
A. Keeps clinical supervision separate from management supervision				
B. Maintains the boundary between clinical supervision & counselling				
C. Is reliable: sticks to appointments & is on time				
D. Helps me to finish the session on time				
E. Protects the space: ensures no interruptions e.g. telephones or people walking in				
F. Seems settled: able to focus on me when we start the session				
G. Helps me to feel at ease with the clinical supervision process				
H. Helps to make clinical supervision a constructive learning experience for me				
I. Has clarified to me what s/he expects of me in clinical supervision & has agreed ground rules or contract with me				
J. Maintains confidentiality (although I realize s/he would have to make an exception in instances of unsafe practice that I'm not addressing)				
K. I can trust that if my clinical supervisor had to break confidentiality, s/he would first inform me.				
L. Sticks to the other ground rules we made				
M. Encourages me to decide which topics I want to bring to clinical supervision				

Part 2   *Please note that the scale has changed*

My clinical supervisor....	Not at all	A little	Just right	A bit too much	Much too much	Don't know
1. Gives me space to tell my story in my own way & listens attentively						
2. Supports me non-verbally						
3. Supports me verbally, explicitly						
4. Encourages me to express & explore my opinions						
5. Encourages me to express & explore my feelings						
6. Enables me to discuss personal concerns affecting my concentration at work						

(continued)

Table 9.15 Clinical Supervision Skills Evaluation Tool No. 4: Feedback from supervisee to clinical supervisor (*Continued*)

7. Enables me to reflect in an intuitive, unstructured way & helps me clarify my emerging issues, insights & my own intuitive solutions							
8. Helps me to focus when I go off the point							
9. Enables me (by prompting & questioning) to analyse my topic logically							
10. Enables me to explore my professional strengths, knowledge & competencies							
11. Helps me to clarify objectives							
12. Prompts me to think of my own solutions to problems							
13. Enables me to explore my professional weaknesses, mistakes & limitations							
14. Enables me to explore my personal strengths & qualities & how these influence my work							
15. Enables me to explore my personal limitations & vulnerabilities & how these influence my work							
16. Helps me to identify themes which emerge over many sessions							
17. Enables me to explore implications & consequences of my actions							
18. Challenges me if I do not stick to the ground rules							
19. Seeks & accepts my feedback of her/his performance as a clinical supervisor							
20. Challenges me to explore topics or aspects of my work that I avoid talking about							
21. Lets me know if s/he thinks I have made a mistake							
22. Gives her/his own opinion							
23. Challenges me to stretch myself by tackling something difficult or learning something new							
24. Makes suggestions or gives guidelines							
25. Provides information							
26. Enables me to work out action plans							
27. Enables me to clarify questions to reflect upon after a session.							
28. Challenges me to carry out my action plans							
29. Takes me & my issues seriously							
30. Uses humour appropriately							
31. Is open about her/his own feelings about how we are working together							
32. Maintains objectivity about my own work situation							
33. Maintains optimism							
34. (*Space to add any other criteria for being an effective clinical supervisor*)							

Any other comments

not seem to matter what criteria were in the boxes, as long as there were some! You may have guessed that tick boxes are not our favourite tools, but we put together these questionnaires, tested them ourselves, as did our supervisees and some course participants, and were surprised how very useful they were in our own supervision and for others.

It is not intended that anyone else would have access to these completed documents. The discussion, which emerges from comparing the completed forms, is part of the confidential clinical supervision relationship, unless the individuals choose to use them, perhaps in their professional portfolio or as evidence of learning for staff appraisal with their manager. The tools are for use after at least three sessions of clinical supervision with the same clinical supervisor and supervisee, and subsequently about every three to six sessions. They can be used as checklists, or for those who are uncomfortable with tick boxes, as a list of ideas for discussion. To use them as checklists, the first step is for the supervisee to complete Tool 1: 'Supervisee self-assessment' (Table 9.12) and then ask the clinical supervisor to complete the second form shown in Table 9.13: 'Feedback to the supervisee'. When both have completed the forms, they get together to compare notes: laying the forms out together will quickly show any differences. Treat these differences as interesting areas for discussion, rather than trying to prove who is 'right'. The very act of completing the forms will have raised some interesting thoughts which will be useful to explore with each other. There is no need to discuss every simple item on the forms: just use them to pinpoint areas for discussion.

Then the process continues with the clinical supervisor completing the third tool shown in Table 9.14 assessing her clinical supervision skills with regard to this particular supervisee. The supervisee completes the fourth tool, in Table 9.15, and they meet to compare and discuss emerging points of interest. Plans are made concerning how to develop the way they work together.

Establish and monitor

The evaluations may indicate a need to redesign your clinical supervision system. When you have clarified and implemented this redesign, you will need to adapt some of your evaluation methods to use as monitoring tools. The all-important sponsorship by a senior manager of the ongoing clinical supervision system needs to continue to be high profile and explicit in its support for the staff, as they continue to refine and develop their clinical supervision.

Summary

In suggesting some practical ways of addressing the organisational dimension of clinical supervision with the intended outcome of setting up, maintaining and developing clinical supervision, we emphasise the need to design a system which creates the conditions required for trust to develop within the working alliance (the relationship between the clinical supervisor and the supervisee) and to ensure that clinical supervision is secure place for in-depth reflection by developing it as a distinct entity separate from and in addition to line management supervision. We have offered some evaluation tools which focus on the skills of clinical supervision and of building the working alliance. We have pointed towards the importance of considering the ethics of facilitating in-depth reflection and therefore the self-disclosure that accompanies it, and the next chapter elaborates on this ethical dimension.

10 A picture of the future

Finally we want to take a look into the future to suggest ways that clinical supervision could support or fuel strategies for change that will empower nurses to have a stronger profile and be at the centre-stage of health care delivery. We focus on two main issues:

- the way that clinical supervision can complement clinical leadership in nursing;
- the need for an ethical code of practice to complement high quality, compassionate care.

Leadership in nursing

Clinical leadership occurs at all levels of patient care, and is essential to clinical governance. It encompasses both a set of attributes required to lead and inspire others such as enthusiasm, openness, flexibility, aptitude for reflection and change, and the ability to orchestrate a set of actions that improve the delivery of client care, such as the ability to prioritize, focus, communicate and enact values and ethical care.

The road to leadership may start by becoming a supervisor (and of course, before that a supervisee, who very early on is able to evaluate the role models they would like to emulate later in the supervision they receive). This makes the choosing of supervisors particularly important. The Commission on the Future of Nursing and Midwifery in England (2010) highlights the importance of developing the ward sister and equivalent clinical lead, and has ideas for fast-tracking those with potential. However, broad organizational change over many years has taken its toll on nursing in the form of massive restructuring, workforce attrition, and the felt and actual reduction in the voice and power of the nurse. How can this be remedied?

We are aware that there have been a number of leadership projects over the past 10 years, notably that of the RCN, which has been extensively evaluated (see Large *et al.* 2003). But we are thinking of something more everyday and ordinary to be monitored and evaluated less ambitiously. We need a greater groundswell of nurses willing to think 'outside the box' and enable others to do the same, mindful of course of what is possible and safe. They need to know where the frame of the picture is. The profession cannot rely on training just for the high-flyers. We repeat, clinical leadership can be at every level, and well managed and supported clinical supervision is the fertile ground where leadership seeds can be sown.

The Commission on the Future of Nursing and Midwifery in England (2010) refers to the earlier radical roots of nursing and midwifery and how one of the biggest workforces in Europe needs to rekindle this potential. It suggests that nurses are ideally placed to influence health from micro to macro level in a wide range of settings. It also states that, 'despite delivering compassionate and effective care, unacceptable variations persist in the standards of care, often associated with systems failure and real or perceived constraints on care' (p. 15). These are the very constraints, both individual and systemic, that we have suggested also get in the way of any new initiative, such as implementing clinical supervision.

There has been a great deal of learning within clinical supervision initiatives about how to achieve systemic change, and this could enable the development of the role of the ward sister and equivalent positions in the community and elsewhere. The process of clinical supervision, with reflective practice at its centre, respectful of the layered complexity of delivering care in complex environments, could offer a pathway to try out those with early leadership potential. They could 'cut their teeth', during the process of supervision, into thinking more creatively, having more confidence in their nursing knowledge and experience, and putting it into practice. The collaborative and enabling aspects of supervision (which are well documented in the studies) can nurture good leadership skills in the future. Leadership also requires an ability to balance autonomy with accountability and to have a repertoire of enabling and challenging skills. To lead well is also to collaborate well, being clear about when to enable and say little, and when to be firm, clear and resolute. We hope that the array of measured and balanced skills you have explored throughout this book will not only prepare you for clinical supervision, but will also pave the way for you as clinical leaders in the future.

Codes of ethics and practice for clinical supervision in nursing

Starting point: compassion and respecting dignity in client care

In order to benefit from the service offered, it is a matter of course that clients are expected to disclose to the practitioners more about themselves than is the social norm between strangers. This disclosure may be physical exposure, emotional exposure, revealing details of lifestyle and social relationships or often all of these areas in which we normally carefully grade our levels of privacy according to the level of intimacy we share with other people. Justifiably, there is increasing pressure from client groups and increasing concern at all levels from government (Department of Health 2010) to practitioners (Baillie *et al.* 2008) that the environment, organization, communication and manner of delivery of health care should strive to maintain clients' dignity by dealing respectfully with the self-disclosure which is required for them to benefit from the care. This is an intrinsic part of compassionate care.

We maintain that in order for practitioners and managers of the service to be in a psychological position to be compassionate and respectful of clients' dignity, they themselves require the experience of being treated with compassion and respect in their workplace. This applies to all areas of their employment and especially to clinical supervision. While the supervisee should be made aware that in order to benefit from clinical supervision they are expected to disclose to the clinical supervisor more about themselves as a person in a professional role than is the social norm between colleagues, their clinical supervision should be structured and provided in a compassionate manner which respects their dignity and the self-disclosure risks they take when reflecting on practice.

We consider this to be an ethical issue and therefore we are proposing here a code of practice in clinical supervision for qualified nurses, in order to open an ethical perspective in the debate about the organization of clinical supervision. There is international interest in this approach from nurses and other non-counseling professionals (Bond 2010). We are curious to know where the debate will go in this regard between the publication of this edition of the book and the next.

First, we need to clarify the ethical basis of a code of practice. A code of practice is a set of standards of professional behaviour, which are underpinned by an ethical code, a set of ethical principles. These standards may be a baseline of acceptable professional behaviour or may be aspirational: for instance, it could be said that the Nursing and Midwifery Council code (2008a) is a combination of both. Here we look first at a code of ethics and then at a code of professional practice as two distinct but related entities.

Table 10.1 For discussion: draft code of ethics for clinical supervision for qualified nurses

---

- Principle A *Priority of clinical supervision*: make the supervisee's care of people the first concern, treating them as individuals and respecting their dignity and to ensure the supervisee provides a high standard of practice and care at all times
- Principle B *Added value*: ensure that the work done in clinical supervision ultimately adds value to the protection and promotion of the health and well-being of those in the supervisee's care, their families and carers, and the wider community
- Principle C *Integrity*: act with integrity and honesty in the organization of clinical supervision, its delivery, training in the clinical supervisor/supervisee relationship and in the monitoring and audit of clinical supervision.
- Principle D *Supervisee well-being*: the supervisee is treated with compassion, respect, lack of discrimination
- Principle E *Sensitivity to supervisee self-disclosure issues* in the organization of clinical supervision, its delivery, training, in the non-managerial nature of the clinical supervisor/supervisee relationship and in the monitoring and audit of clinical supervision.
- Principle F *Supervisee development*: with principles 1 and 2 as the main aims, the focus of clinical supervision sessions is on the support and development of the supervisee
- Principle G *Continuous improvement*: maintain and improve proficiency in the organization of clinical supervision, training for clinical supervision, its delivery, the clinical supervisor/supervisee relationship and in the monitoring and audit of clinical supervision.

Code of ethics

Lee (2003: 74) suggests that 'the adoption of codes of ethics has a clear impact upon the social, economic and performance environment of the organisation', and cites research in the human resources field (Priest 1998). While such a code has not yet been adopted for clinical supervision, discussing the ethics of clinical supervision can have the effect of increased thoughtfulness regarding how to go about it. For instance, this example illustrates an unethical approach to the use of clinical supervision skills can be counter productive:

> In the opening round of 'Why I came on this course', Samantha said: 'I'm the manager of a forensic mental health unit. I need to know how my staff think and feel about their work and I need to know what their childhood histories are, in case they are triggered by the patients' issues. We have patients who have been detained following offences such as paedophilia and murder. As a safety issue I need to know about the mental health of my staff to know if they are up to the job, as I'm concerned about the performance of a few of them. My problem is that I can't get them to open up to me in clinical supervision, so I've come to learn some techniques to do that.'
>
> When the course topics came to the recommendation that staff have clinical supervision from outside their immediate team, Samantha said: 'Oh no, our team is like a family, we've got the rule we have to bring any practice or team issues to the team and get them out in the open, that taking team issues outside breaks the team dynamic.' It was revealed later that the team did not bring team issues to the team meetings: they tended to complain behind their colleagues' backs.
>
> After some carefully structured clinical supervision practice sessions (focusing on real workplace issues, not role-play) in which Samantha took her turn as supervisee and explored something which involved quite a bit of self-disclosure, the course group discussed what they would want from their own clinical supervision and what sort of person they would want as their supervisor. Samantha said, 'I have clinical supervision with my line manager, he's fine but I couldn't do *that* [the self-disclosure] with him.' With some input to prompt the group discussion of the ethics of facilitating/requiring self-disclosure in clinical supervision she suddenly said: 'Ah, I see what you mean about my staff. I need to think about that.'

Lee (2003: 78) goes on say that 'Codes of ethics can be seen as a reflection of society's and of a profession's values, and thus could and should be changed to address changing societal and professional values'. Hence we are testing the water with our proposal: does your organization care enough about its members or employees to have a code of ethics for clinical supervision and if so, what should it be? And what code of practice should it inform? How will that compare to other organizations employing nurses? Could a common code of ethics for clinical supervision emerge? Our draft for discussion is shown in Table 10.1.

Code of practice

Gregory (2006: 4) asserts that:

> Codes of practice are not a substitute for ethical reasoning, which each individual must do for him/herself, but through the sharing of ethical reasoning, people offering the same professional services can agree on some basic ethical principles to apply to their profession. They can also pool their knowledge and skills of best practice in their profession, and from these develop acceptable standards that all can subscribe to.

She goes on to say that 'the imposition of professional codes of practice without a discussion of ethics potentially keeps the person at a lower level of moral development' and cites Kohlberg's six main stages of moral development (Kohlberg and Lickona 1976).

While we fully concur with this approach, we would like to propose a draft code of practice as a trigger for discussion and urge you and your colleagues to

Table 10.2 First of 3 sections of a draft code of practice for clinical supervision for qualified nurses: professional accountability

a) The clinical supervisor and supervisee must be aware of the supervisee's professional code of practice and uphold it at all times.

b) As supervisee, you remain personally accountable for actions and omissions in your practice whatever the content and outcome of the dialogue you have with your clinical supervisor.

c) In the event of unsafe practice being disclosed, as clinical supervisor you have no more or less responsibility than any other professional colleague who becomes aware of unsafe practice: you must disclose information to the appropriate person in authority if the supervisee reveals unsafe practice that is not being dealt with <u>and</u> the supervisee is unable or unwilling to proceed with appropriate haste to deal with it themselves having discussed it with the you. You must keep a record in such a situation and reveal it when/if required.

d) As clinical supervisor you must ensure the supervisee is informed about how and why any information is shared and recorded as above.

e) The clinical supervisor and the supervisee must keep a record of attendance at clinical supervision, showing dates, times and who was present and be willing to share this for monitoring and audit purposes.

f) If requested for monitoring and audit purposes, the clinical supervisor and the supervisee must keep a record of the value or otherwise of the clinical supervision, without breaking supervisee or patient confidentiality.

g) You are not required to keep a record of the content of sessions (exception as above).

h) As clinical supervisor you must not give advice or information on issues outside your own field of expertise (i.e. negligent advice) and you must always be able to justify giving any advice or information.

discuss your own code of ethics and your own emerging code of practice for clinical supervision for qualified nurses. We have observed all the elements shown in Table 10.2, though not all of them in the same organization, so we contend that this draft code is not solely aspirational.

Table 10.3 Second of 3 sections of a draft code of practice for clinical supervision for qualified nurses: the organization of clinical supervision

a) An operational nurse manager is designated to take the lead in developing, maintaining and auditing clinical supervision and an administrator is designated to coordinate the practicalities of maintaining a database of people (not necessarily only nurses) who could be clinical supervisors and of possible venues and booking details. clinical supervision is set up as separate to and does not replace line management or safeguarding supervision.

b) Training in the skills of the supervisee and clinical supervisor is available and attendance is mandatory for those who have not attended either of these courses.

c) Trainers have significant experience in themselves receiving and giving non-managerial clinical supervision and are currently receiving it regularly.

d) Training includes a range of logical, intuitive and emotional models of reflection and after the course, supervisees have the intellectual freedom to choose which, if any, of the models of reflection are used for their in-depth reflection in each of their clinical supervision sessions.

e) Nurses who have been qualified and practised full time for 2 years (or p/t equivalent) are encouraged to attend both supervisee and clinical supervisor skills training and to become clinical supervisors. Incentives are offered to become clinical supervisors or it is made a requirement of employment or of achieving a promotion to a higher band.

f) All qualified nurses are encouraged to attend supervisee skills training and to attend and make good use of clinical supervision and if clinical supervisors are available, it is made a requirement of employment or of achieving a promotion to a higher band.

g) The system must provide for a minimum of 10 clinical supervision sessions per year (or f/t equivalent) for each supervisee, each session providing each supervisee 1 hour minimum of individual time for facilitated in-depth reflection. Total: 10 hours (or f/t equivalent) facilitated in-depth reflection per person per year.

h) In order to avoid compromising anyone's line management authority, and to maintain objectivity and space for the self-disclosure necessary for in-depth reflection, a clinical supervisor is not: i) in the same management line as the supervisee, i.e. is not superior or subordinate in their immediate line of the hierarchy; ii) a colleague of the supervisee within the same day-to-day working team; iii) a close friend or relative. Within those limits, the supervisee must have some choice of clinical supervisor or if no choice available, is explicitly asked to review clinical supervision after 3 sessions and has the choice to terminate working with that clinical supervisor at that or any subsequent point when another clinical supervisor becomes available.

i) All clinical supervisors who currently have supervisees must attend their own concurrent regular clinical supervision.

j) No one can specify what topic a supervisee takes to clinical supervision: the supervisee chooses their own, provided it has some bearing on their work.

(continued)

Table 10.3 Second of 3 sections of a draft code of practice for clinical supervision for qualified nurses: the organization of clinical supervision (*continued*)

---

k) Rooms which afford enough privacy and are not used at particular times are made available to be booked for clinical supervision sessions, e.g. offices, clinics, consulting rooms, small waiting rooms, teaching rooms etc. Strategic managers, including the chief executive, demonstrate support for the clinical supervision lead and the staff by making their offices available when they are at meetings, bookable through their PAs.

l) At strategic level, clinical supervision is included in all initiatives and service contracts. At human resources level, clinical supervision is included in all employment contracts for qualified nurses, both supervisee and clinical supervisor roles.

m) The value of clinical supervision is monitored and audited through the supervisee reporting on its value or otherwise in their line management supervision, appraisal or in completing audit tools. supervisee confidently is respected: it is not required to reveal the content of any sessions (exception listed under 'accountability). All involved must seek to improve the clinical supervision system.

Table 10.4 Third of 3 sections of a draft code of practice for clinical supervision for qualified nurses: the clinical supervisor/supervisee relationship

---

a) The clinical supervisor/supervisee relationship is one of equals, whatever the relative levels in the hierarchy. It is a collaborative endeavour.

b) The clinical supervisor should be fundamentally supportive of the supervisee as an individual while encouraging the supervisee to examine their experiences from another perspective and being rigorous in (supportively) challenging any ethical and performance issues which emerge.

c) Supervisors and supervisees should make explicit the expectations and requirements they have of each other and agree a contract about how they will work together.

d) The clinical supervisor and supervisee should assess the value of working with the other and seek to continually improve how they work together.

e) As clinical supervisor you must treat the supervisee as an individual and respect their dignity and must not discriminate in any way against them. You must treat your supervisee kindly and considerately.

f) You must respect your supervisee's right to confidentiality, in that anything the supervisee discloses during the clinical supervision session is kept confidential between you, unless the supervisee gives permission. The exception is shown under 'accountability'.

g) Except for the above exception, records of clinical supervision sessions must not include any details of what was discussed during the session unless the supervisee gives item-by-item permission, and must never include personal information about the supervisee's private life or emotions, or the names of any patients or colleagues. Records may include aide-memoire summaries of any action plans agreed provided they conform to the previous point.

h) In addition to confidentiality, you must maintain the boundaries of clinical supervision, such as not moving into counselling/psychotherapy, keeping to sexual boundaries, and not have clinical supervision combined with any line management or educational assessment within the same relationship.

By its nature, a code of practice is prescriptive of behaviour, which may seem to contradict the value placed on being facilitative in clinical supervision, but our proposal is prescriptive in order to advocate the establishment of an ethical 'frame' for the clinical supervision relationship, which needs to be sturdy enough to safely facilitate opening up the picture within it.

Summary

In one way it is remarkable what has been achieved in clinical supervision in a little over 10 years since the first edition of this book. Nursing was a long way behind in clinical supervision compared to other professions, and to implement a major change initiative nationally takes much creativity as well as accommodation. Ten years is nothing for a major management of change initiative. It now needs consolidation and further growth.

There may be new opportunities in health care that have not existed before and which could enable more flexibility and ingenuity. Less top-heavy health care delivery systems, such as social enterprises, may provide an opportunity for managers and practitioners to prioritize clinical supervision from the outset: we have seen this happen successfully in one area where district nurses identified protected time for all staff to have clinical supervision as part of their provider contract.

Nursing is increasingly likely to become a profession of autonomous practitioners who, like counsellors and psychotherapists, will become responsible for finding their own professional support and monitoring. In the introduction we quoted Alison Norman's concern that good ideas so often get lost in our profession. She goes on to say that 'to get [clinical supervision] wrong would be a tragedy for nursing and health visiting' (Norman 1995: 25).

Writing a book is one way of emphasizing the importance of trying to get clinical supervision right for the profession of nursing, the individuals within it and their clients – of 'making a bit of a fuss' about it. We would like to believe that in the very near future there will be many more nurses echoing the sentiments of this one, first quoted in Chapter 3:

> What's all the fuss about? What do people mean when they can't see how they'll fit in the time? I've had clinical supervision ever since I started nursing. To me it's as important as my annual leave: if I didn't have it, I'd be less effective at work, in fact I'd be ill. The same with clinical supervision: if I hadn't had it I'd have left nursing by now.

The only sure certainty is that change is here to stay. Effective clinical supervision can provide a secure-enough base from which to find your way, at your own pace, to find your place in this great profession. If you don't lose the heart of it – the value of importance and integrity of relationships at the centre of compassionate, effective care – then you won't lose heart.

References

Ahmad, W. (1992) *The Politics of Race and Health*. Bradford: Bradford University Race Relations Research Unit.

Ainsworth, M., Blehar, M. C., Waters, E. and Wall, S. (1978) *Patterns of Attachment: Assessed in the Strange Situation and at Home*. Hillsdale, NJ: Erlbaum.

Atherton, J. S. (2009) *Learning and Teaching; Experiential Learning*, www.learningandteaching.info/learning/experience.htm, accessed 26 February 2010.

Back, K. and Back, K. (2005) *Assertiveness at Work: A Practical Guide to Handling Awkward Situations*. London: McGraw-Hill.

BACP (British Association for Counselling and Psychotherapy) (2010) *Ethical Framework for Good Practice in Counselling and Psychotherapy*. Lutterworth: British Association for Counselling and Psychotherapy.

Baillie, L., Gallagher, A. and Wainwright, P. (2008) *Defending Dignity: Challenges and Opportunities for Nursing*. London. London: Royal College of Nursing.

Bambling, M. (2003) Clinical supervision: its influence on working alliance and client outcome in the brief treatment of major depression, *Psychotherapy in Australia*, 11(1): 30–5.

Barriball, L., White, A. and Munch, L. (2004) An audit of clinical supervision in primary care, *British Journal of Community Nursing*, 9(9): 389–97.

Bartholomew, K. and Perlman, D. (eds) (1994) *Attachment Processes in Adulthood*. London: Jessica Kingsley.

Begat, I. and Severinsson, E. (2006) Reflection on how clinical nursing supervision enhances nurses' experience of well-being related to their psychosocial work environment, *Journal of Nursing Management*, 14(8): 610–16.

Belbin, R. M. (2010) *Management Teams: Why They Succeed or Fail*, 3rd edn. Oxford: Butterworth Heinemann.

Benner, P. (1984) *From Novice to Expert: Excellence and Power in Clinical Nursing Practice*. Reading, MA: Addison-Wesley.

Bent, A. (1992) The statutory basis to the role of the supervisor, in English National Board, *Preparation of Supervisors of Midwives*. London: English National Board.

Bentley, T. (1994) *Facilitation: Providing Opportunities for Learning*. London: McGraw-Hill.

Berne, E. (2004) *Games People Play: The Basic Handbook of Transactional Analysis*, 40th anniversary edition. New York: Ballantine.

Bion, W. (1967) *Second Thoughts: Selected Papers on Psychoanalysis*. Oxford: Heinemann Medical.

Block, P. (2004) A time to heal: creating healthy conditions for service, *Reflections on Nursing Leadership*, Honor Society of Nursing, Sigma Theta Tau International, Fourth Quarter.

Bluckert, P. (2006) *Psychological Dimensions of Executive Coaching*. Maidenhead: Open University Press.

Bond, M. (1986) *Stress and Self Awareness: A Guide for Nurses*. Oxford: Heinemann.

Bond, M. (1989) Managing emotional energy, in J. Mulligan (ed.) *The Personal Management Handbook*. London: Sphere.

Bond, M. (1991) Setting up support groups: a practical guide, *Nursing Standard*, 21 August, 5(48): 47–51.

Bond, M. and Holland, S. (1992) *Communication in Partnership in Nutrifax*. London: Dairy Council and Community Practitioners and Health Visitors Association.

Bond, M. (2010) In-depth reflection: a requirement for safe practice or doing your head in? Towards a code of practice for clinical supervision in the non-counselling professions, keynote address at the 'Professional Supervision: Common Threads, Different Patterns' conference, Faculty of Education, University of Auckland, New Zealand.

Boore, J. (1978) *Prescriptions for Recovery*. London: Royal College of Nursing.

Booth, K. and Faulkner, A. (1986) Problems encountered in setting up support groups in nursing, *Nursing Today*, 6: 244–51.

Borton, T. (1970) *Reach, Touch and Teach*. London: Hutchinson.

Boud, D. (2010) Relocating reflection in the context of practice, in H. Bradbury *et al.*, *Beyond Reflective Practice*. Abingdon: Routledge.

Boud, D. and Kilty, J. (1983) *Self and Peer Assessment in Higher Education: A Workshop Leader's Manual*. Sydney: Tertiary Education Centre, University of New South Wales.

Boud, D., Keogh, R. and Walker, D. (1985) Promoting reflection in learning: a model, in D. Boud, R. Keogh and D. Walker (eds) *Reflection: Turning Experience into Learning*. London: Kogan Page.

Bowlby, J. (1971) *Attachment and Loss*, vol. 1: *Attachment*. London: Hogarth Press.

Bowlby, J. (1973) *Attachment and Loss*, vol. 2: *Separation: Anxiety and Anger*. London: Hogarth Press.

Bowlby, J. (1980) *Attachment and Loss*, vol. 3: *Loss, Sadness and Depression*. London: Hogarth Press.

Bowlby, J. (1988) *A Secure Base: Clinical Applications of Attachment Theory*. London: Routledge.

Bradbury, H., Frost, N., Kilminster, S. and Zukas, M. (2010) *Beyond Reflective Practice*. Abingdon: Routledge.

Brambling, M. (2004) The developmental model of supervision and contemporary practice *Psychotherapy in Australia*, 11(1): 30–5.

Brockbank, A. and McGill, I. (2006) *Facilitating Reflective Learning Through Mentoring and Coaching*. London: Kogan Page.

Brown, A. and Bourne, I. (1996) *The Social Work Supervisor*. Buckingham: Open University Press.

Brunero, S. and Stein-Parbury, J. (2008) The effectivenss of clinical supervision in nursing: an evidence-based literature review, *Australian Journal of Advanced Nursing*, 25(3).

Burke, B. and Harrison, P. (2010) Anti-oppressive practice, in R. Adams *et al.* (eds) *Social Work*. Basingstoke: Macmillan.

Burnard, P. (1988) Mentors: a supporting act, *Nursing Times*, 83(2): 14–20.

Burnard, P. and Morrison, P. (1988) Nurses' perceptions of their interpersonal skills: a descriptive study using 6-Category Intervention Analysis, *Nurse Education Today*, 8: 272–86.

Butterworth, T. (1992) Clinical supervision . . . as an emerging idea in nursing, in T. Butterworth and J. Faugier (eds) *Clinical Supervision and Mentorship in Nursing*. London: Chapman & Hall.

Butterworth, T. (1995) Introduction to clinical supervision, in Department of Health, *Clinical Supervision – Conference Proceedings*. London: National Health Service Management Executive.

Butterworth, T. (1996) Primary attempts at research-based evaluation of clinical supervision, *Nursing Times Research*, 1(2): 96–101.

Butterworth, T. and Faugier, J. (eds) (1992) *Clinical Supervision and Mentorship in Nursing*. London: Chapman & Hall.

Butterworth, T., Bishop, V. and Carson, J. (1996) First steps towards evaluating clinical supervision in nursing and health visiting: 1. Theory, policy and practice development: a review, *Journal of Clinical Nursing*, 5: 127–32.

Butterworth, T., Carson, J., White, E., Jeacock, J., Clements, A. and Bishop, V. (1997) *It is Good to Talk: Clinical Supervision and Mentorship. An Evaluation Study in England and Scotland*. Manchester: University of Manchester.

Butterworth, T., Bell, L. and Jackson, C. (2008) Wicked spell or magic bullet? A review of the clinical supervision literature 2001–2007, *Nurse Education Today*, 28(3): 264–72.

Buzan, T. (2006) *Use Your Head: Innovative Learning and Thinking Techniques to Fulfil Your Potential*. London: BBC Active.

Calder, D. (2005) *Clinical Supervision for Nurses, Midwives and Health Visitors who Safeguard Children: Best Practice Guidance*. Cardiff: National Public Health Service for Wales.

Campbell, F., Cowley, S. and Buttigieg, M. (1995) *Weights and Measures*. London: Community Practitioners and Health Visitors Association.

Care Quality Commission (2010) *The State of Health Care and Adult Social Care in England – Key Themes and Quality of Services in 2009*. London: The Stationery Office.

Carper, B. (1978) Fundamental ways of knowing in nursing, *Advances in Nursing Science*, 11: 13–23.

Carson, J., Fagin, L. and Ritter, S. A. (eds) (1995) *Stress and Coping in Mental Health Nursing*. London: Chapman & Hall.

Casement, P. (1985) *On Learning From the Patient*. London: Routledge.

Cassidy, J. and Shaver, P. (2008) *Handbook of Attachment Theory, Research and Clinical Application*, 2nd edn. Hove: Guildford Press.

Chavasse, J. (1992) New dimensions of empowerment in nursing, *Journal of Advanced Nursing*, 17: 1–2.

Checkland, P. (1970) *Systems Thinking, Systems Practice*. Chichester: Wiley.

Cherniss, C. and Goleman, D. (2001) *The Emotionally Intelligent Workplace*. San Francisco: Jossey-Bass.

Clulow, C. (1994) Balancing care and control: the supervisory relationship as a focus for promoting organisational health, in A. Obholzer and V.Z. Roberts (eds) *The Unconscious at Work*. London: Routledge.

Cockman, P., Evans, B. and Reynolds, P. (1998) *Consulting for Real People: A Client-Centered Approach for Change Agents and Leaders*. London: McGraw-Hill.

Coleman, D. and Lynch, U. (2006) Professional isolation and the role of clinical supervision in rural and remote communities, *Journal of Community Nursing*, 20(3): 35–7.

Commission on the Future of Nursing and Midwifery in England (2010) *Front Line Care*. London: Commission on the Future of Nursing and Midwifery in England.

Cooper, C. (1981) *The Stress Check: Coping with the Stressors of Life and Work*. Englewood Cliffs, NJ: Spectrum Books.

Corrigall, J. and Wilkinson, H. (2003) *Revolutionary Connections*. London: Karnac.

Cutcliffe, J., Butterworth, T. and Proctor, B. (2001) *Fundamental Themes in Clinical Supervision*. London: Routledge.

Cutcliffe, J. R. and Hyrkas, K. (2006) Multidisciplinary attitudinal positions regarding clinical supervision: a cross-sectional study, *Journal of Nursing Management*, 14(8): 617–27.

Dalal, F. (2002) *Race, Colour and the Processes of Racialisation*. London: Brunner-Routledge.

Dalrymple, J. and Burke, B. (eds) (2006) *Anti-Oppressive Practice*, 2nd edn. Maidenhead: Open University Press.

Damasio, A. (1999) *The Feeling of What Happens: Body, Emotion and the Making of Consciousness*. London: Heinemann.

Dartington, A. (1994) Where angels fear to tread: idealism, despondency and inhibition of thought in hospital nursing, in A. Obholzer and V. Z. Roberts (eds) *The Unconscious at Work*. London: Routledge.

Davies, C. (1995) *Gender and the Professional Predicament in Nursing*. Buckingham: Open University Press.

Department for Children, Schools and Families (2010) *Support for All*. Norwich: The Stationery Office.

Department of Health (1991c) *The Patient's Charter*. London: HMSO.

Department of Health (1991d) *Equal Opportunities for Women in the NHS (Opportunity 2000)*. London: National Health Service Management Executive.

Department of Health (1993a) *A Vision for the Future*. London: National Health Service Management Executive.

Department of Health (1993b) *Ethnic Minority Staff in the NHS: A Programme for Action*. London: National Health Service Management Executive.

Department of Health (1993c) *The Patient's Charter and Primary Health Care*. London: HMSO.

Department of Health (1993d) *A Vision for the Future.* London: National Health Service Management Executive.

Department of Health (1994) *Guideline to Developing a Marketing Action Plan: Coopers and Lybrand/HVA.* London: HMSO.

Department of Health (1995) *Making It Happen: Public Health – the Contribution, Role and Development of Nurses, Midwives and Health Visitors.* London: HMSO.

Department of Health (2003) *Every Child Matters.* London: Department of Health.

Department of Health (2004) *Standards for Better Health.* London: National Health Service Management Executive.

Department of Health (2008a) *Putting People First.* London: Department of Health.

Department of Health (2008b) *High Quality Care for All.* NHS Next Stage Review, final report, CM7432. London: The Stationery Office.

Department of Health (2009) *Nursing Preceptorship Framework.* London: Department of Health.

Department of Health (2010) Privacy and dignity, http://www.dh.gov.uk/en/Managingyourorganisation/Workforce/Leadership/Healthcare environment/DH_4116444, accessed 2 March 2010.

Department of Health, Home Office, Department for Education and Employment (2006) *Working Together to Safeguard Children: A Guide to Inter-agency Working to Safeguard and Promote the Welfare of Children.* London: The Stationery Office.

Dickson, A. (1982) *A Woman in Your Own Right: Assertiveness and You.* London: Quartet.

Dickson, A. (2006) *Difficult Conversations: What to Say in Tricky Situations Without Ruining the Relationship.* London: Piatkus.

Dimond, B. (1990) *Legal Issues in Nursing.* Hemel Hempstead: Prentice-Hall.

Dimond, B. (1998a) Clinical supervision: the legal aspects 1, *British Journal of Nursing,* 7(7): 393–5.

Dimond, B. (1998b) Clinical supervision: the legal aspects 2, *British Journal of Nursing,* 7(7): 487–9.

Driver, C. and Martin, E. (eds) (2005) *Supervision and the Analytic Attitude.* London: Whurr.

Edwards, D., Burnard, P., Hannigan, B., Cooper, L., Adams, J. and Jugessur, T. (2000) *The Effectiveness of Clinical Supervion on Burnout in Community Mental Health Nurses in Wales.* Cardiff: University of Cardiff.

Edwards, D. *et al.* (2005) Factors influencing the effectiveness of clinical supervision, *Journal of Psychiatric and Mental Health Nursing,* 12(4): 405–14.

Egan, G. (1975) *The Skilled Helper: International Edition.* Belmont, CA: Wadsworth.

ENB (English National Board) (1992) *Preparation of Supervisors of Midwives.* London: English National Board.

Faugier, J. (1992) The supervisory relationship, in T. Butterworth and J. Faugier (eds) *Clinical Supervision and Mentorship in Nursing.* London: Chapman & Hall.

Faugier, J. (1995) Introduction to clinical supervision, in Department of Health, *Clinical Supervision – Conference Proceedings,* November 1994. London: National Health Service Management Executive.

Ferguson, K. (1992) Position paper on in-patient psychiatric nursing. London: Department of Health (unpublished).

Fernando, S. (ed.) (1995) *Mental Health in a Multi-Ethnic Society.* London: Routledge.

Fineman, S. (1993a) Organisations as emotional arenas, in S. Fineman (ed.) *Emotions in Organisations.* London: Sage.

Fineman, S. (ed.) (1993b). *Emotions in Organisations.* London: Sage.

Fish, D., Twinn, S. and Purr, B. (1989) *How to Enable Learning through Professional Practice.* London: West London Press.

Fonagy, P., Gergely, G., Jurist, E. J. and Target, M. (2002) *Affect Regulation, Mentalization and the Development of the Self.* New York: Other Press.

Fook, J. (2010) A learning practice: conceptualising professional lifelong learning for the healthcare sector, in H. Bradbury *et al., Beyond Reflective Practice.* Abingdon:Routledge.

Fowler, J. (1996) The organisation of clinical supervision within the nursing profession: a review of the literature, *Journal of Advanced Nursing,* 23: 471–8.

Freud, S. (1915) The unconscious, *SE* 14: 166–204. London: Hogarth Press.

Gibbs, G. (1988) *Learning by Doing: A Guide to Teaching and Learning Methods.* Oxford: Further Education Unit, Oxford Brookes University.

Gobet, F. and Chassy, P. (2008) Towards an alternative to Benner's theory of expert intuition in nursing: a discussion paper, *International Journal of Nursing Studies,* 45(1): 129–39.

Goldberg, D. P., Williams, P., (1988). *The Users Guide to the General Health Questionnaire.* Windsor: nfer-Nelson.

Goldberg, N. (1986) *Writing Down the Bones: Freeing the Writer Within.* Boston, MA: Shambala.

Goldberg, N. (2001) *Thunder and Lightning: Cracking Open the Writer's Craft.* New York: Bantam.

Goodwin, I. (2003) The relevance of attachment theory to the philosophy, organization and practice of adult mental health care, *Clinical Psychology Review,* 23(1): 35–56.

Gregory, J. (1989) Self and peer assessment, *Welling, Kent Nurse Training Resource Interest Group Newsletter,* 1(April).

Gregory, J. (1996) *The Psychosocial Education of Nurses.* Aldershot: Avebury.

Gregory, J. (2006) Ethics and professional practice in coaching., unpublished MSc paper.

Grossman, K., Grossman, K. E., Spangler, G., Suess, G. and Unzer, J. (1985) Maternal sensitivity and newborns' orientation responses as related to quality of attachment in northern Germany, in I. Bretherton and E. Waters (eds) *Growing Points of Attachment Theory and Research, Monographs of the Society for Research in Child Development,* 50(1–2), No. 209.

Guggenbuhl Craig, A. (1971) *Power in the Helping Professions.* Dallas, TX: Spring Publications.

Gullick, J. and Shimadry, B. (2008) Using patient stories to improve quality of care, *Nursing Times,* 104(10): 33–4.

Halton, W. (1994) Some unconscious aspects of organisational life, in A. Obholzer and V. Z. Roberts (eds) *The Unconscious at Work*. London: Routledge.

Ham, C. (2003) Improving the performance of health services: the role of clinical leadership, *The Lancet*, 361(9373): 1978–80.

Handy, C. (1990) *Inside Organisations*. Harmondsworth: Penguin.

Hart, E. and Bond, M. (1993) *Action Research for Health and Social Care: A Guide to Practice*. Buckingham: Open University Press.

Hawkins, P. and Shohet, R. (1989) *Supervision in the Helping Professions*. Milton Keynes: Open University Press.

Hawkins, P. and Shohet, R. (2006) *Supervision in the Helping Professions*, 3rd edn. Maidenhead: Open University Press.

Hawkins, P. and Smith, N. (2006) *Coaching, Mentoring and Organizational Consultancy Supervision and Development*. Maidenhead: Open University Press.

Hay, J. (2007) *Reflective Practice and Supervision for Coaches*. Maidenhead: Open University Press.

Hayward, J. (1975) *Information: A Prescription Against Pain*. London: Royal College of Nursing.

Hearn, J. (1993) Emotive subjects; organisational men, organisational masculinities and the (de)construction of 'emotions', in S. Fineman (ed.) *Emotions in Organisations*. London: Sage.

Heron, J. (1972) *The Concept of a Peer Learning Community*. Guildford: Human Potential Resource Group, University of Surrey.

Heron, J. (1981) *Assessment*. Guildford: Human Potential Resource Group, University of Surrey.

Heron, J. (1983) *Education of the Affect*. Guildford: Human Potential Resource Group, University of Surrey.

Heron, J. (1999) *The Complete Facilitator's Handbook*. London: Kogan Page.

Heron, J. (2001) *Helping the Client*. London: Sage.

Hill, J. (1989) Supervision in the caring professions: a literature review, *Community Psychiatric Nursing Journal*, 9(5): 9–15.

Hingley, P., Cooper, C. L. and Harris, P. (1986) *Stress in Nurse Managers*. London: King's Fund.

Holmes, J. (2001) *The Search for a Secure Base*. Hove: Brunner-Routledge.

Holland, S. (1987) *Stress in Nursing*. London: Distance Learning Centre, South Bank University.

Holland, S. (1991) *Accountability in Health Visiting*. London: Community Practitioners and Health Visitors Association.

Holland, S. (1994) Returning to practice, *Health Visitor*, 67(3): 82–3.

Houston, G. (1990) *Supervision and Counselling*. London: Rochester Foundation.

Huffington, C., Armstrong, D., Halton, W., Hoyle, L. and Pooley, J. (eds) (2004) *Working Below the Surface: The Emotional Life of Contemporary Organizations*. London: Karnac.

HVA (Health Visitors Association) (1994) *Action for Health: Marketing, Skill Mix, Campaigning*. London: Health Visitors Association.

Jacques, D. (2000) *Learning in Groups*, 3rd edn. London: Routledge Falmer.

James, N. (1993) Divisions of emotional labour: disclosure and cancer, in S. Fineman (ed.) *Emotions in Organisations*. London: Sage.

Jarvis, P. (1983) *Professional Education*. Beckenham: Croom Helm.

Jenkins, P. (2006) Supervising workplace counsellors: accountability and duty of care, *Counselling at Work*, winter, www.bacpworkplace.org.uk/journal_pdf/acw_winter06_c.pdf, accessed 26 February 2010.

Johns, C. (1994) Guided reflection, in A. Palmer *et al.* (eds) *Reflective Practice in Nursing*. Oxford: Blackwell Science.

Johnson, D. R. and Johnson, F. P. (2008) *Joining Together: Group Theory and Group Skills: International Edition*, 10th edn. London: Pearson.

Johnson, P. (1995) The community services view, in Department of Health, *Clinical Supervision – Conference Proceedings*. London: National Health Service Management Executive.

Jones, J. and Partington, K. (2007) *Blazing the Trail of Clinical Supervision on the Western Front*. Sydney: South West Sydney Area Health Service.

Jung-Beeman M., and Bowden EM, Haberman J., Frymiare J. L., Arambel-Liu S., et al. (2004) *Neural Activity When People Solve Verbal Problems with Insight*. PLoS Biol 2(4): e97. doi: 10.1371 journal.pbio.0020.

Kadushin, A. (1992) *Supervision in Social Work*, 3rd edn. New York: Columbia University Press.

Kareem, J. and Littlewood, J. (eds) (1992) *Intercultural Therapy*. Oxford: Blackwell Scientific.

Kavanagh, D., Spence, S., Wilson, J. and Crow, N. (2002) Achieving effective supervision, *Drug and Alcohol Review*, 21(3): 247–52.

Kelly, B., Long, A. and McKenna, H. (2001) A survey of community mental health nurses' perceptions of clinical supervision in Northern Ireland, *Journal of Psychiatric and Mental Health Nursing*, 8(1): 33–44.

Kendall, S. (1991) An analysis of health visitor/client interaction: the influence of the HV process on client participation, unpublished PhD thesis, King's College, London.

Kilty, J. (1977) Experiential learning: teaching sessions and handouts on the Community Health Nurse Teachers course at the University of Surrey.

King's Fund (1997) *London's Mental Health: The Report to the King's Fund Commission*. London: King's Fund Centre.

Kohlberg, L. and Lickona, T. (eds) (1976) *Moral Stages and Moralization: The Cognitive-developmental Approach. Moral Development and Behavior: Theory, Research and Social Issues*. New York: Rinehart & Winston.

Kohner, N. (1994) *Clinical Supervision in Practice*. London: King's Fund Centre.

Kolb, D. A. (1984) *Experiential Learning: Experience as the Source of Learning and Development*. Englewood Cliffs, NJ: Prentice Hall.

Kolb, D. A. and Fry, R. (1975) Towards an applied theory of experiential learning, in C. L. Cooper (ed.) *Theories of Group Processes*. Chichester: Wiley.

Kraemer, S. and Roberts, J. (eds) (1996) *The Politics of Attachment*. London: Free Association Books.

Kramer, M. (1974) *Reality Shock: Why Nurses Leave Nursing*. St Louis, MI: C. V. Mosby.

Large, S., Macleod, A., Cunningham, G. and Kitson, A. (2003) *A Multiple Case Study Evaluation of the RCN Clinical Leadership Programme in England*. London: Royal College of Nursing.

Lee, M. (2003) On codes of ethics: the Individual and performance, *Performance Improvement Quartlery*, 16(2): 72–89.

Lewin, K. (1951) *Field Theory in Social Science*. London: Harper.

Lewin, K. (1972) Need, force and valence in psychological fields, in E. P. Hollander and R.G. Hunt (eds) *Classic Contributions to Social Psychology*. London: Oxford University Press.

Main, M. (1994) A move to the level of representation in the study of attachment organisation: implications for psychoanalysis, Annual Research Lecture to the British Psycho-Analytical Society, July 1994.

Main, M. and Goldwyn, R. (1985) Adult attachment classification and rating system, unpublished manuscript, Berkeley, CA:University of California.

Malin, N. (2000) Evaluating clinical supervision in community homes and teams serving adults with learning disabilities, *Journal of Advanced Nursing*, 231(3): 548–57.

Maroda, K. J. (1991) *The Power of Countertransference*. Chichester: Wiley.

Marris, P. (1996) The management of uncertainty, in S. Kraemer and J. Roberts (eds) *The Politics of Attachment*. London: Free Asscociation Books.

Maslach Jackson (1981). *The Maslach Burnout Inventory*. Palo Alto, CA: Consulting Psychologists Press.

Mattinson, J. (1975) *The Reflection Process in Casework Supervision*. London: Institute of Marital Studies.

Menzies, I. (1959) A case study in the functioning of social systems as a defence against anxiety: a report on a study of the nursing service of a general hospital, *Human Relations*, 13: 95–121.

Menzies-Lyth, I. (1988) *Containing Anxiety in Institutions*. London: Free Association Books.

Miyake, K., Chen, S. and Campos, J. (1985) Infant temperament, mother's mode of interaction, and attachment in Japan: an interim report, in I. Bretherton and E. Waters (eds) *Growing Points of Attachment Theory and Research (Monographs of the Society for Research in Child Development)*, 50(1–2), No. 209.

Morgan, H. (2007) The effects of difference of race and colour in supervision, in A. Petts and B. Shapley (eds) *On Supervision*. London: Karnac.

Morton-Cooper, A. and Palmer, A. (1993) *Mentoring and Preceptorship: A Guide to Support Roles in Clinical Practice*. Oxford: Blackwell Scientific Publications.

Morton-Cooper, A. and Palmer, A. (2000) *Mentoring and Preceptorship: A Guide to Support Roles in Clinical Practice*, 2nd edn. Oxford: Blackwell Scientific Publications.

Mosse, J. and Roberts, V. Z. (1994) Finding a voice: differentiation, representation and empowerment in organisations under threat, in A. Obholzer and V. Z. Roberts (eds) *The Unconscious at Work*. London: Routledge.

Mullarkey, K., Keeley, P. and Playle, J. F. (2001) Multiprofessional clinical supervision: challenges for mental health nurses, *Journal of Psychiatric and Mental Health Nursing*, 8: 205–11.

Nash, R. and Young, D. (2009) *Quality and Service Improvement Tools: Force Field Analysis*. Warwick: NHS Institute for Innovation and Improvement, www.institute.nhs.uk/quality_and_service_improvement_tools/quality_and_ service_ improvement_tools/force_field_analysis.html, accessed 26 February 2010.

National Centre for Education and Training on Addiction (NCETA) (2005) *Clinical Supervision Resource Kit*. Adelaide: Alcohol Education and Rehabilitation Foundation.

National Council for the Professional Development of Nursing and Midwifery (NCNM) (2008) Clinical Supervision: A Structured Approach to Best Practice, discussion paper 1, September. Dublin: NCNM.

NHS Confederation (2009) *Reforming Leadership Development*, www.nhsconfed. org/Publications/Documents/Debate%20paper%20%20Future%20of% 20leadership.pdf, accessed 28 February 2010.

Norman, A. (1995) Summing up of plenary session, in Department of Health, *Clinical Supervision – Conference Proceedings*. London: National Health Service Management Executive.

Nursing and Midwifery Council (NMC) (2008a) *The Code: Standards of Conduct, Performance and Ethics for Nurses and Midwives*. London: NMC.

Nursing and Midwifery Council (NMC) (2008b) *Clinical Supervision for Registered Nurses*, www.nmc-uk.org/aDisplayDocument.aspx?documentID=4022, accessed 28 February 2010.

Obholzer, A. and Roberts, V. Z. (eds) (1994) *The Unconscious at Work*. London: Routledge.

Parkes, C. M., Hinde, J. and Marris, P. (eds) (1991) *Attachment Across the Life Cycle*. London: Routledge.

Parkin, W. (1993) The public and the private: gender, sexuality and emotion, in S. Fineman (ed.) *Emotions in Organisations*. London: Sage.

Parkinson, J. (1992) Supervision versus control: can managers provide both managerial and professional supervision? in C. Cloke and J. Naish (eds) *Key Issues in Child Protection for Health Visitors and Nurses*. Harlow: Longman.

Pearson, A. (1988) Therapeutic nursing, unpublished PhD thesis, Burford and Oxford Nursing Development Unit.

Pedler, M., Burgoyne, J. and Boydell, T. (1991) *The Learning Company*. London: McGraw-Hill.

Platt-Koch, L. M. (1986) Clinical supervision for psychiatric nurses, *Journal of Psycho-Social Nursing* (January), 26(1): 7–15.

Priest, J. (1998) Why we bend the rules, *The Journal Record*, 24 July.

Proctor, B. (1986) Supervision: a co-operative exercise in accountability, in M. Marken and M. Payne (eds) *Enabling and Ensuring*. Leicester: National Youth Bureau for Education in Youth and Community Work.

Putnam, L. and Mumby, D. (1993) Organisations, emotion and the myth of rationality, in S. Fineman (ed.) (1993) *Emotions in Organisations*. London: Sage.

Rafferty, A. M. (1993) *Leading Questions: A Discussion Paper on Issues of Nurse Leadership*. London: King's Fund Centre.

Rafferty, A. M. (2008) Creative care, presentation at King's College, 10 February.

Rafferty, M., Jenkins, E. and Parke, S. (2003) Developing a provisional standard for clinical supervision in nursing and health visiting: the methodological trail, *Qualitative Health Research*, 13(10): 1432–52.

Randall, R. and Southgate, J. (1980) *Cooperative and Community Group Dynamics*. London: Barefoot Books.

Reason, P. (1988) *Human Inquiry in Action: Developments in New Paradigm Research*. London: Sage.

Reason, P. and Rowan, J. (1981) *Human Inquiry*. Chichester: Wiley.

Revans, R. W. (1982) *The Origins and Growth of Action Learning*. Bromley: Chartwell-Bratt.

Roberts, V. Z. (1994) Till death us do part: caring and uncaring in work with the elderly, in A. Obholzer and V.Z. Roberts (eds) *The Unconscious at Work*. London: Routledge.

Robertson, J. and Robertson, J. (1989) *Separation and the Very Young*. London: Free Association Books.

Robinson, K. (1992) The nursing workforce: aspects of inequality, in J. Robinson, A. Gray and R. Elkan (eds) *Policy Issues in Nursing*. Buckingham: Open University Press.

Rogers, J. (2008) *Coaching Skills: a Handbook*, 2nd edn. Maidenhead: Open University Press.

Royal College of Nursing (RCN) (2003) *Nursing Care of Lesbian and Gay Male Patients and Clients: Guidance for Nursing Staff*. London: RCN.

Sagi, A., Lamb, E., Lewkowicz, S., Shoham, R., Dvir, R. and Estes, D. (1985) Security of infant, mother, father and metapelet attachments among kibbutz reared Israeli children, in I. Bretherton and E. Waters (eds) *Growing Points of Attachment Theory and Research* (*Monographs of the Society for Research in Child Development*), 50(1–2), No. 209.

Saltiel, D. (2010) *Judgement, Narrative and Discourse: A Critique of Reflective Practice*, in H.Bradbury *et al.*, *Beyond Reflective Practice*. Abingdon: Routledge.

Salvage, J. (1985) *The Politics of Nursing*. Oxford: Heinemann.

Salvage, J. (1992) The new nursing: empowering patients or empowering nurses? in J. Robinson, A. Gray and R. Elkan (eds) *Policy Issues in Nursing*. Buckingham: Open University Press.

Schön, D. (1983) *The Reflective Practitioner*. New York: Basic Books.

Schön, D. (1987) *Educating the Reflective Practitioner*. San Francisco: Jossey-Bass.

Searles, H.F. (1955) The informational value of the supervisor's emotional experience, in *Collected Papers on Schizophrenia and Related Subjects*. London: Hogarth Press, 1965.

Shaw, E. (2004) The 'pointy' end of clinical supervision: ethical, legal and performance issues, *Psychotherapy in Australia*, 10(2).

Skelton, R. (1994) Nursing and empowerment: concepts and strategies, *Journal of Advanced Nursing*, 19: 415–23.

Sloan, G. (2006) *Clinical Supervision in Mental Health Nursing.* Chichester: Whurr.

Smith, R. (1992) *The Emotional Labour of Nursing.* London: Macmillan.

Sperling, M. and Herman, W. (1994) *Attachment in Adults.* New York: Guilford Press.

Sroufe, L. A., Egeland, B. and Kreutzer, T. (1990) The fate of early experience following developmental change: longitudinal approaches to individual adaptation in childhood, *Child Development,* 61: 1363–73.

Starr, J. (2008) *The Coaching Manual,* 2nd edn. Harlow: Pearson Education.

Stein, H. (1985) *The Psycho-dynamics of Medical Practice: Unconscious Factors in Patient Care.* Los Angeles: University of California Press.

Stern, D. (1985) *The Interpersonal World of the Infant.* New York: Basic Books.

Stern, D. (1995) *The Motherhood Constellation: A Unified View of Parent-Infant Psychotherapy.* New York: Basic Books.

Stuart, C. (2007) *Assessment, Supervision & Support in Clinical Practice: A Guide for Nurses, Midwives & Other Health Professionals.* Philadelphia, PA: Churchill Livingstone/Elsevier.

Swain, G. (1995) *Clinical Supervision: The Principles and Process.* London: Community Practitioners and Health Visitors Association.

Taylor, D. (2007) The supervision triangle in *On Supervision,* in A. Petts and B. Shapley (eds) *On Supervision: Psychoanalytic and Jungian Perspectives.* London: Karnac.

Teasdale, K., Brocklehurst, N. and Thom, N. (2001) Clinical supervision and support for nurses: an evaluation study, *Journal of Advanced Nursing,* 33(2): 216–24.

Thomas, B. (1995) Clinical supervision in mental health nursing, in Department of Health, *Clinical Supervision – Conference Proceedings,* November 1994. London: National Health Service Management Executive.

Thomas, M. (2005) Through the looking glass: creativity in supervision in C. Driver, and E. Martin (eds) *Supervision and the Analytic Attitude.* London: Whurr.

Tosey, P. and Gregory, J. (2002) *Dictionary of Personal Development.* London: Whurr.

UKCC (United Kingdom Central Council for Nursing Midwifery and Health Visiting) (1989) *Exercising Accountability – A Framework to Assist Nurses, Midwives and Health Visitors to Consider Ethical Aspects of Professional Practice,* 3rd edn. London: UKCC.

UKCC (United Kingdom Central Council for Nursing Midwifery and Health Visiting) (1992) *The Scope of Professional Practice.* London: UKCC.

UKCC (United Kingdom Central Council for Nursing Midwifery and Health Visiting) (1993) *The Future of Professional Practice: The Council's Standards for Education and Practice Following Registration.* London: UKCC.

UKCC (United Kingdom Central Council for Nursing Midwifery and Health Visiting) (1996) *Position Statement on Clinical Supervision for Nursing and Health Visiting.* London: UKCC.

Van Ooijen, E. (2003) *Clinical Supervision Made Easy.* Edinburgh: Churchill Livingstone.

Victoria Healthcare Association (2006) *Clinical Supervision and Leadership in Community Health.* Melbourne: Victoria Healthcare Association.

Victoria Healthcare Association (2008) *Clinical Governance Project*. Melbourne: Victoria Healthcare Association.

Watkins, S. (1993) Working together for better health, *Health Visitor*, 66(12): 436–7.

Watt, D. (2003) Psychotherapy in an age of neuro-science: bridges to affective neuro-science, in J. Corrigall and H. Wilkinson (eds) *Revolutionary Connections*. London: Karnac.

White, E. (1990) *The Third Quinquennial National Community Psychiatric Nursing Survey Report*. Manchester: University of Manchester.

White, E., Butterworth, T., Bishop, V., Carson, J., Jeacock, J. and Clements, A. (1998) Clinical supervision: insider reports of a private world, *Journal of Advanced Nursing*, 28(1): 185–92.

Williams, B., French, B. and Higgs, J. (2005) Clinical supervision: community nurses' experience, *Primary Health Care*, 15(6): 35–9.

Winnicott, D. W. (1991) *The Maturational Processes and the Facilitating Environment*. London: Hogarth.

Winstanley, J. (2000) *Clinical Supervision: development of an evaluation instrument*. Unpublished PhD thesis, Faculty of Medicine, Dentistry Nursing. University of Menchester.

Wolsey, P. and Leach, L. (1997) Clinical supervision: a hornet's nest? *Nursing Times*, 93(44).

Wood, H. (2007) Boundaries and confidentiality in supervision, in A. Petts and B. Shapley (eds) *On Supervision: Psychoanalytic and Jungian Perspectives*. London: Karnac.

Woodhouse, D. and Pengelly, P. (1991) *Anxiety and the Dynamics of Collaboration*. Aberdeen: Aberdeen University Press.

Woods, D. (1992) The therapeutic use of self in clinical supervision, in T. Butterworth and J. Faugier (eds) *Clinical Supervision and Mentorship in Nursing*. London: Chapman & Hall.

Wright, S. (1997) *Changing Nursing Practice*. London: Hodder Arnold.

Wynne, T. (1994) The burden facing women carers today, *Health Visitor*, 67(7): 241–2.

Index